Mayo
Antimicrobial Therapy

Second Edition

Mayo Clinic
Antimicrobial Therapy
Quick Guide

Second Edition

Editors

John W. Wilson, MD

Consultant
Division of Infectious Diseases, and
Assistant Professor of Medicine
College of Medicine, Mayo Clinic
Rochester, Minnesota

Lynn L. Estes, PharmD

Clinical Pharmacy Specialist
Assistant Professor of Pharmacy
College of Medicine, Mayo Clinic
Rochester, Minnesota

MAYO CLINIC SCIENTIFIC PRESS

OXFORD UNIVERSITY PRESS

MAYO
CLINIC

The triple-shield Mayo logo and the words MAYO, MAYO CLINIC, and MAYO CLINIC SCIENTIFIC
PRESS are marks of Mayo Foundation for Medical Education and Research.

OXFORD
UNIVERSITY PRESS

Oxford University Press, Inc., publishes works that further
Oxford University's objective of excellence in research, scholarship, and education.

Oxford   New York
Auckland   Cape Town   Dar es Salaam   Hong Kong   Karachi   Kuala Lumpur   Madrid
Melbourne   Mexico City   Nairobi   New Delhi   Shanghai   Taipei   Toronto

With offices in
Argentina   Austria   Brazil   Chile   Czech Republic   France   Greece
Guatemala   Hungary   Italy   Japan   Poland   Portugal   Singapore
South Korea   Switzerland   Thailand   Turkey   Ukraine   Vietnam

Library of Congress Cataloging-in-Publication Data
Wilson, John W., 1967-
Mayo Clinic antimicrobial therapy : quick guide / John W. Wilson, Lynn L. Estes. — 2nd ed.
    p. ; cm.
Antimicrobial therapy
Rev. ed. of: Mayo Clinic antimicrobial therapy. c2008.
Includes bibliographical references and index.
ISBN 978-0-19-979778-3 (pbk.)
1. Anti-infective agents—Handbooks, manuals, etc. 2. Communicable diseases—Chemotherapy—
Handbooks, manuals, etc. I. Estes, Lynn L. II. Mayo Clinic. III. Mayo Clinic antimicrobial therapy. IV. Title.
V. Title: Antimicrobial therapy.
    [DNLM: 1. Anti-Infective Agents—therapeutic use—Handbooks. 2. Communicable Diseases—drug
therapy—Handbooks. QV 39]
RM262.M377 2012
615'.1—dc23   2011018569

Mayo Foundation does not endorse any particular products or services, and the reference to any products
or services in this book is for informational purposes only and should not be taken as an endorsement by
the authors or Mayo Foundation. Care has been taken to confirm the accuracy of the information
presented and to describe generally accepted practices. However, the authors, editors, and publisher are
not responsible for errors or omissions or for any consequences from application of the information in this
book and make no warranty, express or implied, with respect to the contents of the publication. This book
should not be relied on apart from the advice of a qualified health care provider.

The authors, editors, and publisher have exerted efforts to ensure that drug selection and dosage set forth
in this text are in accordance with current recommendations and practice at the time of publication.
However, in view of ongoing research, changes in government regulations, and the constant flow of
information relating to drug therapy and drug reactions, readers are urged to check the package insert for
each drug for any change in indications and dosage and for added wordings and precautions. This is
particularly important when the recommended agent is a new or infrequently employed drug.

Some drugs and medical devices presented in this publication have US Food and Drug Administration
(FDA) clearance for limited use in restricted research settings. It is the responsibility of the health care
providers to ascertain the FDA status of each drug or device planned for use in their clinical practice.

9 8 7 6 5 4 3 2 1

Printed in United States of America
on acid-free paper

We dedicate this book to the patients under our care and to our families, who continue to support us in our work.

About the Cover

The cover image illustrates the "journey to wellness" that patients and their health care providers make through the appropriate use of antimicrobial therapy for infectious diseases. Health care providers and scientists worldwide have an opportunity and growing responsibility, through microbial epidemiology and antimicrobial stewardship, to collectively work toward optimal diagnosis and management of infectious diseases.

Preface

The medical management of infectious diseases and antimicrobial therapy can be a daunting task for health care professionals. Although expansive textbooks and online resources are available, we believe that a more simplified, quick reference guide is needed for the day-to-day office and hospital clinical practice. This book is designed to provide information about infectious diseases and antimicrobial therapy in a format that is readily accessible and easily applicable to the clinical environment.

Highlights of this book include simplified and thorough drug dosing recommendations for renal function and renal replacement therapies, drugs of choice for specific organisms (including bacteria, fungi, and viruses), and simplified antimicrobial and management recommendations for specific infectious syndromes.

We hope this book will assist health care providers in the management of infectious diseases and in the selection of appropriate antimicrobial therapy in a time-efficient manner. This book is not meant to serve as a comprehensive review of all infectious diseases topics. Instead, readers are encouraged to seek supplemental information from additional published resources and from the prescribing information provided by pharmaceutical manufacturers.

Contents

Contributors

Salvador Alvarez, MD

Larry M. Baddour, MD

Ritu Banerjee, MD, PhD

Elie F. Berbari, MD

Mark J. Enzler, MD

Lynn L. Estes, PharmD

W. Charles Huskins, MD

Mary J. Kasten, MD

William F. Marshall, MD

Julio C. Mendez, MD

Robert Orenstein, DO

Douglas R. Osmon, MD

Raymund R. Razonable, MD

Irene G. Sia, MD

Ronald M. Sieve, PharmD, RPh

M. Rizwan Sohail, MD

James M. Steckelberg, MD

Rodney L. Thompson, MD

Abinash Virk, MD

Mark P. Wilhelm, MD

John W. Wilson, MD

Abbreviations

AC	arterial catheter
ACIP	Advisory Committee on Immunization Practices
Admin	administration
AFB	acid-fast bacillus
ALT	alanine aminotransferase
Antistaph	antistaphylococcal
AUC	area under the curve
BCG	bacille Calmette-Guérin
bid	2 times a day
BMT	bone marrow transplant
BP	blood pressure
BV	bacterial vaginosis
C	Celsius
CA-MRSA	community-acquired methicillin-resistant *Staphylococcus aureus*
cap	capsule
CAP	community-acquired pneumonia
CBC	complete blood cell count
CCR5	cysteine chemokine receptor 5
CDC	Centers for Disease Control and Prevention
CD4	CD4 T-cell
CF	cystic fibrosis
CFU	colony-forming units
CHD	congenital heart disease
CHF	congestive heart failure
CI	clinically insignificant
CK	creatine kinase
Cl_{Cr}	creatinine clearance
CLSI	Clinical and Laboratory Standards Institute
CMV	cytomegalovirus
CNPA	chronic necrotizing pulmonary aspergillosis
CNS	central nervous system
CPK	creatine kinase
CQ	chloroquine
CRBSI	catheter-related bloodstream infection
CRRT	continuous renal replacement therapy
CSF	cerebrospinal fluid

cSSSI	complicated skin and skin structure infection
CT	computed tomogram; computed tomography
CVC	central venous catheter
CVD	cardiovascular disease
CYP	cytochrome P450
DEET	N,N-diethyl-meta-toluamide
DM	diabetes mellitus
DOT	directly observed therapy
DS	double strength
DTaP	diphtheria and tetanus toxoids and acellular pertussis
DW	dosing weight
EC	enteric coated
ECG	electrocardiogram
ECM	erythema chronicum migrans
EIEC	enteroinvasive *Escherichia coli*
ELISA	enzyme-linked immunosorbent assay
ERCP	endoscopic retrograde cholangiopancreatography
ESBL	extended-spectrum β-lactamase–producing
ESLD	end-stage liver disease
ETEC	enterotoxigenic *Escherichia coli*
F	Fahrenheit
FDA	US Food and Drug Administration
F_{IO_2}	fraction of inspired oxygen
gen	generation
GI	gastrointestinal
GNB	gram-negative bacteria
GU	genitourinary
h	hour
HAART	highly active antiretroviral therapy
HACEK	*Haemophilus parainfluenzae, H aphrophilus, H paraphrophilus, H influenzae, Actinobacillus actinomycetemcomitans, Cardiobacterium hominis, Eikenella corrodens,* and *Kingella kingae*
HAV	hepatitis A virus
HBeAg	hepatitis B e antigen
HBIG	hepatitis B immune globulin
HBs	hepatitis B surface (antigen)
HBsAg	hepatitis B surface antigen
HBV	hepatitis B virus
HCP	health care provider
HCV	hepatitis C virus

HD	hemodialysis
HDCV	human diploid cell vaccine
HDV	hepatitis D virus
HepA	hepatitis A
HepB	hepatitis B
HEV	hepatitis E virus
HGA	human granulocytic anaplasmosis
HGE	human granulocytic ehrlichiosis
Hib	*Haemophilus influenzae* type b conjugate vaccine
HIDA	hepatobiliary iminodiacetic acid
HIV	human immunodeficiency virus
HLA	human leukocyte antigen
HME	human monocytic ehrlichiosis
HPF	high-power field
HPLC	high-performance liquid chromatography
HPV	human papillomavirus
HPV2	human papillomavirus bivalent vaccine
HPV4	human papillomavirus quadrivalent vaccine
HSV	herpes simplex virus
IBW	ideal body weight
ICU	intensive care unit
IE	infective endocarditis
IFN	interferon
IgA	immunoglobulin A
IgG	immunoglobulin G
IgE	immunoglobulin E
IgM	immunoglobulin M
IGRA	interferon-γ release assay
IM	intramuscular
Inh	inhalation
IP	intraperitoneal
IPV	inactivated poliovirus
IV	intravenous
JE-VAX	Japanese encephalitis virus vaccine
KOH	potassium hydroxide
KPC	*Klebsiella pneumoniae* carbapenemase
LAIV	live, attenuated influenza vaccine
LD	loading dose
LFT	liver function test
LGV	lymphogranuloma venereum

LTBI	latent tuberculosis infection
MAC	*Mycobacterium avium-intracellulare* complex
MALT	mucosa-associated lymphoid tissue
max	maximum
MCV4	meningococcal conjugate vaccine, quadrivalent
MD	maintenance dose
MDR	multidrug resistant
MIC	minimal inhibitory concentration
min	minute
misc	miscellaneous
MMR	measles, mumps, and rubella
mo	month
MPSV4	meningococcal polysaccharide vaccine
MRSA	methicillin-resistant *Staphylococcus aureus*
MRSE	methicillin-resistant *Staphylococcus epidermidis*
MSSA	methicillin-sensitive *Staphylococcus aureus*
MSSE	methicillin-susceptible *Staphylococcus epidermidis*
MTD	*Mycobacterium tuberculosis* direct test
MTT	methylthiotetrazole
NA	not applicable
NAA	nucleic acid amplification
ND	no data
NDM-1	New Delhi metallo β-lactamase
NGT	nasogastric tube
NGU	nongonococcal urethritis
NNRTI	non-nucleoside or non-nucleotide reverse transcriptase inhibitor
NRTI	nucleoside or nucleotide reverse transcriptase inhibitor
NSAID	nonsteroidal anti-inflammatory drug
NTM	nontuberculosis mycobacteria
oz	ounce
PAIR	puncture, aspiration, injection, reaspiration
PaO_2	partial pressure of arterial oxygen
PCECV	purified chick embryo cell vaccine
PCP	*Pneumocystis jiroveci* pneumonia (previously known as *Pneumocystis carinii* pneumonia)
PCR	polymerase chain reaction
PCV	pneumococcal conjugate vaccine
PCV7	7-valent pneumococcal polysaccharide vaccine
PCV13	13-valent pneumococcal polysaccharide vaccine
pen	penicillin

PEP	postexposure prophylaxis
PI	protease inhibitor
PID	pelvic inflammatory disease
POHS	presumed ocular histoplasmosis
PPD	purified protein derivative
PPI	proton pump inhibitor
PPSV	pneumococcal polysaccharide vaccine
PSA	prostate-specific antigen
q	every
QFT-GIT	QuantiFERON-TB Gold In-Tube
qid	4 times a day
RNA	ribonucleic acid
RTI	respiratory tract infection
RV	rotavirus
SBP	spontaneous bacterial peritonitis
SCr	serum creatinine; serum creatinine concentration in mg/dL
SDD	susceptible dose-dependent
SLED	sustained low-efficiency dialysis
SQ	subcutaneous
SS	single strength
S&S	swish and swallow
SSTI	skin and soft tissue infection
STARI	southern tick-associated illness
STD	sexually transmitted disease
syn	synergistic
tab	tablet
TB	tuberculosis
TBE	tick-borne encephalitis
TBEV	tick-borne encephalitis virus
Td	tetanus and diphtheria toxoids
Tdap	tetanus and diphtheria toxoids and acellular pertussis
TEE	transesophageal echocardiography
tid	3 times a day
TIV	trivalent inactivated influenza vaccine
TMP	trimethoprim
TMP-SMX	trimethoprim-sulfamethoxazole
TSH	thyroid-stimulating hormone
TST	tuberculin skin test
TTE	transthoracic echocardiography
UDP	uridine diphosphate
US	United States

USDHHS	US Department of Health and Human Services
USSR	Union of Soviet Socialist Republics
UTI	urinary tract infection
VAERS	Vaccine Adverse Event Reporting System
Vd	volume of distribution
VISA	vancomycin intermediate-resistant *Staphylococcus aureus*
VL	viral load
VRE	vancomycin-resistant enterococci
VRSA	vancomycin-resistant *Staphylococcus aureus*
VZV	varicella-zoster virus
WBC	white blood cell count
wk	week
XL	extended release
XR	extended release
y	year

Antimicrobial Dosing—Adult

Adult Antimicrobial Dosing

Table 1 Dosing Information for Antimicrobials in Adult Patients

	Usual Dose[a]	Dose Adjustment
Medication	Cl_{cr} >80 mL/min	Cl_{cr} 50-80 mL/min
abacavir	300 mg bid or 600 mg daily	Unchanged
abacavir/lamivudine (Epzicom)	600 mg abacavir plus 300 mg lamivudine (1 tab) daily	Unchanged
abacavir/lamivudine/ zidovudine (Trizivir)	300 mg abacavir plus 150 mg lamivudine plus 300 mg zidovudine (1 tab) bid	Unchanged
acyclovir IV		
Mucocutaneous disease	5 mg/kg q8h	Unchanged
HSV encephalitis	10 mg/kg q8h	Unchanged
Varicella-zoster virus (immuno-compromised patients)	10-12 mg/kg q8h	Unchanged
acyclovir oral		
Genital herpes	400 mg tid or 800 mg bid or 200 mg 5×/day	Unchanged
Varicella-zoster virus	600-800 mg 5×/day for 7 days or 1,000 mg q6h for 5 days	Unchanged
Chronic suppression for recurrent infection	400 mg bid (or 400-800 mg bid or tid for HIV)	Unchanged
albendazole	400 mg daily or bid	Unchanged

for Renal Impairment[b,c]

Cl$_{Cr}$ 10-49 mL/min	Cl$_{Cr}$ <10 mL/min (or Anuric)	Intermittent HD Dosing[d] (See also CRRT dosing information on page 40)
Unchanged	Unchanged	No data; probably not affected
Use agents individually; see dosing instructions for individual drugs		
Use agents individually; see dosing instructions for individual drugs		
Cl$_{Cr}$ 25-49: 5 mg/kg q12h Cl$_{Cr}$ 10-24: 5 mg/kg q24h	2.5 mg/kg q24h	2.5 mg/kg q24h; on dialysis days, give after HD
Cl$_{Cr}$ 25-49: 10 mg/kg q12h Cl$_{Cr}$ 10-24: 10 mg/kg q24h	5 mg/kg q24h	5 mg/kg q24h; on dialysis days, give after HD
Cl$_{Cr}$ 25-49: 10 mg/kg q12h Cl$_{Cr}$ 10-24: 10 mg/kg q24h	5 mg/kg q24h	5 mg/kg q24h; on dialysis days, give after HD
Cl$_{Cr}$ 25-49: Unchanged Cl$_{Cr}$ 10-24: 200 mg tid	200 mg bid	200 mg bid; on dialysis days, schedule 1 dose after HD
Cl$_{Cr}$ 25-49: Unchanged Cl$_{Cr}$ 10-24: 800 mg tid	800 mg bid	800 mg bid; on dialysis days, schedule 1 dose after HD
Unchanged	200 mg bid	200 mg bid; on dialysis days, schedule 1 dose after HD
Unchanged	Unchanged	No data; probably not affected

(Continues)

Table 1 Dosing Information for Antimicrobials in Adult Patients (*Cont'd.*)

Medication	Usual Dose[a] Cl_cr >80 mL/min	Dose Adjustment Cl_cr 50-80 mL/min
amantadine	Aged <65 y: 100 mg bid	Unchanged
	Aged ≥65 y: 100 mg daily	
amikacin	15-20 mg/kg q24h or 7.5 mg/kg q12h	See Tables 5-7 "Aminoglycoside Adult Dosing and Monitoring"
amoxicillin	250-500 mg tid or 875 mg bid	Unchanged
	Helicobacter pylori: 1 g bid	
	UTI: 500 mg bid	
amoxicillin/ clavulanate	250-500 mg tid or 875 mg bid; if XR give 2,000 mg bid	Unchanged
amphotericin B deoxycholate	0.5-1.5 mg/kg q24h; dose based on indication	Not eliminated renally but may need to reduce dose or dose every other day to reduce risk of further nephrotoxicity
	Yeasts: 0.5-1 mg/kg q24h	
	Aspergillus and other filamentous fungi: 1-1.5 mg/kg q24h	
amphotericin B lipid complex	5 mg/kg q24h; higher or lower doses based on indication	Not significantly cleared renally so dose adjustment not needed for renal dysfunction
amphotericin B liposomal	Empiric therapy: 3 mg/kg q24h	Not significantly cleared renally so dose adjustment not needed for renal dysfunction
	Known systemic infection: 3-5 mg/kg q24h	
	Cryptococcal meningitis HIV (patients): 3-4 mg/kg q24h	
ampicillin IV	1-2 g q4-6h	Unchanged

for Renal Impairment[b,c]

Cl_{cr} 10-49 mL/min	Cl_{cr} <10 mL/min (or Anuric)	Intermittent HD Dosing[d] (See also CRRT dosing information on page 40)
Cl_{cr} 30-49: 100 mg daily	200 mg 1×/wk	200 mg 1×/wk
Cl_{cr} 10-29: 100 mg every other day		
See Tables 5-7 "Aminoglycoside Adult Dosing and Monitoring"		Up to 66% removed; adjust dose based on serum levels
Cl_{cr} 30-49: Unchanged	250-500 mg daily	250-500 mg daily; on dialysis days, give dose after HD or give 250-mg supplement after HD
Cl_{cr} 10-29: 250-500 mg bid		
Do **NOT** use 875-mg tab with Cl_{cr} <30		
Cl_{cr} 30-49: Unchanged	250-500 mg daily	250-500 mg daily; on dialysis days, give dose after HD or give 250-mg supplement after HD
Cl_{cr} 10-29: 250-500 mg bid	Do **NOT** use XR	
Do **NOT** use 875-mg tab or XR with Cl_{cr} <30		
Not eliminated renally but may need to reduce dose or dose every other day to reduce risk of further nephrotoxicity		Not affected
Not significantly cleared renally so dose adjustment not needed for renal dysfunction		Not affected
Not significantly cleared renally so dose adjustment not needed for renal dysfunction		Unknown but probably not affected
Cl_{cr} 30-49: Unchanged	1-2 g q12-24h	1-2 g q12-24h; on dialysis days, schedule after HD
Cl_{cr} 10-29: 1-2 g q8-12h		

(Continues)

Table 1 Dosing Information for Antimicrobials in Adult Patients (*Cont'd.*)

Medication	Usual Dose[a] Cl$_{cr}$ >80 mL/min	Dose Adjustment Cl$_{cr}$ 50-80 mL/min
ampicillin/ sulbactam	1.5-3 g q6-8h	Unchanged
anidulafungin	Candidemia or candidiasis: 200 mg once then 100 mg q24h	Unchanged
	Esophageal candidiasis: 100 mg once then 50 mg q24h	
atazanavir	400 mg daily	Unchanged
atazanavir plus ritonavir	300 mg atazanavir plus 100 mg ritonavir daily	Unchanged
atovaquone oral suspension	750 mg bid or 1,500 mg daily	Unchanged
atovaquone/ proguanil (take with high-fat meals)	Malaria prophylaxis: 250 mg/100 mg (1 tab) daily, from 1-2 days before travel to endemic area to 7 days after return	Unchanged
	Malaria treatment: 1 g/400 mg (4 tab) daily for 3 days	
azithromycin IV	PID or RTI: 500 mg q24h; may switch to oral after 1-2 days	Unchanged
azithromycin oral	RTI: 500 mg daily as follow-up to azithromycin IV	Unchanged
	Mild RTI: 500 mg on day 1 then 250 mg on days 2-5 (XR oral suspension: 2 g once)	
	PID: 250 mg daily as follow-up to azithromycin IV	
	MAC prophylaxis: 1,200 mg/wk	
	Chlamydia trachomatis, chancroid, or NGU: 1 g once	

for Renal Impairment[b,c]

Cl_{cr} 10-49 mL/min	Cl_{cr} <10 mL/min (or Anuric)	Intermittent HD Dosing[d] (See also CRRT dosing information on page 40)
Cl_{cr} 30-49: Unchanged Cl_{cr} 15-29: 1.5-3 g q12h Cl_{cr} 10-14: 1.5-3 g q24h	1.5-3 g q24h	1.5-3 g q24h; on dialysis days, schedule after HD
Unchanged	Unchanged	Not affected
Unchanged	Unchanged	No data; probably not significantly affected
Unchanged	Unchanged	No data; probably not significantly affected
Unchanged	Probably unchanged	No data; probably not affected
Cl_{cr} 30-49: Unchanged Cl_{cr} <30: Not recommended	Cl_{cr} <10: Not recommended	Not recommended
Unchanged	Unchanged	Unchanged
Unchanged	Unchanged	Unchanged

(Continues)

Table 1 Dosing Information for Antimicrobials in Adult Patients (*Cont'd.*)

Medication	Usual Dose[a] Cl$_{cr}$ >80 mL/min	Dose Adjustment Cl$_{cr}$ 50-80 mL/min
aztreonam	0.5-2 g q6h, q8h, or q12h depending on organism and severity	Unchanged
bocepravir	800 mg tid	Unchanged
caspofungin	70 mg once then 50 mg q24h (or 70 mg q24h with concomitant enzyme inducers and in nonresponders)	Unchanged
cefadroxil	500 mg to 1 g bid	Unchanged
cefazolin	1-2 g q8h	Unchanged
cefdinir	300 mg bid (or 600 mg daily for pharyngitis or sinusitis)	Unchanged
cefditoren	200-400 mg bid	Unchanged
cefepime	Most infections: 1-2 g q12h	Cl$_{cr}$ ≥60: Usual dose Cl$_{cr}$ 50-59: 1-2 g q24h
	Consider 2 g q8h for life-threatening infections, systemic pseudomonal infections, or neutropenic fever	Cl$_{cr}$ ≥60: Usual dose Cl$_{cr}$ 50-59: 2 g q12h
cefixime	400 mg q24h or 200 mg bid	Unchanged
cefotaxime	1-2 g q4-12h (usually 1-2 g q8h)	Unchanged
cefotetan	1-2 g q12h	Unchanged

for Renal Impairment[b,c]

Cl_{cr} 10-49 mL/min	Cl_{cr} <10 mL/min (or Anuric)	Intermittent HD Dosing[d] (See also CRRT dosing information on page 40)
Cl_{cr} 30-49: Unchanged Cl_{cr} 10-29: 2 g once then 50% of usual dose q6h, q8h, or q12h	1-2 g once then 25% of dose q8h (125-500 mg q8h)	0.5-2 g once then 125-500 mg q8h; on dialysis days, schedule 1 dose after HD
Unchanged	Unchanged	Unchanged
Unchanged	Unchanged	Unchanged
Cl_{cr} 25-49: 500 mg bid Cl_{cr} 10-24: 500 mg daily	500 mg daily or every other day	500 mg daily or every other day; on dialysis days, schedule after HD
Cl_{cr} 30-49: Unchanged Cl_{cr} 10-29: 1-2 g q12h	1 g q24h	1 g q24h; on dialysis days, give after HD; alternately, give 2 g after HD on dialysis days only
Cl_{cr} 30-49: Unchanged Cl_{cr} <30: 300 mg daily	300 mg daily	300 mg every other day; on dialysis days, schedule after HD
Cl_{cr} 30-49: 200 mg bid Cl_{cr} 10-29: 200 mg daily	Unknown; consider 200 mg daily	Unknown; consider 200 mg daily; on dialysis days, give after HD
Cl_{cr} 30-49: 1-2 g q24h Cl_{cr} 10-29: 500 mg to 1 g q24h	250-500 mg q24h	250-500 mg q24h; on dialysis days, give after HD; alternately, give 2 g after HD on dialysis days only
Cl_{cr} 30-49: 2 g q12h Cl_{cr} 10-29: 2 g q24h	1 g q24h	1 g q24h; on dialysis days, give after HD; alternatively give 2 g after HD on dialysis days only
Cl_{cr} 20-49: 300 mg q24h Cl_{cr} <20: 200 mg q24h	200 mg q24h	300 mg q24h; on dialysis days, give after HD
Cl_{cr} 10-49: 1-2 g q8-12h	1-2 g q24h	1-2 g q24h; on dialysis days, give after HD
Cl_{cr} 10-49: 50% of usual dose q12h or usual dose q24h	1-2 g q48h	Give 50% of usual dose q24h; on dialysis days, schedule after HD

(Continues)

Table 1 Dosing Information for Antimicrobials in Adult Patients (*Cont'd.*)

Medication	Usual Dose[a] Cl$_{cr}$ >80 mL/min	Dose Adjustment Cl$_{cr}$ 50-80 mL/min
cefoxitin	1-2 g q6-8h	Unchanged
cefpodoxime proxetil	100-400 mg bid	Unchanged
cefprozil	250-500 mg bid	Unchanged
ceftazidime	1-2 g q8h	Unchanged
ceftibuten	400 mg daily	Unchanged
ceftriaxone	Most indications: 1-2 g q24h CNS infection: 2 g q12h	Unchanged
cefuroxime IV	750 mg or 1.5 g q8h (or 1.5 g q6h for serious infection)	Unchanged
cefuroxime oral	125-500 mg bid	Unchanged
cephalexin	250 mg to 1 g qid	Unchanged
chloramphenicol	50-100 mg/kg/24h divided q6h (4 g q24h max)	Unchanged; monitor serum levels
chloroquine	Malaria prophylaxis: 300 mg/wk (base) Malaria treatment: 1.5 g (base) over 3 days	Unchanged

for Renal Impairment[b,c]

Cl_{cr} 10-49 mL/min	Cl_{cr} <10 mL/min (or Anuric)	Intermittent HD Dosing[d] (See also CRRT dosing information on page 40)
Cl_{cr} 30-49: 1-2 g q8-12h Cl_{cr} 10-29: 1-2 g q12-24h	1-2 g q24-48h	1-2 g q24-48h; on dialysis days, schedule after HD
Cl_{cr} 30-49: Unchanged Cl_{cr} 10-29: 100-400 mg daily	100-400 mg daily	100-400 mg 3×/wk after HD
Cl_{cr} 30-49: Unchanged Cl_{cr} 10-29: 125-250 mg bid	250 mg daily	250 mg daily; on dialysis days, schedule after HD
Cl_{cr} 30-49: 1-2 g q12h Cl_{cr} 10-29: 1-2 g q24h	500 mg to 1 g q24-48h	1-g to 2-g load then 1 g after HD
Cl_{cr} 30-49: 200 mg daily Cl_{cr} 10-29: 100 mg daily	100 mg daily	Consider 400 mg after HD on dialysis days only
Unchanged	Unchanged	1-2 g q24h or 2 g q12h for CNS infection; on dialysis days, give after HD
Cl_{cr} 20-49: Unchanged Cl_{cr} 10-19: 750 mg q12h	750 mg q24h	750 mg q24h; on dialysis days, schedule after HD
Unchanged	250-500 mg daily	250-500 mg daily; on dialysis days, schedule after HD
Cl_{cr} 30-49: Unchanged Cl_{cr} 10-29: Usual dose bid or tid	250-500 mg bid or daily	250-500 mg daily; on dialysis days, schedule after HD
Unchanged; monitor serum levels	Unchanged; monitor serum levels	Schedule 1 dose after HD; monitor serum levels
Unchanged	Give 50% of usual dose	Not appreciably affected; give 50% of usual dose

(Continues)

Table 1 Dosing Information for Antimicrobials in Adult Patients (*Cont'd.*)

Medication	Usual Dose[a] Cl$_{Cr}$ >80 mL/min	Dose Adjustment Cl$_{Cr}$ 50-80 mL/min
cidofovir (must give with probenecid and fluids)	Induction: 5 mg/kg/wk twice Maintenance: 5 mg/kg q2wk	Reduce dose to 3 mg/kg if SCr increases 0.3-0.4 mg/dL above baseline; discontinue if SCr increases ≥0.5 mg/dL above baseline or with urine protein ≥300 mg/dL (≥3+ proteinuria); contraindicated if Cl$_{Cr}$ ≤55, SCr ≥1.5 mg/dL, or urine protein ≥100 mg/dL (2+ proteinuria)
ciprofloxacin IV[e]	200-400 mg q12h Severe infection (eg, nosocomial pneumonia): 400 mg q8h	Unchanged
ciprofloxacin oral[e]	250-750 mg bid (or XR 500-1,000 mg daily)	Unchanged
clarithromycin	250-500 mg bid (or XL 1,000 mg daily)	Unchanged
clindamycin IV	300-900 mg q6-8h	Unchanged
clindamycin oral	150-450 mg qid	Unchanged
clotrimazole lozenges	10 mg 5×/day	Unchanged
colistin IM or IV (as colistimethate)	5 mg/kg/24h in 2 divided doses	2.5-3.8 mg/kg/24h in 2 divided doses
colistin Inh (as colistimethate)	75-150 mg bid; use after bronchodilator	Unchanged
cotrimoxazole[e]**: See trimethoprim-sulfamethoxazole**		
dalfopristin/ quinupristin	7.5 mg/kg actual body weight q8-12h	Unchanged

for Renal Impairment[b,c]

Cl$_{Cr}$ 10-49 mL/min	Cl$_{Cr}$ <10 mL/min (or Anuric)	Intermittent HD Dosing[d] (See also CRRT dosing information on page 40)
Reduce dose to 3 mg/kg if SCr increases 0.3-0.4 mg/dL above baseline; discontinue if SCr increases ≥0.5 mg/dL above baseline or with urine protein ≥300 mg/dL (≥3+ proteinuria); contraindicated if Cl$_{Cr}$ ≤55, SCr ≥1.5 mg/dL, or urine protein ≥100 mg/dL (2+ proteinuria)		
Cl$_{Cr}$ 30-49: Unchanged Cl$_{Cr}$ 10-29: 200-400 mg q18-24h	200-400 mg q18-24h	200-400 mg q24h; on dialysis days, give after HD
250-500 mg bid (or XR 500 mg daily)	250-500 mg q18-24h (or XR 500 mg daily)	250-500 mg daily (or XR 500 mg daily); on dialysis days, give after HD
Cl$_{Cr}$ 30-49: Unchanged Cl$_{Cr}$ 10-29: 500-mg load then give 50% of dose or double the interval	250 mg daily	250 mg daily; on dialysis days, give after HD
Unchanged	Unchanged	Unchanged
Unchanged	Unchanged	Unchanged
Unchanged	Unchanged	Unchanged
2.5 mg/kg q24h	1.5 mg/kg q24h	1.5 mg/kg q24h; or 2-3 mg/kg after HD on dialysis days only
Unchanged	Unchanged	Unchanged
Unchanged	Unchanged	Not likely to be affected

(*Continues*)

Table 1 Dosing Information for Antimicrobials in Adult Patients (*Cont'd.*)

Medication	Usual Dose^a Cl_{cr} >80 mL/min	Dose Adjustment Cl_{cr} 50-80 mL/min
dapsone	50-100 mg daily	Unchanged
daptomycin	cSSSI: 4 mg/kg q24h	Unchanged
	Bacteremia or endocarditis (and consider for bone or joint infections): 6 mg/kg q24h	
darunavir (give with ritonavir)	Naive or no resistence mutations: 800 mg (plus ritonavir 100 mg) once daily	Unchanged
	At least 1 resistence mutation: 600 mg (plus ritonavir 100 mg) both given bid	
delavirdine	400 mg tid	Unchanged
dicloxacillin	125-500 mg qid	Unchanged
didanosine EC	If >60 kg: 400 mg daily	Cl_{cr} ≥60: Unchanged
	If ≤60 kg: 250 mg daily	Cl_{cr} 50-59: If >60 kg: 200 mg daily If ≤60 kg: 125 mg daily
diethylcarbamazine	Varies by indication (see *Micromedex*)	Unchanged
dirithromycin	500 mg daily	Unchanged
doripenem	500 mg q8h	Unchanged
doxycycline^e IV or oral	200 mg then 100 mg bid	Unchanged
efavirenz	600 mg daily	Unchanged

for Renal Impairment[b,c]

Cl$_{cr}$ 10-49 mL/min	Cl$_{cr}$ <10 mL/min (or Anuric)	Intermittent HD Dosing[d] (See also CRRT dosing information on page 40)
Unchanged	Insufficient data	Insufficient data; not likely to be affected
Cl$_{cr}$ 30-49: Unchanged Cl$_{cr}$ 10-29: Usual dose q48h	Usual dose q48h	Usual dose q48h; on dialysis days, give after HD. Some data support 3×/wk dosing after HD; if this is done, consider giving a 50% higher dose prior to the 72-hour nondialytic period
Cl$_{cr}$ 30-49: Unchanged Cl$_{cr}$ 10-29: Limited data; consider usual dose	Limited data; consider usual dose	Limited data; consider usual dose
Unchanged	Unchanged	Unknown; probably not affected
Unchanged	Unchanged	Unchanged

If >60 kg:
 	
  Cl$_{cr}$ 30-49: 200 mg daily
 	
  Cl$_{cr}$ 10-29: 125 mg daily
 	
If ≤60 kg:
 	
  Cl$_{cr}$ 30-49: 125 mg daily
 	
  Cl$_{cr}$ 10-29: 100 mg daily
	If >60 kg: 125 mg daily
	
	If ≤60 kg: 75 mg daily
		If >60 kg: 125 mg daily
		
		If ≤60 kg: 75 mg daily

Dose reduction needed but specific recommendations lacking		
Unchanged	Unchanged	Unchanged
Cl$_{cr}$ 30-49: 250 mg q8h Cl$_{cr}$ 10-29: 250 mg q12h	Unknown	Unknown but about 50% removed
Unchanged	Unchanged	Unchanged
Unchanged	Unchanged	Unknown but probably not affected

(Continues)

Table 1 Dosing Information for Antimicrobials in Adult Patients (*Cont'd.*)

Medication	Usual Dose[a] Cl$_{cr}$ >80 mL/min	Dose Adjustment Cl$_{cr}$ 50-80 mL/min
emtricitabine	200 mg daily	200 mg daily
emtricitabine plus tenofovir (Truvada)	200 mg emtricitabine plus 300 mg tenofovir (1 tab) daily	Unchanged
emtricitabine plus tenofovir plus efavirenz (Atripla)	200 mg emtricitabine plus 300 mg tenofovir plus 600 mg efavirenz (1 tab) daily	Unchanged
enfuvirtide	90 mg SQ bid	Unchanged
ertapenem	1 g q24h	Unchanged
erythromycin IV	500 mg to 1 g q6h	Unchanged
erythromycin oral (base)	250-500 mg qid	Unchanged
ethambutol	15-25 mg/kg q24h (max 2.5 g q24h) or DOT 50 mg/kg oral 2×/wk or DOT 25-30 mg/kg oral 3×/wk	Unchanged
famciclovir		
Herpes zoster	500 mg tid	Unchanged
Recurrent orolabial or genital herpes (HIV patients)	500 mg bid	Unchanged

for Renal Impairment[b,c]

Cl$_{cr}$ 10-49 mL/min	Cl$_{cr}$ <10 mL/min (or Anuric)	Intermittent HD Dosing[d] (See also CRRT dosing information on page 40)
Cl$_{cr}$ 30-49: 200 mg every 2 days Cl$_{cr}$ 15-29: 200 mg every 3 days Cl$_{cr}$ 10-14: 200 mg every 4 days	200 mg every 4 days	200 mg every 4 days; on dialysis days, give after HD
Cl$_{cr}$ 30-49: 1 tab every other day Cl$_{cr}$ 10-29: Use individual agents separately	Use individual agents separately	Use individual agents separately
Use individual agents separately	Use individual agents separately	Use individual agents separately
Cl$_{cr}$ 35-49: Usual dose Cl$_{cr}$ 15-34: No data	No data	No data
Cl$_{cr}$ 30-49: 1 g q24h Cl$_{cr}$ 10-29: 500 mg q24h	500 mg q24h	500 mg q24h; on dialysis days, give after HD
Unchanged	Give 50-75% of usual dose at normal intervals	Not affected; give 50-75% of usual dose at normal intervals
Unchanged	Give 50-75% of usual dose at normal intervals	Not affected; give 50-75% of usual dose at normal intervals
15 mg/kg q24-36h	15 mg/kg q48h	15-25 mg/kg after HD on dialysis days only
Cl$_{cr}$ 40-49: 500 mg bid Cl$_{cr}$ 20-39: 500 mg daily Cl$_{cr}$ <20: 250 mg daily	250 mg daily	250 mg after HD on dialysis days only
Cl$_{cr}$ 40-49: Unchanged Cl$_{cr}$ 20-39: 500 mg daily Cl$_{cr}$ <20: 250 mg daily	250 mg daily	250 mg after HD on dialysis days only

(Continues)

Table 1 Dosing Information for Antimicrobials in Adult Patients (*Cont'd.*)

Medication	Usual Dose[a] Cl$_{cr}$ >80 mL/min	Dose Adjustment Cl$_{cr}$ 50-80 mL/min
Recurrent orolabial or genital herpes (non-HIV patients)	125 mg bid	Unchanged
Suppression of recurrent genital herpes	250 mg bid	Unchanged
fidaxomicin	200 mg bid	Unchanged
fluconazole[e] **IV or oral**	200-800 mg q24h for most indications (consider load of 2 times maintenance dose)	Unchanged
	Mucocutaneous infection or UTI: 100-200 mg q24h	
	Candidemia or systemic candidiasis: 400-800 mg q24h; use higher doses for SDD isolates	
flucytosine	25 mg/kg q6h	Unchanged; adjust dose based on serum levels
fosamprenavir	Treatment-naive patients: 1,400 mg bid	Unchanged
fosamprenavir plus ritonavir	Treatment-naive patients: 1,400 mg fosamprenavir plus 200 mg ritonavir daily	Unchanged
	Treatment-experienced patients: 700 mg fosamprenavir plus 100 mg ritonavir bid	Unchanged
foscarnet	Induction: 60 mg/kg q8h or 90 mg/kg q12h for 2-3 weeks	See product labeling
	Maintenance: 90-120 mg/kg q24h	See product labeling
fosfomycin	Uncomplicated lower UTI: 3 g once	Unchanged
	Complicated lower UTI: 3 g every 2-3 days	Unchanged

for Renal Impairment[b,c]

Cl$_{cr}$ 10-49 mL/min	Cl$_{cr}$ <10 mL/min (or Anuric)	Intermittent HD Dosing[d] (See also CRRT dosing information on page 40)
Cl$_{cr}$ 40-49: Unchanged Cl$_{cr}$ 20-39: 125 mg daily Cl$_{cr}$ <20: 125 mg daily	125 mg daily	125 mg after HD on dialysis days only
Cl$_{cr}$ 40-49: Unchanged Cl$_{cr}$ 20-39: 125 mg bid Cl$_{cr}$ <20: 125 mg daily	125 mg daily	125 mg after HD on dialysis days only
Unchanged	Unchanged	Unchanged
Load then 50% of usual dose q24h	Load then 25% of usual dose q24h	Give usual dose after HD on dialysis days only
25 mg/kg q12-24h; adjust dose based on serum levels	25 mg/kg q24-48h; adjust dose based on serum levels	25 mg/kg q24-48h; on dialysis days, give after HD; adjust dose based on serum levels
Unchanged	Unchanged	Unchanged
Unchanged	Unchanged	Unchanged
Unchanged	Unchanged	Unchanged
See product labeling	Not recommended	No specific data; consider 45-60 mg/kg after HD
See product labeling	Not recommended	No specific data; consider 45-60 mg/kg after HD
Unchanged	Consider avoiding due to reduced urinary levels	Consider avoiding due to reduced urinary levels
Consider 3 g every 3 days	Consider avoiding due to decreased urinary levels	Consider avoiding: if used, redose after HD

(Continues)

Table 1 Dosing Information for Antimicrobials in Adult Patients (*Cont'd.*)

Medication	Usual Dose[a] Cl$_{cr}$ >80 mL/min	Dose Adjustment Cl$_{cr}$ 50-80 mL/min
ganciclovir IV	Induction: 5 mg/kg q12h	Cl$_{cr}$ 70-80: Unchanged
		Cl$_{cr}$ 50-69: 2.5 mg/kg q12h
	Maintenance: 5 mg/kg q24h	Cl$_{cr}$ 70-80: Unchanged
		Cl$_{cr}$ 50-69: 2.5 mg/kg q24h
ganciclovir oral	1 g tid	Cl$_{cr}$ 70-80: Unchanged
		Cl$_{cr}$ 50-69: 1,500 mg daily or 500 mg tid
gentamicin	3-7 mg/kg/24h in divided doses or daily as pulse dosing; monitor serum levels	See Tables 5-7 ("Aminoglycoside Adult Dosing and Monitoring"); monitor serum levels
imipenem/cilastatin	500 mg q6h (usual) Serious infections with moderately susceptible organisms: Up to 3-4 g per day in divided doses	500 mg q6-8h
indinavir (or indinavir plus ritonavir)	800 mg q8h (or 600-800 mg indinavir plus 100-200 mg ritonavir bid)	Unchanged
iodoquinol	630-650 mg tid	Unchanged
isoniazid	5 mg/kg q24h (max 300 mg q24h) or DOT 15 mg/kg 2-3×/wk (max 900 mg q24h)	Unchanged
itraconazole cap or oral solution	200 mg daily or 200 mg bid; higher doses may be used based on levels	Unchanged
ivermectin	50-200 mcg/kg once	Unchanged
ketoconazole	200-400 mg daily	Unchanged

for Renal Impairment[b,c]

Cl_{cr} 10-49 mL/min	Cl_{cr} <10 mL/min (or Anuric)	Intermittent HD Dosing[d] (See also CRRT dosing information on page 40)
Cl_{cr} 25-49: 2.5 mg/kg q24h Cl_{cr} 10-24: 1.25 mg/kg q24h	1.25 mg/kg 3×/wk	1.25 mg/kg 3×/wk; on dialysis days, give after HD
Cl_{cr} 25-49: 1.25 mg/kg q24h Cl_{cr} 10-24: 0.625 mg/kg q24h	0.625 mg/kg 3×/wk	0.625 mg/kg 3×/wk; on dialysis days, give after HD
Cl_{cr} 25-49: 1 g daily or 500 mg bid Cl_{cr} 10-24: 500 mg daily	500 mg 3×/wk	500 mg 3×/wk; on dialysis days, give after HD
See Tables 5-7 ("Aminoglycoside Adult Dosing and Monitoring"); monitor serum levels		About 60% removed; adjust dose based on serum levels
500 mg q8-12h	250-500 mg q12h	250-500 mg q12h; on dialysis days, schedule 1 dose after HD or give supplement after HD
Unchanged	Unchanged	No data; probably not affected
Unchanged	No data	No data; probably not affected
Unchanged	Unchanged; can give 50% of dose in slow acetylators	Unchanged; can give 50% of dose in slow acetylators; on dialysis days, give after HD
Unchanged	Unchanged	Unchanged
Unchanged	No data; probably unchanged	No data; probably not affected
Unchanged	Unchanged	Unchanged

(*Continues*)

Table 1 Dosing Information for Antimicrobials in Adult Patients (*Cont'd.*)

Medication	Usual Dose[a] Cl$_{Cr}$ >80 mL/min	Dose Adjustment Cl$_{Cr}$ 50-80 mL/min
lamivudine		
HBV	100 mg daily	Unchanged
HIV	150 mg bid (2 mg/kg if <50 kg) or 300 mg daily	Unchanged
lamivudine/ zidovudine (Combivir)	150 mg lamivudine plus 300 mg zidovudine (1 tab) bid	Unchanged
levofloxacin[e] IV or oral	250-750 mg q24h Nosocomial pneumonia, cSSSI, or 5-day CAP therapy: 750 mg q24h Most other indications: 500 mg q24h Uncomplicated UTI: 250 mg q24h	Unchanged

for Renal Impairment^{b,c}

Cl_{cr} 10-49 mL/min	Cl_{cr} <10 mL/min (or Anuric)	Intermittent HD Dosing^d (See also CRRT dosing information on page 40)
Cl_{cr} 30-49: 100-mg load then 50 mg daily	Cl_{cr} 5-9: 35-mg load then 15 mg daily	35-mg load then 10 mg daily
Cl_{cr} 15-29: 100-mg load then 25 mg daily	Cl_{cr} <5: 35-mg load then 10 mg daily	
Cl_{cr} 10-14: 35-mg load then 15 mg daily		
Cl_{cr} 30-49: 150 mg daily	Cl_{cr} 5-9: 150-mg load then 50 mg daily	50-mg load then 25 mg daily
Cl_{cr} 15-29: 150-mg load then 100 mg daily	Cl_{cr} <5: 50-mg load then 25 mg daily	
Cl_{cr} 10-14: 150-mg load then 50 mg daily		
Use agents individually; see dosing instructions for individual drugs		
Cl_{cr} 20-49: Nosocomial pneumonia, cSSSI, or 5-day CAP therapy: 750 mg q48h	Nosocomial pneumonia, cSSSI, or 5-day CAP therapy: 750-mg load then 500 mg q48h	Not affected; dose as for Cl_{cr} <10
Most other indications: 500-mg load then 250 mg q24h	Most other indications: 500-mg load then 250 mg q48h	
Uncomplicated UTI: 250 mg	Uncomplicated UTI: 250 mg q48h	
Cl_{cr} 10-19: Nosocomial pneumonia, cSSSI, or 5-day CAP therapy: 750-mg load then 500 mg q48h		
Most other indications: 500-mg load then 250 mg q48h		
Uncomplicated UTI: 250 mg q48h		

(Continues)

Table 1 Dosing Information for Antimicrobials in Adult Patients (*Cont'd.*)

Medication	Usual Dose[a] Cl$_{cr}$ >80 mL/min	Dose Adjustment Cl$_{cr}$ 50-80 mL/min
linezolid[e] **IV or oral**	600 mg q12h	Unchanged
lopinavir/ritonavir	400 mg/100 mg (2 tab) bid	Unchanged
	Treatment-naive patients: 800 mg/200 mg (4 tab) once daily	
maraviroc	150-600 mg bid depending on concomitant drugs (see prescribing information)	Unchanged
mebendazole	Pinworms: 100 mg once; may repeat in 3 weeks	Unchanged
	Whipworms, roundworms, and hookworms: 100 mg bid for 3 days; may repeat in 3-4 weeks	
	Capillariasis: 200 mg bid for 20 days	
mefloquine	Mild or moderate malaria: 1,250 mg once	Unchanged
	Multidrug-resistant falciparum malaria: 15 mg/kg once then 10 mg/kg 8-24h later	
	Malaria prophylaxis: 250 mg/wk	
meropenem	1 g q8h	Unchanged
	500 mg q6h	500 mg q6h
metronidazole[e] **IV or oral**	15 mg/kg once then 7.5 mg/kg (500 mg) q8-12h	Unchanged
micafungin	Esophageal candidiasis: 150 mg q24h	Unchanged
	BMT prophylaxis: 50 mg q24h	
	Systemic infection: 100 mg q24h	

for Renal Impairment[b,c]

Cl_{Cr} 10-49 mL/min	Cl_{Cr} <10 mL/min (or Anuric)	Intermittent HD Dosing[d] (See also CRRT dosing information on page 40)
Unchanged	Unchanged	Unchanged; on dialysis days, schedule 1 dose after HD or give 200-mg supplement after HD
Unchanged	Unchanged	No data; probably not affected
Unchanged	Unchanged	Unknown
Unchanged	Unchanged	Not significantly affected
Unchanged	No data	No data; probably not affected
Cl_{Cr} 26-49: 1 g q12h Cl_{Cr} 10-25: 500 mg q12h	500 mg q24h	500 mg q24h; on dialysis days, give after HD
Cl_{Cr} 26-49: 500 mg q8h Cl_{Cr} 10-25: 500 mg q12h	Same as above	Same as above
Unchanged	Consider 500 mg q12h or 50% of dose at normal intervals	Consider 500 mg q12h; on dialysis days, schedule at least 1 dose after HD
Unchanged	Unchanged	Unchanged

(Continues)

Table 1 Dosing Information for Antimicrobials in Adult Patients (*Cont'd.*)

Medication	Usual Dose[a] Cl_{cr} >80 mL/min	Dose Adjustment Cl_{cr} 50-80 mL/min
minocycline[e] IV or oral	200-mg load then 100 mg bid	Unchanged
moxifloxacin[e] IV or oral	400 mg q24h	Unchanged
nafcillin	1-2 g q4-6h	Unchanged
nelfinavir	750 mg tid or 1,250 mg bid	Unchanged
nevirapine	200 mg daily for 14 days then either 200 mg immediate release bid or 400 mg extended release daily	Unchanged
nitazoxanide	500 mg bid	Unchanged
nitrofurantoin	50-100 mg qid	Unchanged
nitrofurantoin monohydrate macrocrystals	100 mg bid	Unchanged
nystatin lozenges	200,000-400,000 units 5×/day	Unchanged
nystatin S&S	0.4-1 million units 3-5×/day	Unchanged
oseltamivir	Treatment: 75 mg bid Prophylaxis: 75 mg daily	Unchanged
oxacillin IV	500 mg to 2 g q4-6h	Unchanged

for Renal Impairment[b,c]

Cl_{cr} 10-49 mL/min	Cl_{cr} <10 mL/min (or Anuric)	Intermittent HD Dosing[d] (See also CRRT dosing information on page 40)
Unchanged	Unchanged or consider 200-mg load then 100 mg q24h	Not affected by HD; unchanged or consider 200-mg load then 100 mg q24h
Unchanged	Unchanged	Unchanged
Unchanged	Unchanged	Unchanged
Unchanged	No data; probably not unchanged	No data; probably not affected
Unchanged	Unchanged	No data; probably not affected
Unchanged	No data	No data
Avoid	Avoid	Avoid
Avoid	Avoid	Avoid
Unchanged	Unchanged	Unchanged
Unchanged	Unchanged	Unchanged

Cl_{cr} 30-49: Unchanged
 	
Cl_{cr} 10-29
 	
  Treatment: 75 mg daily
 	
  Prophylaxis: 75 mg q48h or 30 mg daily
	No data; suggest dosing similar to that for Cl_{cr} 10-29	Limited data; suggest 30 mg after every other HD session

Unchanged	Unchanged	Unchanged

(*Continues*)

Table 1 Dosing Information for Antimicrobials in Adult Patients (*Cont'd.*)

Medication	Usual Dose[a] Cl$_{cr}$ >80 mL/min	Dose Adjustment Cl$_{cr}$ 50-80 mL/min
paromomycin	Intestinal amebiasis: 25-35 mg/kg/24h in 3 divided doses	Unchanged
	Cryptosporidium: 1.5-2.5 g/24h in 3-6 divided doses	
	Tapeworm: 1 g q15min for 4 doses	
penicillin G IV	5-24 million units per day divided q4h or as continuous infusion (give load of 3-5 million units for serious infections)	Unchanged
penicillin V oral	250-500 mg tid or qid	Unchanged
pentamidine Inh	300 mg/mo	Unchanged
pentamidine IV	3-4 mg/kg q24h	Unchanged
piperacillin	3-4 g q4-6h	Unchanged
piperacillin/ tazobactam	Most indications: 3.375 g q6h	Unchanged
	Nosocomial pneumonia: 4.5 g q6h	Unchanged
posaconazole	Prophylaxis: 200 mg tid	Unchanged
	Oropharyngeal candidiasis: 100 mg bid on day 1 then 100 mg q24h	

for Renal Impairment[b,c]

Cl_{cr} 10-49 mL/min	Cl_{cr} <10 mL/min (or Anuric)	Intermittent HD Dosing[d] (See also CRRT dosing information on page 40)
Unchanged	No data; avoid if possible	No data
Normal load then 75% of usual dose q4-6h (or 75% of usual daily dose as continuous infusion)	Normal load then 25-50% of usual dose q4-6h (or 25-50% of usual daily dose as continuous infusion)	Normal load then 25-50% of usual dose q4-6h (or 25-50% of usual daily dose as continuous infusion); on dialysis days, schedule at least 1 dose after HD
Unchanged	250 mg tid or qid	250 mg tid or qid; on dialysis days, schedule at least 1 dose after HD or give 250-mg supplement after HD
Unchanged	Unchanged	Unchanged
Unchanged	Probably unchanged	Probably not affected
Cl_{cr} 40-49: Unchanged Cl_{cr} 20-39: 3-4 g q8h Cl_{cr} 10-19: 3-4 g q12h	3-4 g q12h	2 g q8h; on dialysis days, schedule at least 1 dose after HD or give 1-g supplement after HD
Cl_{cr} 40-49: Unchanged Cl_{cr} 20-39: 2.25 g q6h Cl_{cr} 10-19: 2.25 g q8h	2.25 g q8h	2.25 g q12h; on dialysis days, schedule at least 1 dose after HD or give 0.75-g supplement after HD
Cl_{cr} 40-49: Unchanged Cl_{cr} 20-39: 3.375 g q6h Cl_{cr} 10-19: 2.25 g q6h	2.25 g q6h	2.25 g q8h; on dialysis days, schedule at least 1 dose after HD or give 0.75-g supplement after HD
Unchanged	Unchanged but variability in AUC noted; monitor serum levels for efficacy	Not expected to be affected

(Continues)

Table 1 Dosing Information for Antimicrobials in Adult Patients (*Cont'd.*)

Medication	Usual Dose[a] Cl$_{cr}$ >80 mL/min	Dose Adjustment Cl$_{cr}$ 50-80 mL/min
posaconazole (continued)	*Zygomycetes* and other filamentous fungi: 200 mg qid or 400 mg bid; adjust dose based on serum levels	
praziquantel	Varies by indication (see *Micromedex*)	Unchanged
primaquine	Malaria: 15-mg base daily or 45-mg/wk base	Unchanged
pyrazinamide	15-30 mg/kg daily (max 2 g per dose); or 50-70 mg/kg (max 4 g per dose) DOT 2×/wk; or 50-70 mg/kg (max 3 g per dose) DOT 3×/wk	Unchanged
pyrimethamine	25-100 mg daily based on indication	Unchanged
quinidine gluconate IV	Malaria: 10 mg/kg load then 0.02 mg/kg/min for 72 hours; or 24 mg/kg over 4-hour load then 12 mg/kg over 4 hours q8h for 7 days (modify based on clinical response, ECG, BP, and serum levels)	Unchanged
quinine	Malaria: 648 mg tid	Unchanged
raltegravir	400 mg bid	Unchanged
rifabutin	300 mg q24h or 150 mg bid or 300-450 mg DOT 2×/wk	Unchanged
rifampin	Mycobacterial infection: 600 mg q24h; or 600 mg DOT 2-3×/wk Staphylococcal infection: 600-1,200 mg q24h in 2-3 divided doses (do not use as monotherapy)	Unchanged

for Renal Impairment[b,c]

Cl_cr 10-49 mL/min	Cl_cr <10 mL/min (or Anuric)	Intermittent HD Dosing[d] (See also CRRT dosing information on page 40)
Unchanged	No data	No data; probably not affected
Unchanged	No data	No data
Unchanged	12-20 mg/kg daily	25-35 mg/kg after HD
Unchanged	Unchanged	Unchanged
Unchanged	Consider 75-100% of dose (modify based on clinical response, ECG, BP, and serum levels)	Dose as for Cl_cr <10; 5-20% removed
Not well defined; consider 648 mg bid or tid	648-mg load then 324 mg bid	Dose as for Cl_cr <10; on dialysis days, schedule after HD
Unchanged	Unchanged	Unchanged
Unchanged	No data	No data
Unchanged	Give 50-100% of usual dose	Not affected; give 50-100% of usual dose

(Continues)

Table 1 Dosing Information for Antimicrobials in Adult Patients (*Cont'd.*)

Medication	Usual Dose[a] Cl$_{cr}$ >80 mL/min	Dose Adjustment Cl$_{cr}$ 50-80 mL/min
rifaximin	Traveler's diarrhea due to *Escherichia coli*: 200 mg tid	Unchanged
rimantadine	Aged <65 y: 100 mg bid	Unchanged
	Aged ≥65 y: 100 mg daily	
ritonavir	600 mg bid (boosting doses of 100-200 mg q24h have been given with other protease inhibitors)	Unchanged
saquinavir	1,200 mg tid	Unchanged
saquinavir plus ritonavir	1,000 mg saquinavir plus 100 mg ritonavir bid	Unchanged
stavudine	If <60 kg: 30 mg bid	30 mg bid
	If ≥60 kg: 40 mg bid	40 mg bid
streptomycin	7.5 mg/kg q12h	7.5 mg/kg q24h; adjust dose based on serum levels
telapravir	750 mg tid	Unchanged
telavancin	10 mg/kg q24h	Unchanged
tenofovir	300 mg daily	Unchanged
tetracycline	250-500 mg qid	250-500 mg tid or bid
ticarcillin/ clavulanate	3.1 g q4-6h	Unchanged

for Renal Impairment[b,c]

Cl$_{cr}$ 10-49 mL/min	Cl$_{cr}$ <10 mL/min (or Anuric)	Intermittent HD Dosing[d] (See also CRRT dosing information on page 40)
Unchanged	No data; probably unchanged	Probably not affected
Unchanged	100 mg daily	100 mg daily
No data; probably unchanged	No data; probably unchanged	No data; probably not affected
No data; probably unchanged	No data; probably unchanged	No data; probably not affected
No data; probably unchanged	No data; probably unchanged	No data; probably not affected
Cl$_{cr}$ 26-49: 15 mg bid Cl$_{cr}$ 10-25: 15 mg q24h	15 mg q24h	15 mg q24h; on dialysis days, give after HD
Cl$_{cr}$ 26-49: 20 mg bid Cl$_{cr}$ 10-25: 20 mg daily	20 mg daily	20 mg daily; on dialysis days, give after HD
7.5 mg/kg q24-72h; adjust dose based on serum levels	7.5 mg/kg q72-96h; adjust dose based on serum levels	50-75% removed by HD; adjust dose based on serum levels
Unchanged	Unchanged	Unchanged
Cl$_{cr}$ 30-49: 7.5 mg/kg q24h Cl$_{cr}$ 10-29: 10 mg/kg q48h	No dosing recommendations, but consider further reduction in dose	No dosing recommendations; only about 6% removed by HD
Cl$_{cr}$ 30-49: 300 mg every other day Cl$_{cr}$ 10-29: 300 mg 2×/wk	300 mg 1×/wk	300 mg 1×/wk; on dialysis days, give after HD
doxycycline preferred; or use tetracycline 250-500 mg bid or daily	doxycycline preferred; or use tetracycline 250-500 mg daily	Use doxycycline
3.1-g load then: Cl$_{cr}$ 30-49: 2 g q4h Cl$_{cr}$ 10-29: 2 g q8h	3.1-g load then 2 g q12h	Dose as for Cl$_{cr}$ <10; on dialysis days, schedule dose after HD or give 3.1-g supplement after HD

(Continues)

Table 1 Dosing Information for Antimicrobials in Adult Patients (*Cont'd.*)

Medication	Usual Dose[a] Cl_{cr} >80 mL/min	Dose Adjustment Cl_{cr} 50-80 mL/min
tigecycline	100-mg load then 50 mg q12h	Unchanged
tipranavir plus ritonavir	500 mg tipranavir plus 200 mg ritonavir bid	Unchanged
tobramycin Inh	CF: 300 mg bid for 28-day cycle Non-CF: Usually 300 mg bid or 60-80 mg tid	Unchanged
tobramycin IV	3-7 mg/kg/24h in divided doses or daily as pulse dosing; monitor serum levels	See Tables 5-7 ("Aminoglycoside Adult Dosing and Monitoring"); monitor serum levels
trimethoprim	100 mg bid or 200 mg daily	Unchanged
trimethoprim-sulfamethoxazole[e] (cotrimoxazole)		
Non-PCP (IV)	8-10 mg/kg/24h TMP component in 2-4 divided doses	Unchanged
PCP or *Nocardia* (IV)	15-20 mg/kg/24h TMP component in 3-4 divided doses	Unchanged
PCP prophylaxis (oral)	1 DS daily or 3×/wk or 1 SS daily	Unchanged
Most other indications (oral)	1 DS bid	Unchanged

for Renal Impairment[b,c]

Cl$_{Cr}$ 10-49 mL/min	Cl$_{Cr}$ <10 mL/min (or Anuric)	Intermittent HD Dosing[d] (See also CRRT dosing information on page 40)
Unchanged	Unchanged	Unchanged
Unchanged	Unchanged	No data; probably not affected
Unchanged	Unchanged	Unchanged
See Tables 5-7 ("Aminoglycoside Adult Dosing and Monitoring"); monitor serum levels		About 60% removed; adjust dose based on serum levels
Cl$_{Cr}$ 30-49: Unchanged Cl$_{Cr}$ 15-29: 100 mg daily or 50 mg bid	Avoid or consider further reducing dose	Avoid
Cl$_{Cr}$ 30-49: Unchanged Cl$_{Cr}$ 15-29: Consider usual dose for 1-2 days then 4-6 mg/kg/24h in 1-2 doses Cl$_{Cr}$ 10-14: 8-12 mg/kg q48h or 4-6 mg/kg/24h in 1-2 doses	Avoid; or 4-6 mg/kg/24h in 1-2 doses	Dose as for Cl$_{Cr}$ <10; on dialysis days, schedule after HD
Cl$_{Cr}$ 30-49: Unchanged Cl$_{Cr}$ 15-29: 5 mg/kg q6-8h for 48 hours then 3.5-5 mg/kg q12h	7-10 mg/kg/24h in 1-2 doses	Dose as for Cl$_{Cr}$ <10; on dialysis days, schedule after HD
1 SS daily or 3×/wk	1 SS daily or 3×/wk	1 SS tab daily or 3×/wk; on dialysis days, schedule after HD
DS q24h or SS bid	Avoid if possible or 1 DS q48h	Dose as for Cl$_{Cr}$ <10; on dialysis days, schedule after HD

(Continues)

Table 1 Dosing Information for Antimicrobials in Adult Patients (*Cont'd.*)

Medication	Usual Dose[a] Cl$_{Cr}$ >80 mL/min	Dose Adjustment Cl$_{Cr}$ 50-80 mL/min
valacyclovir		
Herpes zoster	1 g tid	Unchanged
First episode genital herpes	1 g bid	Unchanged
Recurrent genital herpes	500 mg bid	Unchanged
Suppression of genital herpes (non-HIV patients)	Less frequent recurrences: 500 mg daily	Unchanged
	Frequent recurrences: 1 g daily	Unchanged
Suppression of genital herpes (HIV patients)	500 mg bid	Unchanged
valganciclovir	Induction or preemptive treatment: 900 mg bid	Cl$_{Cr}$ ≥60: Unchanged Cl$_{Cr}$ 50-59: 450 mg bid
	Maintenance therapy or CMV prophylaxis: 900 mg daily	Cl$_{Cr}$ ≥60: Unchanged Cl$_{Cr}$ 50-59: 450 mg daily
vancomycin IV	15-20 mg/kg q12h; consider load; monitor serum levels	See Table 3 and Table 4 ("Vancomycin Adult Dosing and Monitoring"); monitor serum levels
vancomycin oral	*Clostridium difficile*: 125-500 mg qid (not systemically absorbed)	Unchanged

for Renal Impairment[b,c]

Cl_{Cr} 10-49 mL/min	Cl_{Cr} <10 mL/min (or Anuric)	Intermittent HD Dosing[d] (See also CRRT dosing information on page 40)
Cl_{Cr} 30-49: 1 g bid Cl_{Cr} 10-29: 1 g daily	500 mg daily	Dose as for Cl_{Cr} <10; on dialysis days, schedule after HD
Cl_{Cr} 30-49: Unchanged Cl_{Cr} 10-29: 1 g daily	500 mg daily	Dose as for Cl_{Cr} <10; on dialysis days, schedule after HD
Cl_{Cr} 30-49: Unchanged Cl_{Cr} 10-29: 500 mg daily	500 mg daily	Dose as for Cl_{Cr} <10; on dialysis days, schedule after HD
Cl_{Cr} 30-49: 500 mg daily Cl_{Cr} 10-29: 500 mg every other day	500 mg every other day	Dose as for Cl_{Cr} <10; on dialysis days, schedule after HD
Cl_{Cr} 30-49: 1 g daily Cl_{Cr} 10-29: 500 mg daily	500 mg daily	Dose as for Cl_{Cr} <10; on dialysis days, schedule after HD
Cl_{Cr} 30-49: Unchanged Cl_{Cr} 10-29: 500 mg daily	500 mg daily	Dose as for Cl_{Cr} <10; on dialysis days, schedule after HD
Cl_{Cr} 40-49: 450 mg bid Cl_{Cr} 25-39: 450 mg q24h Cl_{Cr} 10-24: 450 mg q48h	Not recommended	Not recommended
Cl_{Cr} 40-49: 450 mg daily Cl_{Cr} 25-39: 450 mg every other day Cl_{Cr} 10-24: 450 mg 2×/wk	Not recommended	Not recommended
See Table 3 and Table 4 ("Vancomycin Adult Dosing and Monitoring"); monitor serum levels		20-25 mg/kg; monitor serum levels; 25-40% removed by high-flux HD (not appreciably affected by traditional HD)
Unchanged	Unchanged	Unchanged

(Continues)

Table 1 Dosing Information for Antimicrobials in Adult Patients (*Cont'd.*)

Medication	Usual Dose[a] Cl$_{cr}$ >80 mL/min	Dose Adjustment Cl$_{cr}$ 50-80 mL/min
voriconazole IV	6 mg/kg q12h for 2 doses then 3-4 mg/kg q12h (reduce to 3 mg/kg if not tolerated)	Unchanged
voriconazole oral	If ≥40 kg: 200 mg bid (increase to 300 mg bid if response inadequate) If <40 kg: 100 mg bid (increase to 150 mg bid if response inadequate)	Unchanged
zanamivir	10 mg bid	Unchanged
zidovudine	200 mg tid or 300 mg bid	Unchanged

[a] Usual doses are for most common indications. Doses may differ for meningitis, atypical or serious infections, or atypical organisms. Doses may need to be modified for patients with hepatic dysfunction.

[b] Loading doses generally should not be modified in patients with renal dysfunction. Subsequent (maintenance) doses or dosing intervals should be adjusted.

[c] Serum creatinine levels may be deceptively low in elderly, malnourished, or debilitated patients because of reduced muscle mass, which can artificially increase the calculated creatinine clearance.

[d] For conventional (not high-flux) hemodialysis. Dosing does not apply to patients receiving continuous renal replacement therapy.

[e] Serum levels are similar with oral and intravenous therapy. Use oral route when possible.

for Renal Impairment[b,c]

Cl_{cr} 10-49 mL/min	Cl_{cr} <10 mL/min (or Anuric)	Intermittent HD Dosing[d] (See also CRRT dosing information on page 40)
Cl_{cr} <50: Avoid IV unless benefit justifies risk because of accumulation of IV vehicle sulfobutyl ether β-cyclodextrin (consequences of accumulation in humans not known)		
Unchanged	Unchanged	Unchanged
Unchanged	Unchanged	Unchanged
Cl_{cr} 25-49: Unchanged Cl_{cr} <25: 100 mg tid	100 mg tid	100 mg tid; not significantly affected

Adult Dosing for Continuous Renal Replacement Therapy (CRRT)

Table 2 Adult Dosing for Continuous Renal Replacement Therapy (CRRT)

Medication[a]	CRRT Empiric Dosing[b,c]
acyclovir	5-10 mg/kg q12-24h[d]
	Mucocutaneous infection: 5 mg/kg
	CNS infection: 10 mg/kg
amphotericin products	Unlikely to be affected by CRRT
	Use usual dose
anidulafungin	Unlikely to be affected by CRRT due to high protein binding and fairly large volume of distribution
	Use usual dose[d]
azithromycin	Unlikely to be affected by CRRT
	Use usual dose
aztreonam	1 g q8h or 2 g q12h
caspofungin	Unlikely to be affected by CRRT
	Use usual dose; adjust for hepatic dysfunction if pertinent[d]
cefazolin	1-2 g q12h[d]
cefepime	1-2 g q12h
ceftazidime	1-2 g q12h
ceftriaxone	Use usual dose
	Non-CNS infection: 1-2 g q24h
	CNS infection: 2 g q12h
ciprofloxacin	400 mg q12-24h
clindamycin	Unlikely to be affected by CRRT
	Use usual dose
colistin (as colistimethate)	2.5 mg/kg q12-24h[d]

Table 2 Adult Dosing for Continuous Renal Replacement Therapy (CRRT) (*Cont'd.*)

Medication[a]	CRRT Empiric Dosing[b,c]
dalfopristin/quinupristin	Use usual dose: 7.5 mg/kg q8-12h (adjust for hepatic dysfunction if pertinent)
daptomycin	Use usual dose for renal failure: 6-8 mg/kg q48h (with close monitoring)[d]
ertapenem	Unlikely to be affected by CRRT
	Use usual dose for renal failure: 500 mg q24h (with close monitoring)[d]
fluconazole	Use about double the daily dose with CRRT compared with usual dose in patients with normal renal function for specific infection type
ganciclovir	Induction: 2.5 mg/kg q12h (also consider 5 mg/kg q24h)[d]
	Maintenance: 2.5 mg/kg q24h
gentamicin	Use usual conventional dose: 1-2.5 mg/kg (depending on type of infection), but with initial dosing interval of about q24h
	Monitor serum levels and adjust dose accordingly
	No data for pulse dosing
imipenem/cilastatin	500 mg q6-8h
levofloxacin	500-mg load then 250 mg q24h
	Severe or nosocomial infection: Consider 500 mg q24h when targeting levels similar to 750 mg q24h in healthy patients[d]
linezolid	Use usual dose: 600 mg q12h
	Studied with lower flow rates of 1.5-3 L/h; consider 800 mg q12h or 600 mg q8h with higher flow rates or more resistant organisms
meropenem	1 g q8-12h
metronidazole	500 mg q6-8h[d]
	Adjust dose for hepatic dysfunction if pertinent
micafungin	Unlikely to be affected by CRRT
	Use usual dose[d]
moxifloxacin	Use usual dose: 400 mg q24h[d]

(*Continues*)

Table 2 Adult Dosing for Continuous Renal Replacement Therapy (CRRT) (*Cont'd.*)

Medication[a]	CRRT Empiric Dosing[b,c]
penicillin G	Consider about 6 million units per day divided q8-12h or as continuous infusion (comparable to 20 million units when renal function is normal)[d]
piperacillin/tazobactam	2.25-3.375 g q6h[d] or 4.5 g q8h[d]
posaconazole	Unlikely to be affected by CRRT
	Use usual dose, but oral absorption may be suboptimal in CRRT patients; monitor serum levels
tigecycline	Unlikely to be affected by CRRT[d]
	Use usual dose: 100-mg load then 50 mg q12h (with close monitoring)
trimethoprim-sulfamethoxazole (TMP-SMX)	Consider 5 mg/kg TMP q8-12h[d]
	Monitor serum levels and adjust dose accordingly
vancomycin	25-mg/kg load then 15-20 mg/kg q24-48h
	Monitor serum levels and adjust dose accordingly
voriconazole	Use usual dose but adjust for hepatic dysfunction if pertinent[d]
	CRRT appears to remove vehicle

[a] For drugs not included, equations can be used (even in the absence of good studies) to make predictions about how they might be affected by CRRT.

[b] Dosing recommendations apply to total CRRT flow rates of 3-4 L/h. Other forms of CRRT (eg, SLED) or use of higher or lower flow rates may have different dosing needs.

[c] Assuming minimal residual renal function, normal liver function, and total flow rates of 3-4 L/h.

[d] Support in the medical literature is unavailable or limited; monitor serum levels when possible to confirm dose.

Vancomycin Adult Dosing and Monitoring

(Note: Several vancomycin dosing and monitoring protocols exist; this is the one used at Mayo Clinic.)

Usual Dose

- **Loading dose:** Consider 20-30 mg/kg, especially in critically ill patients with serious infections such as meningitis, health care–associated pneumonia, or endocarditis.
- **Maintenance dose:** Give 15-20 mg/kg based on actual body weight for most patients (20 mg/kg is reasonable when aiming for a trough range of 15-20 mcg/mL). Adjust based on serum levels. See also the following sections on hemodialysis and continuous renal replacement therapy.

Dosing Interval

The dosing frequency depends on renal function (see Table 3 on "Dosing Interval Based on Creatinine Clearance Estimation"). If a measured creatinine clearance (Cl_{Cr}) is not available, the estimated Cl_{Cr} can be calculated with the equation below. The estimated or measured Cl_{Cr} can then be used to choose the appropriate dosing interval.

Creatinine Clearance (Cl_{Cr}) Estimation:

$$\text{Males:} \frac{(140 - \text{age [y]}) \times (\text{weight [kg]})}{\text{SCr [mg/dL]} \times 72}$$

$$\text{Females :} \frac{0.85 \times (140 - \text{age [y]}) \times (\text{weight [kg]})}{\text{SCr [mg/dL]} \times 72}$$

Table 3 Dosing Interval Based on Creatinine Clearance Estimation

Cl_{Cr}, mL/min	Vancomycin Dosing Interval, h[a]
≥60	q12h; for Cl_{Cr} >90 mL/min, consider q8h initial dose and adjust as needed based on levels
35-59	q24h; for severe infections,[a] consider q12h initial dose for Cl_{Cr} >50 mL/min[a] and adjust as needed based on levels
21-34	Approximately q48h; for severe infections,[a] consider q24h initial dose and adjust as needed based on levels
<20	q48-72h; adjust as needed based on serum levels
Hemodialysis	Give 25 mg/kg[b] and monitor serum levels for when to redose (see section below on patients receiving intermittent hemodialysis)

[a] For severe infections with higher trough goals, including meningitis and nosocomial pneumonia, a shorter dosing interval or a larger dose may be necessary when initiating therapy. Serum levels should be measured to determine necessary dosage modifications because the drug will likely accumulate over time.

[b] Patients on hemodialysis typically have higher volumes of distribution.

Infusion Rate

Since infusion-related side effects can occur when infusions are given rapidly, the infusion rate table below can be used as a general guide. If an infusion is poorly tolerated, it can be further extended.

Table 4 Vancomycin Infusion Rate

Dose	Minimum Infusion Time[a]
≤1 g	60 min
1.1-1.5 g	90 min
1.6-2.0 g	120 min
>2 g	About 1 g per hour

[a] In some instances, it may be appropriate to infuse more rapidly if the patient can tolerate it.

Monitoring

Renal Function

- Serum creatinine (SCr) should be measured and Cl_{Cr} should be measured or calculated at the start of therapy (baseline).
- In stable hospitalized patients, SCr monitoring should be done every 3-5 days.
- In patients with critical illness, changing renal function, or concomitant exposure to nephrotoxic agents, SCr monitoring should be done more frequently (ie, every 1-3 days).

Serum Levels

- Serum levels do **NOT** need to be checked if initial dosing relies on the nomogram above, if renal function is stable, and if the expected duration of therapy is <5 days.
- Trough levels correlate better with efficacy than do peak levels. Trough level–only monitoring can be done in most patients.
- Peak levels do not correlate well with efficacy and thus do not need to be checked in most patients. Checking peak levels may be reasonable in the special patient populations described below.
- For patients with severe renal dysfunction, drawing 2 levels after the same dose at least 1 half-life apart allows for calculation of Ke, half-life, and the time needed for the level to drop to the desired value. This information is useful for determining the appropriate time to redose without requiring daily random levels.

Trough Level–Only Monitoring
(See also the following sections on peak and trough monitoring, first-dose levels, hemodialysis, and continuous renal replacement therapy.)
- **Timing**
  - Draw trough level at steady state (4-5 half-lives) immediately before dose
  - Half-life can be estimated with the following equation:

$$Ke = 0.0044 + (0.00083 \times Cl_{Cr}); \text{ half-life} = 0.693/Ke;$$
$$\text{steady state occurs after 4-5 half-lives}$$

- **Goal trough levels**
  - 10-15 mcg/mL for most patients (with the exception of patients with one of the infectious syndromes noted below)
  - 15-20 mcg/mL for meningitis and staphylococcal hospital-acquired or ventilator-associated pneumonia
  Note: These trough-level guidelines are based on consensus opinion rather than on randomized controlled studies. There is little information about the optimal vancomycin trough levels for nonstaphylococcal organisms, and target troughs may be lower when treating more susceptible organisms. Some data support a higher risk of nephrotoxicity with higher trough levels, so more frequent renal function monitoring is reasonable.
- **Level frequency:** Draw trough level at steady state and at least once per week thereafter. More frequent monitoring is needed in patients with serious infections, concurrent nephrotoxins, or changing renal function.

Peak and Trough Monitoring in Special Patient Populations

Vancomycin displays time-dependent (peak-independent) antimicrobial activity. Thus peak levels do not correlate well with efficacy. In addition, toxicity is typically not seen until peak levels are >80 mcg/mL. Since peak levels are unlikely to be in the toxic range if trough levels are appropriate, trough-level monitoring can be used in most patients. However, in some patients, peak and trough levels may be appropriate to ensure penetration and/or to allow for pharmacokinetic analysis and individualization of the dosing regimen.

- Steady-state peak and trough levels may be reasonable at least once in special patient populations to ensure penetration and/ or to individualize dosing based on pharmacokinetic calculations. Subsequently, these patients can often be followed with trough-only monitoring.
- If peak levels are used, they should be drawn at least 1 hour after the end of infusion, and up to 2-3 hours after the end of infusion in patients with renal dysfunction, to ensure complete distribution.
- Special patient populations for whom peak and trough monitoring may be reasonable:
  - Patients with infections such as meningitis, for whom penetration should be ensured
  - Obese patients in whom doses >4 g per day are used
  - Patients who are critically ill or are expected to have large volumes of distribution
  - Patients with considerable renal dysfunction, rapidly changing renal function, or renal function that is difficult to estimate

First-Dose Levels

In select patients, drawing 2-3 levels after the first dose may allow for rapid dose individualization based on pharmacokinetic parameters. Levels drawn after the first dose can be used to determine pharmacokinetic parameters, estimated steady-state levels, and dosing needs. This approach allows for rapid dose adjustment rather than waiting for steady state.

First-dose levels may be reasonable in patients with meningitis; in patients with serious infections and unpredictable renal function; in very obese or fluid-overloaded patients; and in patients on hemodialysis or continuous renal replacement therapy. Optimally, levels should be scheduled at least 1.5 half-lives apart.

- Estimated half-life calculation:

$$Ke = 0.0044 + (0.00083 \times Cl_{cr}); \text{ half-life} = 0.693/Ke$$

Patients Receiving Intermittent Hemodialysis

Removal by Hemodialysis

The newer high-flux hemodialysis filters used at Mayo Clinic and in many other treatment centers remove about 25-40% of vancomycin (amount removed by filters used at other hospitals may differ). Thus dosing intervals should be more frequent than the previous interval of every 5-7 days typically used with conventional, lower-efficiency hemodialysis filters. For institutions **NOT** using high-flux hemodialysis filters, vancomycin removal by hemodialysis is insignificant.

- **Dosing**
  - Because of the higher than usual volume of distribution in end-stage renal failure patients, a loading dose of 25-30 mg/kg should be used initially. Doses and intervals can be modified on the basis of serum levels.
  - One empiric option for patients getting high-flux hemodialysis every 2-3 days is a 25-mg/kg loading dose, followed by approximately 7-10 mg/kg after each dialysis session. (A couple of small studies support a load followed by 500 mg at the end of high-flux hemodialysis.) Levels should be done to confirm that appropriate target levels are obtained.
  - Another empiric option is 25 mg/kg after every 2-3 hemodialysis sessions. Levels should be done to confirm that appropriate target levels are obtained.
- **Serum levels:** Consider obtaining an initial serum level 6 hours after the first dose, a predialysis level, and a 6-hour post-hemodialysis level to individualize dosing, determine kinetic variables, and determine the percentage of drug removed by dialysis. Alternatively, a predialysis level (assuming about 30% removal) can be used to monitor ongoing therapy, and redosing can typically occur when the postdialysis level is anticipated to be in the target trough range, depending on the type of infection.

Patients Receiving Continuous Renal Replacement Therapy

Loading Dose

An initial dose of 25 mg/kg of actual body weight can be used.

Subsequent Empiric Dosing

Requirements in patients on continuous renal replacement therapy will vary, depending on flow rates. Empiric dosing of about 15-20 mg/kg every 24-48 hours is reasonable to start with, and adjustments can be based on serum levels. When trying to achieve higher trough levels (15-20 mcg/mL), start with q24h dosing and base adjustments on serum levels.

Serum Levels

Draw levels after the first dose to allow for individualization of the dosing interval. Check an initial level 2 hours after the first dose and a random level about 24 hours after the first dose. Consult with a pharmacist for assistance in calculating doses based on pharmacokinetic analysis (eg, half-life, volume of distribution). Trough-level monitoring can be done subsequently.

Aminoglycoside Adult Dosing and Monitoring

Empiric Conventional Aminoglycoside Dosing and Monitoring Guidelines in Adults

Several protocols exist, but this is the one used at Mayo Clinic. (See also guidelines that follow for pulse [extended-interval or once-daily] dosing.)

Creatinine clearance (Cl_{Cr}) calculation:

$$\text{Males}: \frac{(140 - \text{age [y]}) \times (\text{weight [kg]})}{\text{SCr [mg/dL]} \times 72}$$

$$\text{Females}: 0.85 \times \frac{(140 - \text{age [y]}) \times (\text{weight [kg]})}{\text{SCr [mg/dL]} \times 72}$$

For obese patients (>20% of ideal body weight [IBW]), use dosing weight (DW) rather than actual body weight for calculating mg/kg dosing per Table 5 below.

Dosing weight = IBW + 0.4 (actual body weight − IBW):

IBW calculation:

Males: 50 kg + 2.3 kg/inch >60 inches

Females: 45.5 kg + 2.3 kg/inch >60 inches

Table 5 Conventional Maintenance Dosing[a,b,c]

Indication	gentamicin and tobramycin		amikacin	
	Desired Concentration, mcg/mL	Dose, mg/kg (see Table 6 on "Empiric Dosing Interval Selection")	Desired Concentration, mcg/mL	Dose, mg/kg (see Table 6 on "Empiric Dosing Interval Selection")
Cystic fibrosis	Peak: ≥10-12 mcg/mL	2.5-3.0 mg/kg	Peak: 25-35 mcg/mL	7-8 mg/kg
	Trough: 0.6-1.2 mcg/mL		Trough: 2.5-8.0 mcg/mL	
Pneumonia, septic shock, life-threatening infection	Peak: 7-10 mcg/mL	1.7-2.5 mg/kg (may need higher dose with high estimated Vd)	Peak: 25-35 mcg/mL	7-8 mg/kg
	Trough: 0.6-1.2 mcg/mL		Trough: 2.5-8.0 mcg/mL	
Bacteremia, SSTI, pyelonephritis	Peak: 6-8 mcg/mL	1.5-2.0 mg/kg	Peak: 20-30 mcg/mL	6 mg/kg
	Trough: 0.6-1.2 mcg/mL		Trough: 2.5-4.0 mcg/mL	
UTI	Peak: 4-5 mcg/mL	1.0-1.3 mg/kg	Peak: 15-20 mcg/mL	5-6 mg/kg
	Trough: 0.6-1.2 mcg/mL		Trough: 2.5-4.0 mcg/mL	
Gram-positive synergy	Peak: 3-4 mcg/mL	1 mg/kg (gentamicin only)	NA	NA
	Trough: <1 mcg/mL			

[a] Loading dose can be given regardless of renal function to achieve therapeutic levels quickly. Loading doses for gentamicin and tobramycin are typically 2-3 mg/kg for gram-negative infections.

[b] The appropriate dose and resulting serum concentrations depend on the seriousness of the infection and the site of infection.

[c] Fluid status may also affect the required dosing regimen to achieve goal serum levels. Patients with considerably higher than normal fluid status have higher volumes of distribution (Vd) and may require higher doses to achieve desired serum concentrations. With diuresis, subsequent doses may require adjustment.

Table 6 Empiric Dosing Interval Selection: Based on Estimated Creatinine Clearance

Cl$_{cr}$	Dosing Interval
>80 mL/min	q8h (usually q12h for amikacin)
50-80 mL/min	q12h
30-49 mL/min	q12-24h
15-29 mL/min	q24-36h
<15 mL/min	Base on serum levels

Serum Level and Toxicity Monitoring for Conventional Aminoglycoside Therapy

Renal Function and Ototoxicity Monitoring

- Check serum creatinine (SCr) (or Cl$_{cr}$ or both) at baseline.
- Check SCr (or measured Cl$_{cr}$) at least every 4 days in hospitalized patients and more often in patients who have changing renal function or critical illness or who are receiving another nephrotoxic medication.
- Monitor signs and symptoms consistent with ototoxicity (eg, tinnitus, feeling of ear-fullness, hearing loss). Instruct patients to alert their physician if these symptoms occur. Consider audiology or vestibular testing at baseline and periodically for longer-term use.

Aminoglycoside Levels

- If therapy is expected to continue for >72 hours, measure peak and trough serum levels at steady state, which occurs after 4-5 half-lives (usually 3rd or 4th dose), and adjust doses accordingly.
- Estimate the half-life with the following equation:

$$Ke = 0.01 + (0.0024 \times Cl_{cr}); \text{ half-life} = 0.693/Ke;$$
$$\text{steady state occurs after 4-5 half-lives}$$

- Draw peak levels 30 minutes after infusion; draw trough levels immediately before dose.
- In severely ill patients or patients expected to have unusual pharmacokinetics, first-dose or non–steady state levels can help determine pharmacokinetic parameters and dosage requirements more quickly. A pharmacist can assist with scheduling levels and interpretation.
- In patients receiving intermittent hemodialysis (HD), 3 serum levels can be drawn after the first dose as follows: A 2-hour postdose level, a pre-HD level, and a level 2 hours after completion of HD. A pharmacist can assist with interpretation of levels, pharmacokinetic analysis, and dosage calculations. For patients receiving gram-positive

synergy dosing, consider 1 mg/kg after 3×/wk HD; check pre-HD level periodically. Level should be <2 mcg/mL (assuming about 50% removal by HD).

- Monitor fluid status, because fluid shifts can affect dosing requirements and serum levels.

Pulse Dosing Aminoglycoside Therapy Guidelines

Rationale for Pulse Dosing of Aminoglycosides

- Aminoglycosides display concentration- or peak-dependent killing. Goal peak levels are about 10 times the minimum inhibitory concentration (MIC) of the organism.
- Aminoglycosides have postantibiotic and sub-MIC effects that allow for continued activity even after the concentration has fallen below the MIC.
- Pulse dosing may minimize development of adaptive resistance.
- Nephrotoxicity may be decreased or delayed.
- Pulse dosing may reduce costs associated with drug administration and monitoring.

Patients (or Conditions) That May NOT Be Good Candidates for Pulse Dosing (Limited Data)

- **Enterococcal endocarditis:** Evidence suggests that traditional (multiple daily dose) dosing is more effective than pulse dosing for treatment of enterococcal endocarditis. However, data support pulse dosing of aminoglycosides in combination with a β-lactam for treatment of penicillin-susceptible viridans group streptococci.
- **Immunosuppression or neutropenia:** Some studies have shown efficacy in this patient group, but data are limited. The duration of the postantibiotic effect may be shorter in neutropenic patients. If pulse dosing is used, the aminoglycoside should be combined with a broad-spectrum β-lactam or other agent active against suspected or known pathogens.
- **Pediatric patients:** Several studies have shown efficacy with pulse dosing, but pediatric patients may need more frequent dosing because of altered pharmacokinetics. With pulse dosing, it may be advisable to administer aminoglycosides with another active agent and to monitor serum levels to determine whether the dose or interval needs to be modified (q12h dosing may be required).
- **Cystic fibrosis (CF):** These patients generally have an increased volume of distribution and more rapid clearance than other patients. Higher daily doses or q12h dosing may be necessary.
- **Pregnancy or postpartum:** Pharmacokinetic alterations exist in pregnant or postpartum patients. Until more studies are available, caution should be used with pulse dosing in this patient group.
- **Renal insufficiency:** Because of insufficient data about the optimal dosing method and the possibility of increased nephrotoxicity due to

prolonged drug exposure in patients with renal dysfunction, we suggest using traditional dosing in patients with an estimated Cl_{cr} <40 mL/min.

- **Neuromuscular diseases:** Consideration should be given to other antimicrobial choices in patients with neuromuscular diseases (eg, myasthenia gravis) or in patients taking a neuromuscular blocker. These patients may be at higher risk for neuromuscular blockade when given large doses of an aminoglycoside.

- **Other:** Caution should be exercised in patients with serious liver disease or ascites, and in patients with burns covering >20% of their body surface area. The volume of distribution can be altered in these subpopulations as well as in critically ill patients.

Patient Selection for Pulse Dosing of Aminoglycosides

- Most studies have been performed in patients with low failure rates (eg, those with urinary tract infections, abdominal infections, or pelvic infections). These patient groups may be good candidates for pulse dosing.

- It may be advisable, especially in critically ill patients, to use pulse dosing of an aminoglycoside **in combination with** a β-lactam or other agent with gram-negative coverage. Doing so will ensure adequate serum concentrations of an appropriate antibiotic in the event that the postantibiotic or sub-MIC effects of the aminoglycoside are exceeded.

Dosing

Pulse (Extended-Interval) Aminoglycoside Therapy

Cl_{cr} calculation:

$$\text{Males}: \frac{(140 - \text{age [y]}) \times (\text{weight [kg]})}{\text{SCr [mg/dL]} \times 72}$$

$$\text{Females}: 0.85 \times \frac{(140 - \text{age [y]}) \times (\text{weight [kg]})}{\text{SCr [mg/dL]} \times 72}$$

For obese patients (>20% IBW), use DW rather than actual body weight for calculating mg/kg dosing per Table 7 on "Pulse Dosing."
Dosing weight = IBW + 0.4 (actual body weight − IBW):

IBW calculation:

Males: 50 kg + 2.3 kg/inch >60 inches

Females: 45.5 kg + 2.3 kg/inch >60 inches

Table 7 Pulse Dosing: Empiric Dosage Selection for Gram-Negative Organisms (Except Viridans Group Streptococci)

Estimated Cl$_{Cr}$	Dose for gentamicin or tobramycin,[a,b,c] mg/kg	Dose for amikacin,[a,b,d] mg/kg	Dosing Interval, h	Serum Level (mcg/mL) 6-14 h
≥60 mL/min	5-7 mg/kg	15-20 mg/kg	q24h	See nomogram[c]
40-59 mL/min	5-7 mg/kg	15-20 mg/kg	q36h	See nomogram
<40 mL/min	Conventional dosing[e]	NA	Conventional dosing[d]	NA

[a] For obese patients, use DW and IBW for dosage determination: DW = IBW + 0.4 (actual body weight − IBW).

[b] Consider higher dose of 7 mg/kg for gentamicin and tobramycin and 20 mg/kg for amikacin in patients with normal renal function who are septic or critically ill; who are volume overloaded or have ascites; who have hospital-acquired or ventilator-associated pneumonia; or who are suspected of being infected with more resistant organisms (eg, *Pseudomonas aeruginosa*).

[c] For viridans group streptococcal endocarditis dosing, dose per treatment guidelines is 3 mg/kg IV q24h for normal Cl$_{Cr}$. Monitor trough levels, which should be undetectable.

[d] For amikacin use in mycobacterial infections, peak serum levels of 35-45 for a 15-mg/kg once-daily dosing and 65-80 for 25-mg/kg twice-weekly dosing are recommended by Peloquin CA. Drugs. 2002;62(15):2169–83.

[e] At Mayo Clinic, we do not recommend the use of pulse dosing in patients with a Cl$_{Cr}$ <40 mL/min because of the potential for a long duration of relatively high serum levels that may lead to toxicity.

Administration

To minimize the possibility of neuromuscular blockade, give pulse doses of aminoglycoside over 60 minutes.

Renal Function and Ototoxicity Monitoring

- Check SCr (or measured Cl$_{Cr}$) at baseline.
- Check SCr (or measured Cl$_{Cr}$) at least twice weekly in hospitalized patients or more often in patients with changing renal function or who are receiving another nephrotoxic medication.
- Monitor for signs and symptoms consistent with ototoxicity (eg, tinnitus, feeling of ear-fullness, hearing loss). Instruct patients to alert their physician when these symptoms occur. Consider audiology or vestibular testing at baseline and periodically for longer-term use.

Aminoglycoside Levels

- **Stable patients not expected to have abnormal pharmacokinetics:** If anticipated duration of therapy is <4 doses, no serum levels are necessary unless the patient is severely ill or receiving a concomitant nephrotoxin.

- **Hartford or Urban and Craig nomogram:** For most other patients (see "individualized dosing" below for critically ill or volume-overloaded patients), draw a level 6-14 hours after the start of the first infusion and apply the nomogram (Figures 1 and 2).
- Other clinicians have suggested just a periodic trough level to ensure that the drug is not accumulating (goal would be an undetectable trough) in stable patients.
- **Individualized dosing:** In critically ill, septic, or volume-overloaded patients, it may be desirable to individualize dosing at least once. It may be prudent to measure serum levels at 2 hours and then at 8-12 hours after the end of the first dose. These levels can be used to calculate pharmacokinetic parameters (eg, extrapolated peak, trough, half-life) of individual patients so as to optimize the dose. Anticipated extrapolated peaks for gentamicin and tobramycin are typically 20-24 mcg/mL, and peaks for amikacin are about 40-70 mcg/mL. Extrapolated troughs should be undetectable. A pharmacist can assist with pharmacokinetic and dosing calculations.

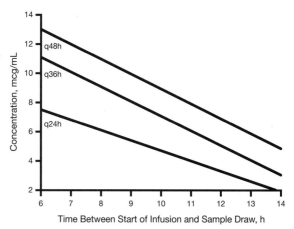

Hartford Pulse-Dosing Nomogram (gentamicin and tobramycin, 7 mg/kg)

Figure 1 (Adapted from Nicolau DP, et al. Antimicrob Agents Chemother. 1995 Mar;39[3]:650-5. Used with permission.)

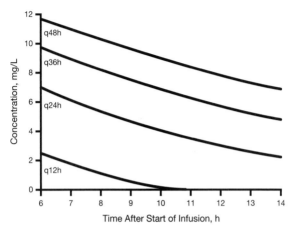

Figure 2 (Adapted from Urban AW, Craig WA. Curr Clin Top Infect Dis. 1997;17:236–55. Used with permission.)

Interpretation of 6- to 14-Hour Level (After Start of Infusion) According to Hartford Nomogram or Urban and Craig Nomogram

If the serum interval level is within the area marked as q24h or q36h, the dosing interval should be every 24 hours and every 36 hours, respectively. At Mayo Clinic, we suggest discontinuing pulse dosing and changing to conventional dosing if the level is above the q36h dosing interval area.

With amikacin, use of the Hartford nomogram has not been validated; however, some authors have suggested dividing the amikacin serum concentration by 2 before plotting on the Hartford nomogram. Consider individualized dosing with peaks/troughs or just monitoring periodic troughs to ensure that the amikacin is not accumulating.

Antimicrobial Dosing—Pediatric

Pediatric Antimicrobial Dosing

Definitions of Age Categories

- Neonate: Full-term newborn 0-4 weeks postnatal age
- Infant: 1 month to 1 year of age
- Child: >1 year to 12 years of age
- Adolescent: 13-18 years of age
- Adult: >18 years of age

Table 8 Creatinine Clearance-Estimating Method[a] in Pediatric Patients With Stable Renal Function

Age	K
≤1 y (low birth weight)	0.33
≤1 y (full term)	0.45
2-12 y	0.55
13-21 y (female)	0.55
13-21 y (male)	0.70

[a] $Cl_{Cr} = K \times L/SCr$; Cl_{Cr} = creatinine clearance in mL/min/1.73 m²; K = age-specific constant of proportionality; L = length in cm; SCr = serum creatinine concentration in mg/dL.

Pediatric Antimicrobial Dosing Guidelines

The following tables do **NOT** apply to the dosing of antimicrobials in neonates. When calculating a pediatric antimicrobial dose, keep the patient's clinical condition in mind and be sure to compare the results with those of the usual adult dose so as not to exceed usual adult-dosing guidelines.

For antiparasitic or antimalarial agents, see Red Book,[a] or consult a pediatric infectious diseases specialist.

---

[a] Red book: 2009 report of the Committee on Infectious Diseases. 28th ed. American Academy of Pediatrics; 2009. p. 784-816 (Tables 4.9, 4.10, and 4.11).

Table 9 Pediatric Antibacterial Dosing Guidelines

Antimicrobial Agents	Usual Daily Dose $Cl_{cr} \geq 50$ mL/min	Max Daily Dose $Cl_{cr} \geq 50$ mL/min
amikacin	15-30 mg/kg/24h divided q8h Monitor serum levels (see recommendations in Table 16 on "Interval Determination" and Table 17 on "Maintenance Dosing for Aminoglycosides")	See aminoglycoside-dosing protocol (Table 16 and Table 17)
amoxicillin	Infants ≤3 mo: 20-30 mg/kg/24h divided q12h	2-3 g/24h
	Infants >3 mo and children: 25-50 mg/kg/24h divided q8-12h	2-3 g/24h
	Acute otitis media, sinusitis, pneumonia: 80-90 mg/kg/24h divided q12h	2-3 g/24h
	Bone or joint infection: 100 mg/kg/24h divided q6h	2-3 g/24h
	Group A streptococcal pharyngitis: 50 mg/kg/24h daily	1,000 mg/24h
amoxicillin/clavulanate	4:1 formulation: 40 mg/kg/24h amoxicillin divided q8h	500 mg q8h
	7:1 formulation: 25-45 mg/kg/24h amoxicillin divided q12h	875 mg q12h
	14:1 formulation (otitis media, sinusitis, pneumonia): 80-90 mg/kg/24h amoxicillin divided q12h	2,000 mg q12h
ampicillin IV	100-200 mg/kg/24h divided q6h	12 g/24h
	Meningitis: 200-400 mg/kg/24h divided q6h	
ampicillin oral	50-100 mg/kg/24h divided q6h	2-3 g/24h

Dose Adjustment for Renal Impairment	
Cl_{Cr} 10-49 mL/min	Cl_{Cr} <10 mL/min or Anuric
See aminoglycoside-dosing protocol (Table 16 and Table 17)	
Cl_{Cr} 31-49: Use usual dose Cl_{Cr} 10-30: 10 mg/kg/dose q12h	10 mg/kg/dose q24h
Cl_{Cr} 31-49: Use usual dose Cl_{Cr} 10-30: 6.25-12.5 mg/kg/dose q12h	20 mg/kg/dose q24h
Cl_{Cr} 31-49: Use usual dose Cl_{Cr} 10-30: 20 mg/kg/dose q12h	20 mg/kg/dose q24h
Cl_{Cr} 31-49: Use usual dose Cl_{Cr} ≤30: 25 mg/kg/dose q12h; do **NOT** use 875-mg tab	25 mg/kg/dose q24h Do **NOT** use 875-mg tab
Cl_{Cr} 31-49: Use usual dose Cl_{Cr} 10-30: 25 mg/kg/dose q24h	12.5 mg/kg/dose q24h
Cl_{Cr} 31-49: Use usual dose Cl_{Cr} 10-30: 10 mg/kg/dose amoxicillin q12h	10 mg/kg/dose amoxicillin q24h
Cl_{Cr} <30: Do **NOT** use 875-mg tab or XR tab	Do **NOT** use 875-mg tab or XR tab
Cl_{Cr} 31-49: Use usual dose Cl_{Cr} 10-30: 20 mg/kg/dose amoxicillin q12h	20 mg/kg/dose amoxicillin q24h
Cl_{Cr} 31-49: Use usual dose Cl_{Cr} 10-30: 50 mg/kg/dose q8-12h	50 mg/kg/dose q12h
Cl_{Cr} 31-49: Use usual dose Cl_{Cr} 10-30: 12.5-25 mg/kg/dose q6-12h	25 mg/kg/dose q12h

(*Continues*)

Table 9 Pediatric Antibacterial Dosing Guidelines (*Cont'd.*)

Antimicrobial Agents	Usual Daily Dose $Cl_{cr} \geq 50$ mL/min	Max Daily Dose $Cl_{cr} \geq 50$ mL/min
ampicillin/sulbactam	Dose based on ampicillin content:	ampicillin 8 g/24h
	Infants: 100-150 mg/kg/24h divided q6h	
	Children: 100-200 mg/kg/24h divided q6h	
	Meningitis (infants): 200-300 mg/kg/24h divided q6h	
	Meningitis (children): 200-400 mg/kg/24h divided q6h	
azithromycin oral	Otitis, pneumonia, or pertussis: 10 mg/kg on day 1 then 5 mg/kg on days 2-5; or for otitis 30 mg/kg as single dose or 10 mg/kg q24h for 3 days	Day 1: 500 mg Days 2-5: 250 mg
	Group A streptococcal pharyngitis: 12 mg/kg q24h for 5 days	500 mg
aztreonam	90-120 mg/kg/24h divided q6-8h	8 g/24h
	CF: 200 mg/kg/24h divided q6h	
cefadroxil	30 mg/kg/24h divided q12-24h	2 g/24h
	Osteomyelitis: 50 mg/kg/24h divided q12h	4 g/24h
cefazolin	60-100 mg/kg/24h divided q8h	12 g/24h
cefdinir	14 mg/kg/24h daily or divided q12h	600 mg/24h
cefepime	100 mg/kg/24h divided q12h	2-6 g/24h
	Meningitis or life-threatening infection: 150 mg/kg/24h divided q8h	

Dose Adjustment for Renal Impairment	
Cl_{cr} 10-49 mL/min	**Cl_{cr} <10 mL/min or Anuric**
Cl_{cr} 30-49: Use usual dose	50 mg/kg/dose ampicillin q24h
Cl_{cr} 10-29: 50 mg/kg/dose ampicillin q12h	
Unchanged	No information
Unchanged	No information
Cl_{cr} 31-49: Use usual dose	7.5-10 mg/kg/dose q8h
Cl_{cr} 10-30: 15-20 mg/kg/dose q8h	
CF: Cl_{cr} 10-30: 25 mg/kg/dose q6h	CF: 12.5 mg/kg/dose q6h
Cl_{cr} 26-49: Use usual dose	15 mg/kg/dose q36h
Cl_{cr} 10-25: 15 mg/kg/dose q24h	
Cl_{cr} 26-49: Use usual dose	25 mg/kg/dose q36h
Cl_{cr} 10-25: 25 mg/kg/dose q24h	
Cl_{cr} 31-49: Use usual dose	25 mg/kg/dose q24h
Cl_{cr} 10-30: 25 mg/kg/dose q12h	
Cl_{cr} 31-49: Use usual dose	7 mg/kg/dose q24h
Cl_{cr} ≤30: 7 mg/kg/dose q24h	
25-50 mg/kg/dose q24h	12.5-25 mg/kg/dose q24h

(Continues)

Table 9 Pediatric Antibacterial Dosing Guidelines (*Cont'd.*)

Antimicrobial Agents	Usual Daily Dose	Max Daily Dose
	$Cl_{cr} \geq 50$ mL/min	$Cl_{cr} \geq 50$ mL/min
cefixime	8 mg/kg/24h divided q12-24h	400 mg/24h
	Cl_{cr} 50-60: 6 mg/kg/dose q24h	
	Acute UTI: 16 mg/kg/24h divided q12h on day 1 then 8 mg/kg q24h	
cefotaxime	100-200 mg/kg/24h divided q6-8h	12 g/24h
	Meningitis: 200-300 mg/kg/24h divided q6h	12 g/24h
cefotetan	40-80 mg/kg/24h divided q12h	6 g/24h
cefoxitin	80-160 mg/kg/24h divided q6-8h	12 g/24h
cefpodoxime proxetil	10 mg/kg/24h divided q12h	800 mg/24h
cefprozil	Group A streptococcal pharyngitis: 15 mg/kg/24h divided q12h	1,000 mg/24h
	Otitis media: 30 mg/kg/24h divided q12h	
	SSTI: 20 mg/kg q24h	
ceftazidime	100-150 mg/kg/24h divided q8h	6 g/24h
	Meningitis: 150 mg/kg/24h divided q8h	
ceftibuten	9 mg/kg/24h divided q24h	400 mg/24h
ceftizoxime	150-200 mg/kg/24h divided q6-8h	12 g/24h
	Cl_{cr} 50-80: 50 mg/kg/dose q8-12h	
ceftriaxone	50-75 mg/kg/24h divided q12-24h	4 g/24h
	Meningitis: 100 mg/kg/24h divided q12-24h	

Dose Adjustment for Renal Impairment	
Cl$_{cr}$ 10-49 mL/min	**Cl$_{cr}$ <10 mL/min or Anuric**
Cl$_{cr}$ 21-49: 6 mg/kg/dose q24h Cl$_{cr}$ ≤20: 4 mg/kg/dose q24h	4 mg/kg/dose q24h
Cl$_{cr}$ 20-49: Use usual dose Cl$_{cr}$ <20: 50 mg/kg/dose q12h	50 mg/kg/dose q24h
Cl$_{cr}$ 20-49: Use usual dose Meningitis: 75 mg/kg/dose q12h	Meningitis: 75 mg/kg/dose q24h
Cl$_{cr}$ 31-49: Use usual dose Cl$_{cr}$ 10-30: 20-40 mg/kg/dose q24h	20-40 mg/kg/dose q48h
Cl$_{cr}$ 30-49: 20-53 mg/kg/dose q8-12h Cl$_{cr}$ 10-29: 20-53 mg/kg/dose q12h	20-53 mg/kg/dose q24h
Cl$_{cr}$ 30-49: Use usual dose Cl$_{cr}$ <30: 5 mg/kg/dose q24h	5 mg/kg/dose q24h
Cl$_{cr}$ 30-49: Use usual dose Cl$_{cr}$ <30: 3.75-7.5 mg/kg/dose q12h	3.75-7.5 mg/kg/dose q12h
SSTI: Cl$_{cr}$ <30: 10 mg/kg/dose q24h	
Cl$_{cr}$ 30-49: 33-50 mg/kg/dose q12h Cl$_{cr}$ 10-29: 33-50 mg/kg/dose q24h	33-50 mg/kg/dose q48h
Cl$_{cr}$ 30-49: 4.5 mg/kg/dose q24h Cl$_{cr}$ 10-29: 2.25 mg/kg/dose q24h	2.25 mg/kg/dose q24h
50 mg/kg/dose q36-48h	50 mg/kg/dose q48-72h
Unchanged for ≤2 g/24h	Unchanged for ≤2 g/24h

(Continues)

Table 9 Pediatric Antibacterial Dosing Guidelines (*Cont'd.*)

Antimicrobial Agents	Usual Daily Dose Cl_{cr} ≥50 mL/min	Max Daily Dose Cl_{cr} ≥50 mL/min
ceftriaxone (continued)	Otitis media: 50 mg/kg/dose once	1 g/dose
cefuroxime IV	75-150 mg/kg/24h divided q8h	6 g/24h
cefuroxime oral	Group A streptococcal pharyngitis: 20 mg/kg/24h divided q12h	1,000 mg/24h
	Otitis media, sinusitis, or impetigo: 30 mg/kg/24h divided q12h	
cephalexin	25-50 mg/kg/24h divided q6-8h	4 g/24h
	Bone or joint infection: 100-150 mg/kg/24h divided q6h	4 g/24h
	Group A streptococcal pharyngitis: 25-50 mg/kg/24h divided q12h	1,000 mg/24h
cephradine	25-50 mg/kg/24h divided q6-12h	4 g/24h
	Otitis media: 75-100 mg/kg/24h divided q6-12h	4 g/24h
chloramphenicol	50-75 mg/kg/24h divided q6h	4 g/24h
	Meningitis: 75-100 mg/kg/dose divided q6h	
ciprofloxacin IV	20-30 mg/kg/24h divided q12h	800 mg/24h
	CF: 30 mg/kg/24h divided q8-12h	CF: 1,200 mg/24h
ciprofloxacin oral	20-30 mg/kg/24h divided q12h	1,500 mg/24h
	CF: 40 mg/kg/24h divided q12h	CF: 2,000 mg/24h
clarithromycin	15 mg/kg/24h divided q12h	1 g/24h

Dose Adjustment for Renal Impairment	
Cl_{cr} 10-49 mL/min	**Cl_{cr} <10 mL/min or Anuric**
Cl_{cr} 21-49: Use usual dose Cl_{cr} 10-20: 25-50 mg/kg/dose q12h	25-50 mg/kg/dose q24h
Cl_{cr} 21-49: Use usual dose Cl_{cr} 10-20: 10-15 mg/kg/dose q12h	10-15 mg/kg/dose q24h
Cl_{cr} 41-49: Use usual dose Cl_{cr} 10-40: 6.25-12.5 mg/kg/dose q8-12h	6.25-12.5 mg/kg/dose q24h
Cl_{cr} 41-49: Use usual dose Cl_{cr} 10-40: 25-37.5 mg/kg/dose q8-12h	25-37.5 mg/kg/dose q24h
Cl_{cr} 41-49: Use usual dose Cl_{cr} 10-40: 6.25-12.5 mg/kg/dose q8-12h	6.25-12.5 mg/kg/dose q24h
3-6.25 mg/kg/dose q6h	12.5-50 mg/kg/dose q36h
9-12.5 mg/kg/dose q6h	12.5-50 mg/kg/dose q36h
Adjust dose based on serum levels	Adjust dose based on serum levels
Cl_{cr} 31-49: Use usual dose Cl_{cr} 10-30: 10-15 mg/kg/dose q18-24h	10-15 mg/kg/dose q24h
Cl_{cr} 31-49: Use usual dose Cl_{cr} 10-30: 15 mg/kg/dose q18-24h	15 mg/kg/dose q24h
Cl_{cr} 31-49: Use usual dose Cl_{cr} 10-30: 10-15 mg/kg/dose q18-24h	10-15 mg/kg/dose q24h
Cl_{cr} 31-49: Use usual dose Cl_{cr} 10-30: 20 mg/kg/dose q18-24h	20 mg/kg/dose q24h
Cl_{cr} 31-49: Use usual dose Cl_{cr} 10-30: 3.75 mg/kg/dose q12h	3.75 mg/kg/dose q12h

(Continues)

Table 9 Pediatric Antibacterial Dosing Guidelines (*Cont'd.*)

Antimicrobial Agents	Usual Daily Dose $Cl_{cr} \geq 50$ mL/min	Max Daily Dose $Cl_{cr} \geq 50$ mL/min
clindamycin IV	25-40 mg/kg/24h divided q6-8h	4.8 g/24h
clindamycin oral	10-30 mg/kg/24h divided q6-8h	1.8 g/24h
	Bone or joint infection: 40 mg/kg/24h divided q6h	
colistin Inh (as colistimethate)	CF: 75 mg nebulized q12h	
colistin IV (as colistimethate)	2.5-5 mg/kg/24h divided q6-12h	480 mg/24h
	CF: 5-8 mg/kg/24h divided q8h (max 160 mg)	
dalfopristin/ quinupristin	VRE infection: 22.5 mg/kg/24h divided q8h	
	cSSSI: 15 mg/kg/24h divided q12h	
dapsone	Leprosy: 1-2 mg/kg q24h	100 mg/24h
	PCP prophylaxis: 2 mg/kg q24h or 4 mg/kg/dose 1 ×/wk	200 mg/dose
daptomycin	4-6 mg/kg/24h daily	
dicloxacillin	25-50 mg/kg/24h divided q6h	2 g/24h
	Bone or joint infection: 100 mg/kg/24h divided q6h	
doxycycline IV or oral	Children >7 y: 2-4 mg/kg/24h divided q12-24h	200 mg/24h
ertapenem	Infants ≥3 mo and children ≤12 y: 30 mg/kg/24h divided q12h	1 g/24h
	Adolescents: 1 g daily	
erythromycin (base) oral	30-50 mg/kg/24h divided q6-8h	2 g/24h
erythromycin IV	15-50 mg/kg/24h divided q6h	4 g/24h

Dose Adjustment for Renal Impairment	
Cl$_{cr}$ 10-49 mL/min	**Cl$_{cr}$ <10 mL/min or Anuric**
Unchanged	Reduce dose with severe renal impairment
Unchanged	Reduce dose with severe renal impairment
Unchanged	Unchanged
SCr 1.3-1.5: 1.25-1.9 mg/kg/dose q12h	SCr 1.3-1.5: 1.25-1.9 mg/kg/dose q12h
SCr 1.6-2.5: 1.25 mg/kg/dose q12h	SCr 1.6-2.5: 1.25 mg/kg/dose q12h
SCr 2.6-4.0: 1.5 mg/kg/dose q36h	SCr 2.6-4.0: 1.5 mg/kg/dose q36h
Dose reduction may be necessary	Dose reduction may be necessary
Unchanged	Necessary, but insufficient information available to make recommendation
Cl$_{cr}$ 30-49: Usual dose Cl$_{cr}$ <30: 4-6 mg/kg/dose q48h	Consult a pediatric infectious diseases specialist
Unchanged	Unchanged
Unchanged	Unchanged
Cl$_{cr}$ 31-49: Use usual dose Cl$_{cr}$ ≤30: 7.5 mg/kg/dose q12h	7.5 mg/kg/dose q12h
Unchanged	Unchanged
Unchanged	Unchanged

(*Continues*)

Table 9 Pediatric Antibacterial Dosing Guidelines (*Cont'd.*)

Antimicrobial Agents	Usual Daily Dose $Cl_{cr} \geq 50$ mL/min	Max Daily Dose $Cl_{cr} \geq 50$ mL/min
gemifloxacin	Little or no information exists on dosing in children; consult a pediatric infectious diseases specialist	
gentamicin	5-7.5 mg/kg/24h divided q8h	See aminoglycoside-dosing protocol (Table 16 and Table 17)
	CF: 7.5-10 mg/kg/24h divided q8h	See aminoglycoside-dosing protocol (Table 16 and Table 17)
	Single daily dosing may be considered in some children; monitor serum levels (see Table 16 on "Interval Determination" and Table 17 on "Maintenance Dosing for Aminoglycosides")	
imipenem-cilastatin	Infants >4 wk and <3 mo: 100 mg/kg/24h divided q6h	4 g/24h
	Infants ≥3 mo: 60-100 mg/kg/24h divided q6h	
	With renal impairment and Cl_{cr} 50-70: 7.5-12.5 mg/kg/dose q6h	
levofloxacin IV or oral	Infants ≥6 mo and children ≤5 y: 20 mg/kg/24h divided q12h	750 mg/24h
	Children >5 y: 10 mg/kg/24h	
linezolid IV or oral	30 mg/kg/24h divided q8h	1,200 mg/24h
lomefloxacin	Little or no information exists on dosing in children; consult a pediatric infectious diseases specialist	
meropenem	60 mg/kg/24h divided q8h	6 g/24h
	Meningitis: 120 mg/kg/24h divided q8h	
metronidazole IV or oral	Anaerobic infection: 30 mg/kg/24h divided q6h	4 g/24h
moxifloxacin IV or oral	Little or no information exists on dosing in children; consult a pediatric infectious diseases specialist	

Dose Adjustment for Renal Impairment	
Cl_{cr} 10-49 mL/min	Cl_{cr} <10 mL/min or Anuric
Little or no information exists on dosing in children; consult a pediatric infectious diseases specialist	
See aminoglycoside-dosing protocol (Table 16 and Table 17)	
See aminoglycoside-dosing protocol (Table 16 and Table 17)	
Cl_{cr} 41-49: 7.5-12.5 mg/kg/dose q6h	7.5-12.5 mg/kg/dose q24h
Cl_{cr} 21-40: 7.5-12.5 mg/kg/dose q8h	Cl_{cr} <5: Do **NOT** give unless patient is on HD
Cl_{cr} 10-20: 7.5-12.5 mg/kg/dose q12h	
Cl_{cr} 20-49: Give initial full dose then 5-10 mg/kg/dose (max 250 mg) q24h	Give initial full dose then 5-10 mg/kg/dose (max 250 mg) q48h
Cl_{cr} 10-19: Give initial full dose then 5-10 mg/kg/dose (max 250 mg) q48h	
No adjustment necessary	Consider dosage adjustment
Little or no information exists on dosing in children; consult a pediatric infectious diseases specialist	
Cl_{cr} 26-49: 20-40 mg/kg/dose q12h	10-20 mg/kg/dose q24h
Cl_{cr} 10-25: 10-20 mg/kg/dose q12h	
Unchanged	Unchanged
Little or no information exists on dosing in children; consult a pediatric infectious diseases specialist	

(Continues)

Table 9 Pediatric Antibacterial Dosing Guidelines (*Cont'd.*)

Antimicrobial Agents	Usual Daily Dose	Max Daily Dose
	Cl$_{cr}$ ≥50 mL/min	Cl$_{cr}$ ≥50 mL/min
nafcillin	Mild to moderate infection: 50-100 mg/kg/24h divided q6h	12 g/24h
	Severe infection: 100-200 mg/kg/24h divided q6h	12 g/24h
nitrofurantoin	Infants >1 mo and children: 5-7 mg/kg/24h divided q6h	400 mg/24h
	Cl$_{cr}$ <60: Avoid	
	UTI prophylaxis: 1-2 mg/kg q24h	
ofloxacin	15 mg/kg/24h divided q12h; consult a pediatric infectious diseases specialist	800 mg/24h
oxacillin IV	Mild to moderate infection: 100-150 mg/kg/24h divided q6h	12 g/24h
	Severe infection: 150-200 mg/kg/24h divided q6h	12 g/24h
penicillin G IV	100,000-250,000 units/kg/24h divided q4-6h	24 million units per day
	Severe infection: 250,000-400,000 units/kg/24h divided q4-6h	24 million units per day
penicillin V oral	25-50 mg/kg/24h divided q6-8h	3 g/24h
	Bone or joint infection: 125 mg/kg/24h divided q6h	3 g/24h
	Prophylaxis of pneumococcal infection/asplenia:	
	Infants and children <3y: 125 mg bid	
	Children ≥3 y and adolescents: 250 mg bid	
	Primary prevention of rheumatic fever (children): 250 mg 2-3 times daily for 10 days	
	Group A streptococcal pharyngitis:	
	Children: 250 mg q12h or q8h	
	Adolescents: 500 mg q12h or q8h	

Dose Adjustment for Renal Impairment	
Cl$_{Cr}$ 10-49 mL/min	Cl$_{Cr}$ <10 mL/min or Anuric
Unchanged	12.5 mg/kg/dose q6h
Unchanged	25 mg/kg/dose q6h
Avoid	Avoid
Cl$_{Cr}$ 20-49: 7.5 mg/kg/dose q24h Cl$_{Cr}$ <20: 3.75 mg/kg/dose q24h	3.75 mg/kg/dose q24h
Unchanged	25 mg/kg/dose q6h
Unchanged	37.5 mg/kg/dose q6h
Cl$_{Cr}$ 31-49: Use usual dose Cl$_{Cr}$ 10-30: 17,000-62,500 units/kg/dose q8-12h	17,000-62,500 units/kg/dose q12-18h
Cl$_{Cr}$ 10-30: 42,000-100,000 units/kg/dose q8-12h	42,000-100,000 units/kg/dose q12-18h
Unchanged	10 mg/kg/dose q8h
Unchanged	30 mg/kg/dose q8h

(Continues)

Table 9 Pediatric Antibacterial Dosing Guidelines (*Cont'd.*)

Antimicrobial Agents	Usual Daily Dose	Max Daily Dose
	Cl$_{cr}$ ≥50 mL/min	Cl$_{cr}$ ≥50 mL/min
piperacillin	200-300 mg/kg/24h divided q6h	24 g/24h
	CF: 350-500 mg/kg/24h divided q4h	24 g/24h
piperacillin/tazobactam	Infants <6 mo: 169-337 mg/kg/24h (150-300 mg/kg/24h piperacillin) divided q6-8h	20 g/24h (18 g/24h piperacillin)
	Children ≥6 mo: 270-337 mg/kg/24h (240-300 mg/kg/24h piperacillin) divided q8h	
	CF: 337-449 mg/kg/24h (300-400 mg/kg/24h piperacillin) divided q6h	20 g/24h (18 g/24h piperacillin)
rifampin	*Haemophilus influenzae* prophylaxis: Infants <1 mo: 10 mg/kg q24h for 4 days Infants ≥1 mo and children: 20 mg/kg q24h for 4 days Meningococcal prophylaxis: Infants <1 mo: 10 mg/kg/24h divided q12h for 2 days Infants ≥1 mo and children: 20 mg/kg/24h divided q12h for 2 days Staphylococcal endocarditis (with standard treatment): 10-20 mg/kg q24h	600 mg/24h
telithromycin	Little or no information exists on dosing in children; consult a pediatric infectious diseases specialist	
tetracycline oral	Children >8 y and adolescents: 25-50 mg/kg/24h divided q6h	3 g/24h
	With renal impairment and Cl$_{cr}$ 50-80: 6-12 mg/kg/dose q8-12h	

Dose Adjustment for Renal Impairment

Cl_{cr} 10-49 mL/min	Cl_{cr} <10 mL/min or Anuric
Cl_{cr} 41-49: Use usual dose	Cl_{cr} <20: 50-75 mg/kg/dose q12h
Cl_{cr} 20-40: 50-75 mg/kg/dose q8h	
CF: Cl_{cr} 41-49: Use usual dose	CF: Cl_{cr} <20: 60-125 mg/kg/dose q12h
CF: Cl_{cr} 20-40: 60-125 mg/kg/dose q8h	
Cl_{cr} 41-49: Use usual dose	28-56 mg/kg/dose (25-50 mg/kg/dose piperacillin) q8h
Cl_{cr} 20-40: 28-56 mg/kg/dose (25-50 mg/kg/dose piperacillin) q6h	
Cl_{cr} <20: 28-56 mg/kg/dose (25-50 mg/kg/dose piperacillin) q8h	
CF: Cl_{cr} 20-40: 56-79 mg/kg/dose (50-70 mg/kg/dose piperacillin) q6h	56-79 mg/kg/dose (50-70 mg/kg/dose piperacillin) q8h
CF: Cl_{cr} <20: 56-79 mg/kg/dose (50-70 mg/kg/dose piperacillin) q8h	
Unchanged	2.5-10 mg/kg/dose q12-24h (give 50% of usual daily dose)

Little or no information exists on dosing in children; consult a pediatric infectious diseases specialist

Cl_{cr} 10-49: 6-12 mg/kg/dose q12-24h	6-12 mg/kg/dose q24h or avoid

(Continues)

Table 9 Pediatric Antibacterial Dosing Guidelines (*Cont'd.*)

Antimicrobial Agents	Usual Daily Dose $Cl_{cr} \geq 50$ mL/min	Max Daily Dose $Cl_{cr} \geq 50$ mL/min
ticarcillin/clavulanate	200-300 mg/kg/24h ticarcillin divided q6h	18-24 g/24h
tobramycin IV	5-7.5 mg/kg/24h divided q8h	See aminoglycoside-dosing protocol (Table 16 and Table 17)
	CF: 7.5-10 mg/kg/24h divided q8h; single daily dosing may be considered in some children; monitor serum levels (see Table 16 on "Interval Determination" and Table 17 on "Maintenance Dosing for Aminoglycosides")	
	Nebulization: ≥6 y: 300 mg nebulized q12h	
trimethoprim	Infants ≥6 mo and children:	200 mg/24h
	Acute otitis media: 10 mg/kg/24h divided q12h	
	UTI: 4-6 mg/kg/24h divided q12h	
trimethoprim-sulfamethoxazole	Children >2 mo: 6-12 mg/kg/24h TMP divided q12h	320 mg/24h TMP
	PCP treatment: 15-20 mg/kg/24h TMP divided q6-8h	PCP dosing: 20 mg/kg/24h TMP
	PCP prophylaxis: 5 mg/kg/24h (or 150 mg/m²/24h TMP) divided q12h for 3 consecutive days per week	
	UTI prophylaxis: 2 mg/kg TMP q24h or 5 mg/kg/dose TMP 2×/wk	
vancomycin IV	60 mg/kg/24h divided q6h	See vancomycin-dosing protocol (Table 13 and Table 15)
	CNS infection: 60 mg/kg/24h divided q6h; monitor serum levels (see Table 13 on "Maintenance Dosing for Vancomycin" and Table 15 on "Infusion Rates for Vancomycin")	
vancomycin oral	*Clostridium difficile*–associated diarrhea (metronidazole is drug of first choice): 40 mg/kg/24h divided q6h	2,000 mg/24h

Dose Adjustment for Renal Impairment	
Cl_{cr} 10-49 mL/min	**Cl_{cr} <10 mL/min or Anuric**
Cl_{cr} 31-49: Use usual dose	50-75 mg/kg/dose q12h
Cl_{cr} 10-30: 50-75 mg/kg/dose q8h	

See aminoglycoside-dosing protocol (Table 16 and Table 17)

Cl_{cr} 31-49: Use usual dose	Avoid
Acute otitis media: Cl_{cr} 15-30: 2.5 mg/kg/dose q12h	
UTI: Cl_{cr} 15-30: 1-1.5 mg/kg/dose q12h	
Cl_{cr} <15: Avoid	
Cl_{cr} 31-49: Use usual dose	Avoid
Cl_{cr} 15-30: Reduce total daily dose 50% and maintain interval as for usual dose; monitor serum levels	
Cl_{cr} <15: Avoid	

See vancomycin-dosing protocol (Table 13 and Table 15)

Unchanged	Unchanged

Table 10 Pediatric Antifungal Dosing Guidelines

Antifungal Agents	Usual Daily Dose $Cl_{cr} \geq 50$ mL/min
amphotericin B deoxycholate	0.25-1 mg/kg q24h; may increase short-term dose to 1.5 mg/kg q24h; consider test dose of 0.1 mg/kg/dose (max 1 mg) at start of therapy
amphotericin B lipid complex	2.5-5 mg/kg q24h
amphotericin B liposomal	3-5 mg/kg q24h; higher doses may be used for CNS or severe or life-threatening infection
anidulafungin	Children 2-11 y: 0.75 mg/kg q24h
	Children and adolescents 12-17 y: 1.5 mg/kg q24h
	Little or no information exists on dosing in children; consult a pediatric infectious diseases specialist
caspofungin	Infants 3 mo to children 17 y: 70 mg/m² on day 1, then 50 mg/m² q24h
clotrimazole lozenges	10 mg 5×/24h (dissolve slowly in mouth)
fluconazole IV or oral	6-12 mg/kg/dose load then 3-12 mg/kg q24h
	Prophylaxis: 3 mg/kg/24h
	Standard infection: 6 mg/kg/24h
	Severe infection: 12 mg/kg/24h
flucytosine	50-150 mg/kg/24h divided q6h; monitor serum levels

Max Daily Dose	**Dose Adjustment for Renal Impairment**	
Cl_{Cr} ≥50 mL/min	Cl_{Cr} 10-49 mL/min	Cl_{Cr} <10 mL/min or Anuric
	May need to reduce dose due to nephrotoxicity	
	May need to reduce dose due to nephrotoxicity	
	May need to reduce dose due to nephrotoxicity	
	Unchanged	Unchanged
Day 1: 70 mg max then 50 mg/24h max; may use a max daily dose of 70 mg if 50 mg/24h is clinically inadequate	Unchanged	Unchanged
Unchanged	Unchanged	Unchanged
800 mg/24h	Cl_{Cr} 21-49: 3-6 mg/kg/ dose load then 1.5-3 mg/kg/dose q24h	1.5-3 mg/kg load then 0.75-1.5 mg/kg/dose q24h
	Cl_{Cr} ≤20: 1.5-3 mg/kg/ dose load then 0.75-1.5 mg/kg/ dose q24h	
	Cl_{Cr} 41-49: Use usual dose	12.5-37.5 mg/kg/dose q24-48h; monitor serum levels
	Cl_{Cr} 20-40: 12.5-37.5 mg/kg/dose q12h	
	Cl_{Cr} 10-19: 12.5-37.5 mg/kg/dose q24h	
	Monitor serum levels	

(Continues)

Table 10 Pediatric Antifungal Dosing Guidelines (*Cont'd.*)

Antifungal Agents	Usual Daily Dose Cl$_{cr}$ ≥50 mL/min
itraconazole	3-10 mg/kg q24h or divided bid
	Recommended starting dose: 5 mg/kg q24h
	Monitor serum levels
micafungin	Infants and children: 1-4 mg/kg/24h most common; some centers use doses up to 12 mg/kg/24h due to clearance higher than that in adults; current dosing data are limited due to short-duration trials and case reports
	Adolescents:
	Candidemia: 100 mg/day
	Esophageal candidiasis: 150 mg/day
	Invasive aspergillosis: 150 mg/day under investigation
	Limited information about dosing in children; consult pediatric infectious diseases specialist
nystatin	Infants: 200,000 units qid
	Children: 200,000-600,000 units qid
posaconazole oral	Patients ≥13 y:
	Prophylaxis of invasive *Aspergillus* or *Candida* infection: 200 mg tid (with full meal)
	Refractory invasive fungal infection: 800 mg/24h divided bid or qid (with full meal)
	Oropharyngeal candidiasis: 100 mg bid on day 1 then 100 mg daily for 13 days
	Refractory oropharyngeal candidiasis: 400 mg bid
voriconazole IV	Children 2-11 y:
	Load: 12 mg/kg/24h divided q12h for day 1
	Maintenance: 8 mg/kg/24h divided q12h
	Children ≥12 y with inadequate response: Increase dose to 300 mg q12h
	Esophageal candidiasis: 200 mg q12h

Max Daily Dose	Dose Adjustment for Renal Impairment	
Cl_{cr} ≥50 mL/min	Cl_{cr} 10-49 mL/min	Cl_{cr} <10 mL/min or Anuric
600 mg/24h; monitor serum levels	Unchanged Cl_{cr} <30: Do **NOT** use injectable dose form	1.5-5 mg/kg/dose q24h; use with caution; do **NOT** use injectable dose form
150 mg/24h	Unchanged	Unchanged
150 mg/24h	Unchanged	Unchanged
	Unchanged	Unchanged
No information available	Unchanged	Unchanged
	Cl_{cr} <50: Change to oral voriconazole because parenteral formulation contains an excipient that accumulates in patients with renal impairment	

(Continues)

Table 10 Pediatric Antifungal Dosing Guidelines (*Cont'd.*)

Antifungal Agents	Usual Daily Dose
	Cl$_{cr}$ ≥50 mL/min
voriconazole IV (continued)	If on concurrent phenytoin therapy and <40 kg: Increase maintenance dose from 100 mg q12h to 200 mg q12h
	If on concurrent phenytoin therapy and ≥40 kg: Increase maintenance dose from 200 mg q12h to 400 mg q12h
voriconazole oral	Limited dosing information available; consult a pediatric infectious diseases specialist
	Some centers use initial maintenance doses of 6-10 mg/kg/24h divided q12h in patients <25 kg
	OR
	Esophageal candidiasis and <40 kg: 100 mg q12h; may increase to 150 mg q12h if response is inadequate
	Esophageal candidiasis and >40 kg: 200 mg q12h; may increase to 300 mg q12h if response is inadequate
	Serious fungal infection (aspergillosis) and <40 kg: 100 mg q12h maintenance dose
	Serious fungal infection (aspergillosis) and ≥40 kg: 200 mg q12h maintenance dose

Max Daily Dose	Dose Adjustment for Renal Impairment	
$Cl_{cr} \geq 50$ mL/min	Cl_{cr} 10-49 mL/min	Cl_{cr} <10 mL/min or Anuric
	No adjustment	No adjustment

Table 11 Pediatric Antimycobacterial Dosing Guidelines

Antimycobacterial Agents	Usual Daily Dose
	Cl_{cr} ≥50 mL/min
ethambutol	15-25 mg/kg q24h or 50 mg/kg/dose 2×/wk (use in patients <13 y only if benefits outweigh risks of therapy)
isoniazid	10-15 mg/kg/24h divided q12-24h or 20-30 mg/kg/dose 2×/wk
	Latent TB: 10 mg/kg/24h daily
pyrazinamide	20-40 mg/kg/24h divided q12-24h
rifampin	10-20 mg/kg q24h
streptomycin	Children with TB:
	Cl_{cr} ≥80: 20-40 mg/kg q24h
	20-40 mg/kg q24h 2×/wk
	Cl_{cr} 50-80: 7.5 mg/kg/dose q24h
	Dose based on serum levels
Agents used for drug-resistant TB (capreomycin, ciprofloxacin, cycloserine, ethionamide, kanamycin, levofloxacin, ofloxacin, para-aminosalicylic acid)	See Red book: 2009 report of the Committee on Infectious Diseases. 28th ed. American Academy of Pediatrics; c2009. p. 692 (Table 3.84), or consult a pediatric infectious diseases specialist.
Agents used for non-TB mycobacterial infection	See Red book: 2009 report of the Committee on Infectious Diseases. 28th ed. American Academy of Pediatrics; c2009. p. 705-6 (Table 3.87), or consult a pediatric infectious diseases specialist.

Max Daily Dose	Dose Adjustment for Renal Impairment	
$Cl_{Cr} \geq 50$ mL/min	Cl_{Cr} 10-49 mL/min	Cl_{Cr} <10 mL/min or Anuric
2.5-g dose	15-25 mg/kg/dose q24-36h	15-25 mg/kg/dose q48h or 7.5-12.5 mg/kg/dose q24h
300 mg/24h or 900-mg dose 2×/wk	Unchanged	5-7.5 mg/kg/dose q24h in slow acetylators
2 g/24h	Cl_{Cr} <50: Avoid or reduce to 12-20 mg/kg/dose q24h	Avoid or reduce to 12-20 mg/kg/dose q24h
600 mg/24h	Unchanged	2.5-10 mg/kg/dose q12-24h (50% of usual daily dose)
1 g/24h or 1.5 g 2×/wk	7.5 mg/kg/dose q24-72h	7.5 mg/kg/dose q72-96h
Dose based on serum levels	Dose based on serum levels	Dose based on serum levels

See Red book: 2009 report of the Committee on Infectious Diseases. 28th ed. American Academy of Pediatrics; c2009. p. 692 (Table 3.84), or consult a pediatric infectious diseases specialist.

See Red book: 2009 report of the Committee on Infectious Diseases. 28th ed. American Academy of Pediatrics; c2009. p. 705-6 (Table 3.87), or consult a pediatric infectious diseases specialist.

Table 12 Pediatric Antiviral Dosing Guidelines[a]

	Usual Daily Dose	Max Daily Dose
Antiviral Agents	**Cl_{cr} ≥50 mL/min**	**Cl_{cr} ≥50 mL/min**
acyclovir IV	Oral, cutaneous, or genital HSV: 15 mg/kg/24h (or 750 mg/m²/24h if ≥1 y) divided q8h	
	Immunocompromised: Consult pediatric infectious diseases specialist; 15-30 mg/kg/24h (or 750-1,500 mg/m²/24h if ≥1 y) divided q8h	
	HSV prophylaxis in immunocompromised: 15 mg/kg/24h (or 750 mg/m²/24h if ≥1 y) divided q8h	
	HSV encephalitis (neonatal): Consult pediatric infectious diseases specialist; 60 mg/kg/24h divided q8h	
	HSV encephalitis (nonneonatal) in infants ≥3 mo and children ≤12 y: 60 mg/kg/24h divided q8h (or 1,500 mg/m²/24h if ≥1 y) divided q8h (larger dose may be indicated)	
	HSV encephalitis (nonneonatal) in children and adolescents >12 y: 30-45 mg/kg/24h divided q8h	
	VZV: 30 mg/kg/24h (or 1,500 mg/m²/24h if ≥1 y) divided q8h	
adefovir	Little or no information exists on dosing in children; consult a pediatric infectious diseases specialist	
amantadine	1-9 y: 5 mg/kg/24h divided q12h	150 mg/24h
	If ≥10 y and <40 kg: 5 mg/kg/24h divided bid	
	If ≥10 y and ≥40 kg: 100 mg bid	200 mg/24h

Dose Adjustment for Renal Impairment

Cl_{Cr} 10-49 mL/min	Cl_{Cr} <10 mL/min or Anuric
Cl_{Cr} 25-49: 5 mg/kg/dose (or 250 mg/m²/dose) q12h	2.5 mg/kg/dose (or 125 mg/m²/dose) q24h
Cl_{Cr} 10-24: 5 mg/kg/dose (or 250 mg/m²/dose) q24h	
Cl_{Cr} 25-49: 10 mg/kg/dose (or 500 mg/m²/dose) q12h	5 mg/kg/dose (or 250 mg/m²/dose) q24h
Cl_{Cr} 10-24: 10 mg/kg/dose (or 500 mg/m²/dose) q24h	
Cl_{Cr} 25-49: 5 mg/kg/dose (or 250 mg/m²/dose) q12h	2.5 mg/kg/dose (or 125 mg/m²/dose) q24h
Cl_{Cr} 10-24: 5 mg/kg/dose (or 250 mg/m²/dose) q24h	
Cl_{Cr} 25-49: 20 mg/kg/dose q12h	10 mg/kg/dose q24h
Cl_{Cr} 10-24: 20 mg/kg/dose q24h	
Cl_{Cr} 25-49: 20 mg/kg/dose (or 500 mg/m²/dose) q12h	10 mg/kg/dose (or 250 mg/m²/dose) q24h
Cl_{Cr} 10-24: 20 mg/kg/dose (or 500 mg/m²/dose) q24h	
Cl_{Cr} 25-49: 10-15 mg/kg/dose q12h	5-7.5 mg/kg/dose q24h
Cl_{Cr} 10-24: 10-15 mg/kg/dose q24h	
Cl_{Cr} 25-49: 10 mg/kg/dose (or 500 mg/m²/dose) q12h	5 mg/kg/dose (or 250 mg/m²/dose) q24h
Cl_{Cr} 10-24: 10 mg/kg/dose (or 500 mg/m²/dose) q24h	
Little or no information exists on dosing in children; consult a pediatric infectious diseases specialist	
Cl_{Cr} 30-49: 5 mg/kg day 1 then 2.5 mg/kg	Cl_{Cr} <15: 5 mg/kg every 7 days
Cl_{Cr} 15-29: 5 mg/kg day 1 then 2.5 mg/kg every other day	
Cl_{Cr} <15: 5 mg/kg every 7 days	

(Continues)

Table 12 Pediatric Antiviral Dosing Guidelines[a] (*Cont'd.*)

Antiviral Agents	Usual Daily Dose Cl_{cr} ≥50 mL/min	Max Daily Dose Cl_{cr} ≥50 mL/min
cidofovir	Accompany with concomitant oral probenecid and IV usual saline (0.9 normal saline) hydration	
	Adenovirus: 1 mg/kg/dose 3×/wk	
	CMV induction: 5 mg/kg/dose once	
	CMV maintenance: 3 mg/kg/dose 1×/wk	
famciclovir	Little or no information exists on dosing in children	1,500 mg/24h
	Adolescents:	
	Genital herpes: 250 mg oral tid	
	Episodic recurrent genital herpes: 125 mg oral bid	
	Daily suppressive therapy: 125-250 mg oral bid for 1 year, then reassess for recurrence	
foscarnet	CMV retinitis:	
	Induction: 180 mg/kg/24h divided q8h	
	Maintenance: 90-120 mg/kg q24h	
	Acyclovir-resistant HSV: 120 mg/kg/24h divided q8-12h	
ganciclovir IV	Induction: 10 mg/kg/24h divided q12h	
	Cl_{cr} 50-69 (with renal impairment): 2.5 mg/kg/dose q12h	
	Maintenance or prophylaxis: 5 mg/kg/dose q24h	
	Cl_{cr} 50-69: 2.5 mg/kg/dose q24h	
ganciclovir oral	Maintenance or prophylaxis: 90 mg/kg/24h divided q8h	1,000 mg q8h
	Cl_{cr} 50-69 (with renal impairment): 15 mg/kg/dose q8h	
oseltamivir oral	Influenza type A and B:	150 mg/24h
	Infants <9 mo: 6 mg/kg/24h divided q12h	
	Infants ≥9 mo to 1 y: 7 mg/kg/24h divided q12h	

Dose Adjustment for Renal Impairment

Cl_{cr} 10-49 mL/min	Cl_{cr} <10 mL/min or Anuric
If SCr increases by 0.3-0.4 mg/dL above baseline, reduce dose by 40%; discontinue therapy with SCr increases ≥0.5 mg/dL above baseline or development of ≥3+ proteinuria	Contraindicated for preexisting renal impairment of SCr >1.5, Cl_{cr} ≤55 mL/min, or ≥2+ proteinuria
See product labeling	See product labeling
See product labeling	Contraindicated
Cl_{cr} 25-49: 2.5 mg/kg/dose q24h Cl_{cr} 10-24: 1.25 mg/kg/dose q24h	1.25 mg/kg/dose 3×/wk after HD
Cl_{cr} 25-49: 1.25 mg/kg/dose q24h Cl_{cr} 10-24: 0.625 mg/kg/dose q24h	0.625 mg/kg/dose 3×/wk after HD
Cl_{cr} 25-49: 15 mg/kg/dose q12h Cl_{cr} 10-24: 7.5 mg/kg/dose q24h	7.5 mg/kg/dose 3×/wk after HD
Cl_{cr} 31-49: Use usual dose Cl_{cr} 10-30: Give dose once daily instead of twice daily	No information available

(*Continues*)

Table 12 Pediatric Antiviral Dosing Guidelines[a] (Cont'd.)

Antiviral Agents	Usual Daily Dose Cl_cr ≥50 mL/min	Max Daily Dose Cl_cr ≥50 mL/min
oseltamivir oral (continued)	Children >1-12 y:	150 mg/24h
	If ≤15 kg: 30 mg bid for 5 days	
	If 16-23 kg: 45 mg bid for 5 days	
	If 24-40 kg: 60 mg bid for 5 days	
	If >40 kg: 75 mg bid for 5 days	
	For prophylaxis, give corresponding treatment dose, but only once daily for 10 days (eg, if patient is >1 y and ≤15 kg, give 30 mg q24h for 10 days)	
ribavirin	See product labeling	
rimantidine	Children 1-9 y and ≥10 y but <40 kg: 5 mg/kg/24h divided bid	150 mg bid
	If ≥10 y and ≥40 kg: 100 mg q12h	200 mg bid
valacyclovir	VZV (immunocompetent):	3 g/24h
	Children and adolescents 2-18 y: 60 mg/kg/24h divided q8h	
	Immuncompromised at risk for HSV or VZV (limited data): 45-90 mg/kg/24h divided q8h	6 g/24h
	Adolescents:	
	Genital HSV: 1,000 mg q12h for 7-10 days	
	Recurrent genital HSV: 500 mg q12h	
	Suppression of genital HSV: 500-1,000 mg q24h	2 g/24h
valganciclovir	Consult a pediatric infectious diseases specialist for dosing formula for infants and children	
	Adolescents or adults:	1,800 mg/24h
	CMV retinitis (induction): 900 mg bid for 21 days	
	CMV retinitis maintenance: 900 mg q24h	
	CMV prophylaxis: 900 mg q24h	

Dose Adjustment for Renal Impairment	
Cl$_{cr}$ 10-49 mL/min	**Cl$_{cr}$ <10 mL/min or Anuric**
Cl$_{cr}$ 31-49: Give usual dose	No information available
Cl$_{cr}$ 10-30: Give dose once daily instead of twice daily	
Prophylaxis: Give dose every other day instead of daily	
See product labeling	
No adjustment	2.5 mg/kg daily
Cl$_{cr}$ 30-49: 20 mg/kg/dose q12h	10 mg/kg/dose q24h
Cl$_{cr}$ 10-29: 20 mg/kg/dose q24h	
Consult a pediatric infectious diseases specialist for dosing formula for infants and children	
Induction:	Contraindicated in HD
Cl$_{cr}$ 40-49: 450 mg bid	
Cl$_{cr}$ 25-39: 450 mg q24h	
Cl$_{cr}$ 10-24: 450 mg q48h	

(Continues)

Table 12 Pediatric Antiviral Dosing Guidelines[a] (Cont'd.)

Antiviral Agents	Usual Daily Dose Cl_{cr} ≥50 mL/min	Max Daily Dose Cl_{cr} ≥50 mL/min
valganciclovir (continued)		
zanamivir Inh	Children ≥7 y: 10 mg (2 Inh) bid for 5 days	

[a] For antiretroviral agents, see AIDSinfo[b] or consult a pediatric infectious diseases specialist.

[b] Guidelines for the use of antiretroviral agents in pediatric HIV infection [Internet]. August 16, 2010; p. 1-219. Available from: http://www.aidsinfo.nih.gov/ContentFiles/PediatricGuidelines.pdf.

Dose Adjustment for Renal Impairment	
Cl_{cr} 10-49 mL/min	Cl_{cr} <10 mL/min or Anuric
Maintenance or prophylaxis:	No information
Cl_{cr} 40-49: 450 mg q24h	
Cl_{cr} 25-39: 450 mg q48h	
Cl_{cr} 10-24: 450 mg 2×/wk	
Unchanged	Unchanged

Pediatric Vancomycin Dosing

Conventional Empiric Pediatric Vancomycin Dosing

Information in the following tables does **NOT** apply to the dosing of anti-microbials in neonates.

Table 13 Maintenance Dosing for Vancomycin

Cl_{cr}	Dose
>90 mL/min	15 mg/kg/dose q6h[a,b] (60 mg/kg/24h; max dose 6 g/24h or as indicated by serum levels)
70-89 mL/min	15 mg/kg/dose q8h
46-69 mL/min	15 mg/kg/dose q12h
30-45 mL/min	15 mg/kg/dose q18h
15-29 mL/min	15 mg/kg/dose q24h
<15 mL/min	Dose intermittently by serum levels

[a] The same total daily dose may be administered using intervals of q8h or q12h for older children and adolescents with normal renal function.

[b] Use 60 mg/kg/24h divided q6h for CNS infection.

Recommendations for Measurement of Vancomycin Serum Levels

- Measure vancomycin serum levels (trough) in cases of:
  - Unstable or changing renal function
  - Administration of other nephrotoxic drugs
  - Positive blood cultures or other cultures
- Consider measuring vancomycin serum levels (peak and trough) to pharmacokinetically optimize dose and interval in cases of:
  - Meningitis infection
  - Osteomyelitis infection

Table 14 Vancomycin Serum Trough Targets

Trough Level (mcg/mL)	Comment
<5	Inadequate
5-10	Acceptable in uncomplicated patients improving clinically
10-15	Normal target goals
15-20	Indicated for very severe infections, including CNS infections, osteomyelitis, nosocomial pneumonia, and infections in which the causative agent (eg, MRSA) has a MIC of 2

Table 15 Infusion Rates for Vancomycin

Dose	Rate
≤1 g	Infuse over 60 min (some patients may require longer infusions due to red man syndrome)
>1 g	Infuse over 90 min

Pediatric Aminoglycoside Dosing

Conventional Empiric Pediatric Aminoglycoside Dosing

The following tables do **NOT** apply to the dosing of antimicrobials in neonates.

Table 16 Interval Determination[a]

Cl$_{cr}$	Interval
≥60 mL/min	q8h
40-59 mL/min	q12h
20-39 mL/min	q24h

[a] Single daily dosing may be considered for some children.

Table 17 Maintenance Dosing for Aminoglycosides[a]

Disease State	gentamicin or tobramycin (mg/kg/dose)	Desired Peak and Trough (mcg/mL)[b]	amikacin (mg/kg/dose)	Desired Peak and Trough (mcg/mL)[b]
CF[c]	2.5-3 mg/kg/dose	Peak: 8-10 mcg/mL	7.5-10 mg/kg/dose	Peak: 25-30 mcg/mL
		Trough: 1-1.5 mcg/mL		Trough: 5-10 mcg/mL
Life-threatening illness, fever neutropenia	2.5 mg/kg/dose	Peak: 7-10 mcg/mL	7.5-10 mg/kg/dose	Peak: 25-30 mcg/mL
		Trough: 1-1.5 mcg/mL		Trough: 5-10 mcg/mL
Bacteremia, SSTI, pyelonephritis	2-2.5 mg/kg/dose	Peak: 6-8 mcg/mL	6-7.5 mg/kg/dose	Peak: 20-25 mcg/mL
		Trough: 0.5-1.5 mcg/mL		Trough: 5-8 mcg/mL
UTI	1.5-2 mg/kg/dose	Peak: 4-6 mcg/mL	5 mg/kg/dose	Peak: 20 mcg/mL
		Trough: 0.5-1 mcg/mL		Trough: 5-8 mcg/mL

Table 17 Maintenance Dosing for Aminoglycosides[a] (*Cont'd.*)

Disease State	gentamicin or tobramycin (mg/kg/dose)	Desired Peak and Trough (mcg/mL)[b]	amikacin (mg/kg/dose)	Desired Peak and Trough (mcg/mL)[b]
Synergy (gram positive endocarditis)	1.5 mg/kg/dose	Peak: 3-4 mcg/mL Trough: 0.6-1.2 mcg/mL	NA	NA

[a] Individualization of dosing and dosing interval is critical due to narrow therapeutic index. Renal function should be assessed before initiation of therapy and periodically thereafter.

[b] Recommendations for measurement of aminoglycoside serum levels (peak and trough) include duration of therapy of at least 5 days, unstable or changing renal function, and administration of other nephrotoxic drugs.

[c] May require q6h dosing interval.

Antimicrobial Agent Fundamentals

Pharmacokinetics of Antimicrobial Agents

Table 18 Pharmacokinetic Highlights of Antimicrobial Agents
(Normal Organ Function)

Medication	Usual Admin. Route	Major Elimination Route (Minor Component)	Usual Half-Life, h
ANTIBACTERIALS			
AMINOGLYCOSIDES			
amikacin	IV	Renal	2-4
gentamicin	IV	Renal	2-4
tobramycin	IV, Inh	Renal	2-4
β-LACTAMS			
Carbapenems			
doripenem	IV	Renal	1
ertapenem	IV	Renal	4
imipenem/ cilastatin	IV	Renal	1
meropenem	IV	Renal	1
Cephalosporins			
cefadroxil	Oral	Renal	1.2-1.7
cefazolin	IV	Renal	1.9
cefepime	IV	Renal	2
cefotaxime	IV	Renal	1.2
cefotetan	IV	Renal	4
cefoxitin	IV	Renal	0.8-1.0
cefpodoxime proxetil	Oral	Renal	2.1-2.8
cefprozil	Oral	Renal	1.3
ceftazidime	IV	Renal	1.9
ceftriaxone	IV	Biliary, renal	5.8-8.7
cefuroxime	IV, oral	Renal	1.2-1.9
cephalexin	Oral	Renal	1

CSF Penetration (Poor, Fair, Good, Unknown)[a]	Urinary Concentration (Poor, Fair, Good, Unknown)	Removal by Conventional HD[b,c,d]
Poor	Good	Yes
Poor	Good	Yes
Poor	Good	Yes
Fair	Good	Yes
Fair	Good	Yes
Fair	Good	Yes
Fair	Good	Yes
Poor	Good	Yes
Poor	Good	Yes
Fair	Good	Yes
Fair	Good	Yes
Poor	Good	Yes
Poor	Good	Yes
Poor	Fair	Yes
Poor	Good	Yes
Fair	Good	Yes
Fair	Good	CI
Fair[e]	Good	Yes
Poor	Good	Yes

(*Continues*)

Table 18 Pharmacokinetic Highlights of Antimicrobial Agents (Normal Organ Function) (*Cont'd.*)

Medication	Usual Admin. Route	Major Elimination Route (Minor Component)	Usual Half-Life, h
Monobactams			
aztreonam	IV	Renal	1.7
Penicillins			
amoxicillin	Oral	Renal	1
amoxicillin/ clavulanate	Oral	Renal	1.0-1.4
ampicillin	IV, oral	Renal	0.7-1.4
ampicillin/ sulbactam	IV	Renal	1
dicloxacillin	Oral	Renal	0.7
nafcillin	IV	Hepatic	0.5-1.0
oxacillin	IV	Hepatic	0.3-0.8
penicillin G	IV	Renal	0.3-0.8
penicillin V	Oral	Renal	0.5
piperacillin	IV	Renal	0.6-1.2
piperacillin/ tazobactam	IV	Renal	0.7-1.2
ticarcillin/ clavulanate	IV	Renal	1.1
FLUOROQUINOLONES			
ciprofloxacin	IV, oral	Renal (hepatic)	4
gemifloxacin	Oral	Fecal, biliary (renal)	7
levofloxacin	IV, oral	Renal	6-8
moxifloxacin	IV, oral	Hepatic	12
MACROLIDES, CLINDAMYCIN, AND KETOLIDES			
azithromycin	IV, oral	Biliary	68 (about 3 days)
clarithromycin	Oral	Hepatic	3-7
clindamycin	IV, oral	Hepatic	2.4
erythromycin	IV, oral	Hepatic	1.4
telithromycin	Oral	Hepatic	10
TETRACYCLINES AND GLYCYLCYCLINE			
doxycycline	IV, oral	Hepatic	18-22

CSF Penetration (Poor, Fair, Good, Unknown)[a]	Urinary Concentration (Poor, Fair, Good, Unknown)	Removal by Conventional HD[b,c,d]
Fair	Good	Yes
Poor	Good	Yes
Poor	Good	Yes
Fair	Good	Yes
Fair	Good	Yes
Poor	Good	CI
Fair	Fair	CI
Poor	Fair	CI
Fair	Good	Yes
Poor	Good	Yes
Fair	Good	Yes
Fair	Good	Yes
Fair	Good	Yes
Fair	Good	CI
Unknown	Fair	CI
Fair	Good	CI
Fair	Poor	CI
Poor	Poor	CI
Poor	Fair	CI
Poor	Fair	CI
Poor	Poor	CI
Poor	Poor	CI
Fair to good	Fair	CI

(*Continues*)

Table 18 Pharmacokinetic Highlights of Antimicrobial Agents
(Normal Organ Function) (*Cont'd.*)

Medication	Usual Admin. Route	Major Elimination Route (Minor Component)	Usual Half-Life, h
TETRACYCLINES AND GLYCYLCYCLINE (Continued)			
minocycline	IV, oral	Hepatic	15.5
tetracycline	IV, oral	Renal	6-12
tigecycline	IV	Biliary, fecal	42
MISC. ANTIBIOTICS			
atovaquone	Oral	Fecal	67-78
colistin	IV, Inh	Renal	2-3
dalfopristin/ quinupristin	IV	Fecal, biliary	0.70/0.85
dapsone	Oral	Renal (hepatic)	28
daptomycin	IV	Renal	8-9
linezolid	IV, oral	Hepatic	4-5
metronidazole	IV, oral	Hepatic (renal)	6-14
nitrofurantoin	Oral	Renal	0.5
telavancin	IV	Renal	8
TMP	IV, oral	Renal	8-10
TMP-SMX	IV, oral	Renal	8-10
vancomycin[f]	IV	Renal	4-6
Antifungals			
amphotericin B	IV	Biliary, fecal	15 days
lipid complex	IV		7 days
liposomal	IV		7 days
anidulafungin	IV	Chemical degradation	40-50
caspofungin	IV	Hepatic	9-11
fluconazole	IV, oral	Renal	30
flucytosine	Oral	Renal	3-6
itraconazole	IV, oral	Hepatic	64
micafungin	IV	Hepatic	14-17
posaconazole	Oral	Hepatic	16-36
voriconazole	IV, oral	Hepatic	6

CSF Penetration (Poor, Fair, Good, Unknown)[a]	Urinary Concentration (Poor, Fair, Good, Unknown)	Removal by Conventional HD[b,c,d]
Fair to good	Fair	CI
Poor	Good	CI
Poor	Fair	CI
Poor	Poor	CI
Poor	Good	CI
Unknown	Fair	CI
Unknown		Yes
Poor	Good	CI
Good	Good	Yes
Good	Good	Yes
Poor	Good	Yes
Poor	Good	CI
Good	Good	Yes
Good	Good	Yes
Poor to fair	Good	CI[g]
Poor	Poor	CI
Poor	Poor	CI
Poor	Poor	CI
Poor	Poor	CI
Poor	Poor	CI
Good	Good	Yes
Good	Good	Yes
Poor	Poor	CI
Poor	Poor	CI
Poor	Poor	CI
Good	Poor	CI

(Continues)

Table 18 Pharmacokinetic Highlights of Antimicrobial Agents (Normal Organ Function) (Cont'd.)

Medication	Usual Admin. Route	Major Elimination Route (Minor Component)	Usual Half-Life, h
SELECT ANTIMYCOBACTERIALS			
ethambutol	Oral	Renal	2.4-4.0
isoniazid	IV, oral	Hepatic	1-4
pyrazinamide	Oral	Hepatic (renal)	9-10
rifabutin	Oral	Hepatic (renal)	45
rifampin	IV, oral	Hepatic	1.5-5.0
Antivirals (Non-HIV)			
acyclovir	IV, oral	Renal	2.5-3.3
cidofovir	IV	Renal	2.5
entecavir	Oral	Renal	About 7 days
famciclovir	Oral	Hepatic (renal)	2-3
foscarnet	IV	Renal	2-4
ganciclovir	IV, oral	Renal	3
oseltamivir	Oral	Hepatic (renal)	6-10
ribavirin	Oral, Inh	Renal	Oral = about 12 days; Inh = 9.5 hours
valacyclovir	Oral	Renal	3
valganciclovir	Oral	Renal	4
zanamivir	Inh	Renal	2.5-5.1

[a] Poor = low penetration into central spinal fluid; fair = moderate penetration or good penetration in presence of meningeal inflammation; good = good penetration, regardless of presence of meningeal inflammation.

[b] Yes, indicates removal of ≥30% of dose.

[c] CI, (clinically insignificant) indicates <30% of dose removed.

[d] Data from Johnson CA. 2009 Dialysis of drugs. CKD Insights, LLC; c2009 (cited 2010 Nov 12). Available from: http://www.ckdinsights.com/downloads/DialysisDrugs2009.pdf.

[e] Fair, but of suboptimal efficacy, so not recommended.

[f] Oral vancomycin formulation available (not absorbed); listed pharmacokinetic data refer to IV form.

[g] Not removed significantly by conventional HD, but can have significant removal with high-flux or high-permeability HD membranes.

CSF Penetration (Poor, Fair, Good, Unknown)[a]	Urinary Concentration (Poor, Fair, Good, Unknown)	Removal by Conventional HD[b,c,d]
Fair	Good	CI
Good	Fair	CI
Good	Good	Yes
Fair	Poor	CI
Fair	Fair	CI
Good	Good	Yes
Poor	Good	Contraindicated
Unknown	Good	CI
Unknown	Good	Yes
Fair	Good	Yes
Good	Good	Yes
Unknown	Unknown	Yes
Unknown	Unknown	CI
Fair	Good	Yes
Good	Good	Yes
Poor	Poor	CI

Antimicrobial Drug Levels

Table 19 Select Antimicrobial Assays: Infusion Times and Timing of Serum Levels

Medication	Route	Infusion Time or Rate	Timing of Levels[a]
amikacin	IV or IM	IV: 30-60 min	Peak: 30 min after IV dose; 1 hour after IM dose
			Trough: Just before dose
chloramphenicol	IV or oral	IV: 15 min	Peak: 1.0-1.5 hours after IV dose; 2-4 hours after oral dose
			Trough: Just before dose
fluconazole	IV or oral	IV: 200 mg per hour	Levels not routinely performed; long half-life makes timing not important; if level desired, consider steady-state (usually in 5-7 days) trough or random level
flucytosine	Oral	NA	Peak: 2 hours after dose
			Trough: Just before dose
fluoroquinolones	IV or oral	IV: 60 min	Levels not routinely performed
			If level desired, consider peak: 1.5-2.0 hours after oral dose; 30 min after IV dose
gentamicin or tobramycin	IV or IM	IV: 30-60 min	Peak for conventional dosing: 30 min after IV dose; 60 min after IM dose
			Trough for conventional dosing: Just before dose
			Pulse dosing: 6- to 14-hour level: Apply to Hartford nomogram or consider periodic trough monitoring (goal undetectable)
			Individualized pulse dosing: 2 hours and 8-12 hours after first dose

Approximate Half-Life[b,c]	Desired Levels, mcg/mL
2-4 hours	Peak for conventional dosing: 20-35 mcg/mL (diagnosis dependent)
	Trough for conventional dosing: <8 mcg/mL
3-4 hours	Peak: 15-25 mcg/mL
	Trough: 5-10 mcg/mL
30 hours	No clearly defined therapeutic range
3-6 hours (trough not routinely indicated)	Peak level: 30-100 mcg/mL; optimal level not clearly defined but increased toxicity with >100 mcg/mL
levofloxacin: 6-8 hours	levofloxacin: Normal steady-state peak after 500-mg dosing is 5.5-6.5 mcg/mL and after 750-mg dosing is 9-12 mcg/mL
ciprofloxacin: 4 hours	ciprofloxacin: Normal steady-state peak after 400-mg IV q8h or q12h is about 4.5 mcg/mL; after 500-mg oral q12h is about 3 mcg/mL; after 750-mg oral q12h is about 3.6 mcg/mL
moxifloxacin: 12 hours	moxifloxacin: Normal steady-state peak after 400-mg IV daily dosing is about 4-6 mcg/mL; after 400-mg oral daily dosing is about 3.5-4.5 mcg/mL
2-3 hours	Peak for conventional dosing: 3-10 mcg/mL for most patients (depending on indication)
	Trough for conventional dosing: <1.2 mcg/mL
	Pulse dosing: Apply 6- to 14-hour level to Hartford nomogram; or, if trough level is measured, it should typically be undetectable

(Continues)

Table 19 Select Antimicrobial Assays: Infusion Times and Timing of Serum Levels (*Cont'd.*)

Medication	Route	Infusion Time or Rate	Timing of Levels[a]
itraconazole	Oral	IV: >1 hour	Because of long half-life, timing is not important; consider steady-state trough or random level (after absorption phase); steady state usually occurs in about 7 days
posaconazole	Oral	NA	Consider trough level (to avoid drug absorption and distribution phase) at steady state
sulfamethoxazole (for TMP-SMX)	IV or oral	IV: 1 hour	Levels usually not indicated except in patients with risk for toxicity, significant or uncertain kidney function, or possible suboptimal oral absorption; also consider in patients being treated for PCP or *Nocardia* infection
			Peak: 1 hour after IV dose or 2-3 hours after oral dose
vancomycin	IV	≤1 g: 60 min	Trough: Just before dose
		1.1-1.5 g: 90 min	Peak: 1 hour after dose (longer with renal dysfunction); trough-only monitoring is appropriate in most patients[d]
		1.6-2.0 g: 2 hours	
		>2 g: 1 g per hour	
voriconazole	IV or oral	Over 1-2 hours (max rate of 3 mg/kg/h)	Trough: Just before dose

[a] Do not draw blood for peak levels through the same line where medication was infused.

[b] With normal organ function.

[c] Drug levels are usually drawn at steady state, which occurs about 3-5 half-lives after starting the drug or after a dose change.

[d] Peak levels not usually recommended.

Approximate Half-Life[b,c]	Desired Levels, mcg/mL
36 hours	No clearly defined therapeutic range but level should be detectable; for serious infections consider target of >1 mcg/mL for itraconazole plus hydroxyitraconazole
36 hours	Not well defined; FDA recommends a level >700 ng/mL
8-12 hours	Supporting data for a target level are limited: 100-150 mcg/mL for PCP or *Nocardia* has been suggested; for other indications, lower levels should be adequate Toxicity has been associated with levels >200 mcg/mL
4-6 hours	Trough: 10-15 mcg/mL (15-20 mcg/mL for select infections; see section on "Vancomycin Adult Dosing and Monitoring" beginning on page 43 for discussion) Peak: 20-45 mcg/mL[d]
6-10 hours	Limited information; goal is steady-state trough level >1-2 mcg/mL and ≤5.5 mcg/mL (efficacy is impaired at lower levels and toxicity increases with levels >5.5 mcg/mL)

Laboratory and Clinical Toxicity Monitoring

Table 20 Laboratory and Clinical Toxicity Monitoring for Antimicrobials[a]

Medication	Select Toxicities
ANTIBACTERIAL AGENTS	
aminoglycosides (eg, gentamicin, tobramycin, amikacin, streptomycin)	Nephrotoxicity, auditory toxicity, vestibular toxicity, neuromuscular blockade
aztreonam	GI effects, hypersensitivity
carbapenems (eg, ertapenem, imipenem, meropenem, doripenem)	Hypersensitivity, GI effects, *Clostridium difficile*, seizures (especially with high dose or doses not adjusted for renal dysfunction)
cephalosporins	GI effects, hypersensitivity reactions, *C difficile*
With MTT side chain (eg, cefotetan, cefmetazole, moxalactam, cefoperazone, cefamandole)	Same as above for cephalosporins plus hypoprothrombinemia and disulfiram-like reactions with alcohol
ceftriaxone	Same as above for cephalosporins plus biliary sludge (especially in young children), gallstones
clindamycin	Diarrhea, *C difficile* colitis, nausea or vomiting
dalfopristin/quinupristin	Pain or inflammation at infusion site, arthralgia or myalgia, hyperbilirubinemia
daptomycin	GI effects, hypersensitivity, headache, elevated CK, myalgia; rarely rhabdomyolysis or eosinophilic pneumonia
fluoroquinolones (eg, ciprofloxacin, ofloxacin, levofloxacin, moxifloxacin, gemifloxacin)	GI effects, arthropathy (especially in pediatric patients), tendon rupture, prolongation of QT interval, hypersensitivity (especially with gemifloxacin), CNS effects (especially with ciprofloxacin)

Minimum Laboratory Monitoring[b,c]	Clinical Monitoring
SCr at least 2×/wk (for dose-adjustment and nephrotoxicity assessments); monitor serum levels if therapy continues >72 hours	Baseline and periodic hearing and vestibular function questioning (audiologic testing with prolonged therapy)
SCr weekly (for dose-adjustment assessment), CBC weekly	Hypersensitivity, diarrhea
SCr weekly (for dose-adjustment assessment), CBC weekly	Hypersensitivity, GI effects, seizures (rare but often seen with renal dysfunction without dose adjustment or with underlying seizure disorder)
For IV cephalopsorins: SCr weekly (for dose-adjustment assessment) except for ceftriaxone, which does not require dose adjustment for renal dysfunction; CBC weekly	Hypersensitivity, diarrhea, other GI effects
Same as above for IV cephalosporins plus INR with prolonged use	Same as above for cephalosporins plus avoid alcohol; bleeding with long-term use; diarrhea
Same as above for IV cephalosporins plus consider LFTs in pediatric patients with prolonged use	Same as above for cephalosporins plus signs of biliary sludge or gallstones
Not routinely indicated	Hypersensitivity, GI effects, photosensitivity
LFTs weekly	Phlebitis, arthralgia, myalgia
CK weekly (twice weekly if on a statin); SCr weekly (for dose-adjustment assessment)	Hypersensitivity, GI effects, myalgia, rhabdomyolysis, new pneumonia symptoms
Consider periodic SCr and LFTs with prolonged use	Hypersensitivity, GI effects, drug-to-drug interactions, prolongation of QT interval with risk factors (avoid use with other QT-prolonging agents or monitor closely), CNS effects, photosensitivity

(Continues)

Table 20 Laboratory and Clinical Toxicity Monitoring for Antimicrobials[a] (Cont'd.)

Medication	Select Toxicities
linezolid	Myelosuppression, diarrhea, nausea, rash, optic neuritis, peripheral neuropathy, rare cases of serotonin syndrome in combination with serotonergic drugs
macrolides (eg, erythromycin, clarithromycin, azithromycin)	GI effects (less likely with clarithromycin and azithromycin), cholestatic jaundice, transient hearing loss (at high doses), prolongation of QT interval or torsades de pointes (primarily with erythromycin or clarithromycin), allergic reaction
metronidazole	Nausea, diarrhea, disulfiram-like reactions with alcohol, metallic taste, reversible neutropenia
penicillins	Hypersensitivity reactions, GI effects (nausea, diarrhea, *C difficile*)
natural penicillins	IV form: Same as above for penicillins plus seizures (with high dose), phlebitis, pain during infusion, excess sodium or potassium (depending on salt form)
aminopenicillins (eg, ampicillin, amoxicillin, amoxicillin/clavulanate, ampicillin/sulbactam)	Same as above for penicillins plus amoxicillin/clavulanate results in greater incidence of diarrhea and hepatitis
penicillinase-resistant penicillins (eg, nafcillin, oxacillin)	Same as above for penicillins plus thrombophlebitis, hepatitis, neutropenia (with prolonged use), interstitial nephritis
carboxypenicillins (eg, ticarcillin, ticarcillin/clavulanate)	Same as above for penicillins plus hypokalemia, hypernatremia, platelet dysfunction, neutropenia
ureidopenicillins (eg, piperacillin, piperacillin/tazobactam)	Same as above for penicillins plus neutropenia or thrombocytopenia (with prolonged use)
telavancin	Nephrotoxicity, taste disturbance, nausea, foamy urine

Minimum Laboratory Monitoring[b,c]	Clinical Monitoring
CBC baseline and weekly; consider periodic LFTs with prolonged use	Hypersensitivity, GI effects, optic or peripheral neuropathy (with prolonged use), drug-to-drug interactions (eg, with serotonergic or adrenergic drugs)
Consider periodic LFTs with prolonged use; baseline SCr for clarithromycin (for dose-adjustment assessment)	Hypersensitivity, GI effects, drug-to-drug interactions, QT prolongation with risk factors (avoid use with other QT-prolonging agents), hearing (especially with high-dose IV erythromycin)
Consider baseline LFTs with known or suspected liver dysfunction (for dose-adjustment assessment)	GI effects (avoid alcohol)
For IV penicillins: SCr weekly (for dose-adjustment assessment except for penicillinase-resistant penicillins), CBC weekly	Hypersensitivity, diarrhea, other GI effects
Same as above for IV penicillins plus sodium or potassium (depending on salt form)	Same as above for penicillins plus phlebitis
Same as above for IV penicillins plus periodic LFTs with prolonged use	Same as above for penicillins plus higher incidence of diarrhea
Same as above for IV penicillins plus weekly LFTs	Same as above for penicillins plus phlebitis
Same as above for IV penicillins plus weekly sodium and potassium	Same as above for penicillins plus bleeding
Same as above for IV penicillins	Same as above for penicillins
SCr baseline and at least weekly (for dose-adjustment and nephrotoxicity assessments), weekly CBC	GI adverse effects, nausea, infusion reactions

(Continues)

Table 20 Laboratory and Clinical Toxicity Monitoring for Antimicrobials[a] (Cont'd.)

Medication	Select Toxicities
tetracyclines (eg, tetracycline, doxycycline, minocycline)	Photosensitivity, permanent staining of developing teeth (avoid in pregnant patients and children <8 y), GI effects, rash, vestibular toxicity (minocycline)
tigecycline	Nausea (higher incidence than comparators), permanent staining of developing teeth (avoid in pregnant patients and children <8 y)
TMP-SMX	Nausea, hypersensitivity reactions, bone marrow suppression, hyperkalemia
vancomycin	Ototoxicity, red man syndrome, nephrotoxicity (usually in combination with other nephrotoxins), phlebitis, reversible neutropenia
ANTITUBERCULAR AGENTS (see also fluoroquinolones and linezolid above)	
isoniazid	Hepatitis, hypersensitivity reactions, lupus-like reactions, peripheral neuropathy
rifamycins (eg, rifampin, rifabutin, rifapentine)	Orange discoloration of body fluids, thrombocytopenia, hepatitis, uveitis (with rifabutin)
pyrazinamide	Hepatitis, hyperuricemia, nausea, anorexia, polyarthralgia
ethambutol	Retrobulbar neuritis, optic neuritis, hyperuricemia
ethionamide	High incidence of GI effects, drowsiness, asthenia, psychiatric effects, hepatitis, hypothyroidism
para-aminosalicylic acid	Rash, GI effects, hypersensitivity, hypothyroidism
cycloserine	CNS toxic effects (somnolence, headache, tremor, psychosis, seizures)

Minimum Laboratory Monitoring[b,c]	Clinical Monitoring
Not routinely needed	Hypersensitivity, diarrhea, other GI effects, drug-to-drug interactions (chelators with oral tetracyclines), vestibular toxicity (minocycline), photosensitivity
LFTs weekly	GI effects
With high dose (15 mg/kg/day TMP): Baseline and weekly SCr (for dose-adjustment and nephrotoxicity assessments), CBC, potassium, and LFTs	Hypersensitivity, GI effects
SCr baseline and at least weekly (for dose-adjustment and nephrotoxicity assessments); CBC weekly; trough serum levels weekly	Phlebitis, hypersensitivity
LFTs monthly in patients with underlying liver dysfunction	Hypersensitivity, neuropathy, drug-to-drug interactions
LFTs monthly in patients with underlying liver dysfunction and in patients with clinical symptoms of liver dysfunction	Uveitis (with rifabutin), flu-like symptoms or myalgia (with rifampin), numerous drug-to-drug interactions, hypersensitivity
LFTs monthly in patients with underlying liver dysfunction; uric acid as indicated	GI effects, hypersensitivity
Not routinely indicated	Baseline vision or color discrimination testing and monthly questioning (repeat testing with prolonged use or with doses >25 mg/kg/day); consider monthly vision or color discrimination testing; GI effects
LFTs in patients with underlying liver dysfunction; TSH baseline and monthly	GI effects, CNS effects
LFTs and TSH at baseline; TSH every 3 months for prolonged use	Hypersensitivity, GI effects
Serum levels may help establish optimum dose	Monthly assessment of neuropsychiatric effects

(*Continues*)

Table 20 Laboratory and Clinical Toxicity Monitoring for Antimicrobials[a] (Cont'd.)

Medication	Select Toxicities
streptomycin, amikacin, kanamycin, capreomycin	Nephrotoxicity, auditory toxicity, vestibular toxicity, neuromuscular blockade
ANTIFUNGAL AGENTS **amphotericin B deoxycholate**	Infusion-related reactions (fever, chills, rigors, nausea, hypertension, hypotension), nephrotoxicity, hypokalemia, hypomagnesemia, reversible anemia
lipid amphotericin products	Lower incidence of nephrotoxicity than with amphotericin B deoxycholate; lower incidence of infusion-related effects than with liposomal amphotericin B
flucytosine	Bone marrow suppression, GI effects, hepatitis
triazoles (eg, fluconazole, itraconazole, posaconazole, voriconazole)	GI effects, hepatitis, prolongation of QT interval, hypersensitivity
itraconazole	Same as above for triazoles plus CHF; high doses can sometimes produce endocrine effects similar to those of ketoconazole
posaconazole	Same as above for triazoles
voriconazole	Same as above for triazoles plus transient visual disturbances, cyclodextrin vehicle accumulation with IV formulation in patients with renal dysfunction (clinical significance of risk vs benefit unknown)
echinocandins (eg, caspofungin, micafungin, anidulafungin)	Facial flushing or swelling (histamine mediated but rare), hypersensitivity, hepatitis
ANTIVIRAL AGENTS CYTOMEGALOVIRUS AGENTS **cidofovir**	Renal impairment, neutropenia, ocular hypotonia, headache, asthenia, alopecia, rash, GI effects

Minimum Laboratory Monitoring[b,c]	Clinical Monitoring
SCr baseline and at least weekly; serum levels if available	Baseline hearing, vestibular, or Romberg testing; monthly questioning about symptoms; repeat testing as indicated
Twice-weekly SCr, potassium, and magnesium; weekly LFTs and CBC	Infusion-related effects, BP check as indicated
Twice-weekly SCr, potassium, and magnesium; weekly LFTs and CBC	Infusion-related effects
Twice-weekly SCr (for dose-adjustment assessment) and CBC; weekly LFTs; periodic serum levels as indicated	Nausea (often associated with elevated serum levels)
Baseline and periodic LFTs and SCr (for dose-adjustment assessment with fluconazole; cyclodextrin vehicle accumulation with IV voriconazole)	GI effects, prolongation of QT interval with risk factors (avoid if possible with other QT-prolonging agents), hypersensitivity, photosensitivity, many drug-to-drug interactions
Same as above for triazoles; consider periodic potassium and sodium; consider serum levels as indicated	Same as above for triazoles plus edema, signs of CHF (uncommon)
Same as above for triazoles, plus check serum levels regularly to ensure absorption	Same as above for triazoles
Same as above for triazoles plus periodic SCr with IV (cyclodextrin vehicle accumulation with renal dysfunction, use oral if possible or consider risk vs benefit); consider serum levels as indicated	Same as above for triazoles plus visual side effects, hallucinations
Baseline and periodic LFTs	Hypersensitivity, a few drug-to-drug interactions (with caspofungin)
SCr (also give saline load and probenecid), WBC, and urinalysis, all at least 1×/wk (within 48 hours before dose on dosing weeks)	GI effects, hypersensitivity (especially with probenecid)

(Continues)

Table 20 Laboratory and Clinical Toxicity Monitoring for Antimicrobials[a] (Cont'd.)

Medication	Select Toxicities
foscarnet	Renal impairment, electrolyte disturbance, seizures, GI effects
ganciclovir or valganciclovir	Myelosuppression, GI effects
INFLUENZA AGENTS	
amantadine	GI effects, CNS effects (especially in elderly or without appropriate dose adjustment)
oseltamivir	GI effects (usually well tolerated)
rimantidine	GI effects, CNS effects (less than with amantadine)
zanamivir	Bronchospasm with underlying lung disease
HERPES VIRUS AGENTS	
acyclovir or valacyclovir	Malaise, nausea, diarrhea; phlebitis (with IV acyclovir); nephrotoxicity and CNS effects more common with high-dose IV therapy
famciclovir	Headache, dizziness, nausea, diarrhea, fatigue

[a] Also monitor for signs and symptoms of infection improvement or worsening.

[b] Monitor more frequently in critically ill patients and in patients with abnormal or changing test results.

[c] For select medications, providers may choose to monitor additional laboratory tests. Institutional laboratory monitoring policies may vary.

For additional information, see Tice et al. Clin Infect Dis. 2004 Jun 15;38(12):1651–72.

Minimum Laboratory Monitoring[b,c]	Clinical Monitoring
SCr 2×/wk (for dose-adjustment and nephrotoxicity assessments); weekly electrolytes, including calcium and phosphorus	GI effects, hypersensitivity
CBC 1-2×/wk; SCr weekly (for dose-adjustment assessment)	GI effects
SCr at baseline with renal dysfunction (for dose-adjustment assessment)	GI and CNS effects
SCr at baseline with renal dysfunction (for dose-adjustment assessment)	GI effects
SCr at baseline with renal dysfunction (for dose-adjustment assessment)	GI and CSF effects
NA	Bronchospasm (avoid in patients with lung injury or asthma)
SCr weekly with IV acyclovir (for dose-adjustment and nephrotoxicity assessments)	Phlebitis, CNS effects (with IV acyclovir), GI effects
SCr at baseline with known renal dysfunction (for dose-adjustment assessment)	GI effects

Treatment of Specific Organisms

Spectrum of Activity

Table 21 Aerobic Gram-Negative Bacteria: Aminoglycosides, Carbapenems, Cephalosporins, Aztreonam, and Fluoroquinolones

| Aerobes | Aminoglycosides | | | Carbapenems | | Cephalosporins[a] 1st Gen | 2nd Gen | |
	amikacin	gentamicin	tobramycin	ertapenem	imipenem, meropenem	cefazolin, cephalexin	cefotetan, cefoxitin	cefuroxime
Acinetobacter	2[f]	1-2[f]	2[f]	0-1	2[f]	0	0-1	0
Aeromonas hydrophila	2	2	2	2	2	0		1
Enterobacter, Citrobacter, Serratia	2	2	2	1-2	2	0	0	1
ESBL (Escherichia coli, Klebsiella)	1-2[d]	1[d]	1[d]	1-2[c]	2[c]	0	0-1	0
E coli (non-ESBL)	2	2	2	2	2	1-2[f]	1-2[f]	1-2
Haemophilus influenzae	2	2	2	2	2	1	1-2	1-2
Klebsiella (non-ESBL)	2	2	2	2	2	1	1	1-2
Legionella	0	0	0	0	0	0	0	0
Moraxella catarrhalis	2	2	2	2	2		1	1-2
Neisseria gonorrhoeae	0	0	0	2	2	1	1	1
N meningitidis	0	0	0	2	2	0	1	1
Proteus mirabilis	2	2	2	2	2	1	1	1-2
Proteus vulgaris, Providencia	2	1-2	1-2	2	2	0	1	0
Pseudomonas aeruginosa	2	1-2	2	0	2	0	0	0
Salmonella				2	2	0		1
Shigella	1	1	1	1	1			1
Stenotrophomonas maltophilia	0	0	0	0	0	0	0	0

| Cephalosporins[a] | | | | Monobactams | Fluoroquinolones | | |
| 3rd Gen | | 4th Gen | Other | | | | |
cefotaxime, ceftriaxone	ceftazidime	cefepime	ceftaroline	aztreonam	ciprofloxacin	levofloxacin	moxifloxacin, gemifloxacin
1	1-2	1-2	0	1	1-2[b]	1-2[b]	1-2[b]
1	1	1		1	2	2	2
1[e]	1[e]	1-2	1	1-2	2	2	2
0	0	0	0	0	1[d]	1[d]	1[d]
2	2	2	2	2	2[c]	2[c]	2[c]
2	2	2	2	2	2	2	2
2	2	2	2	2	2	2	2
0	0	0	0	0	1	2	2
2	2	2	2	2	2	2	2
2	1	1-2	1	1-2	2[f(t)]	2[f(t)]	2[f(t)]
2	1	2	1	2	2	2	2
2	2	2	1-2	2	2	2	2
2	2	2		2	2	2	2
0	2	2	0	2	1-2	1-2	0
2	2	2		2	2[c]	2[c]	2[c]
1	1	1		1	2	2	2
0	0-1	0-1	0	0	1	1-2	1-2

(*Continues*)

Table 21 Aerobic Gram-Negative Bacteria: Aminoglycosides, Carbapenems, Cephalosporins, Aztreonam, and Fluoroquinolones (Cont'd.)

[a] Representative agents; not all-inclusive.

[b] Some treatment centers or geographic regions have high rates of fluoroquinolone resistance in *Acinetobacter*.

[c] Increased resistance may be observed in some local areas.

[d] Coresistance may be found in ESBL-producing organisms.

[e] Use of 3rd-gen cephalosporins for *Enterobacter* or *Citrobacter* is generally not advised, because they can induce resistance during therapy.

[f] Higher fluoroquinolone resistance rates for *N gonorrhoeae* are now being widely reported. As of 2007, the Centers for Disease Control and Prevention no longer recommends routine treatment of gonorrhea with fluoroquinolones.

0 = Little or no activity; 1 = moderate activity, with some resistance noted; 2 = good activity; blank box = inadequate data to rank.

[f] High or increasing rates of resistance reported. Do not use empirically without susceptibility data.

Table 22 Aerobic Gram-Negative Bacteria: Penicillins, Macrolides, Tetracyclines, Tigecycline, and Other Medication Classes

Aerobes	Natural Penicillins — penicillin	Antistaph Penicillins[a] — nafcillin, dicloxacillin	Aminopenicillins — ampicillin, amoxicillin	Aminopenicillins — amoxicillin/ clavulanate, ampicillin/ sulbactam
Acinetobacter	0	0	0	0-2[b]
Aeromonas hydrophila	0	0	0	0-1
Enterobacter, Citrobacter, Serratia	0	0	0	0
ESBL (Escherichia coli, Klebsiella)	0	0	0	0
E coli (non-ESBL)	0	0	1	2[f]
Haemophilus influenzae	0-1	0	1	2
Klebsiella (non-ESBL)	0	0	0	2
Legionella	0	0	0	0
Moraxella catarrhalis	0	0	0	1-2
Neisseria gonorrhoeae	1[f]	0	1[f]	1
N meningitidis	2	0	2	2
Proteus mirabilis	0	0	1	2
Proteus vulgaris, Providencia	0	0	0	1
Pseudomonas aeruginosa	0	0	0	0
Salmonella	0	0	0-1	2
Shigella	0	0	0-1	1
Stenotrophomonas maltophilia	0	0	0	0

[a] Representative agents; not all-inclusive.

[b] For *Acinetobacter*, ampicillin/sulbactam (Unasyn) has activity, whereas amoxicillin/clavulanate (Augmentin) does not.

[c] In vitro or animal models; limited clinical experience.

[d] Colistin is not active against *Serratia*.

0 = Little or no activity; 1 = moderate activity, with some resistance noted; 2 = good activity; blank box = inadequate data to rank.

[f] High or increasing rates of resistance reported. Do not use empirically without susceptibility data.

* Concern exists about antimicrobial tissue penetration related to the most common infectious syndrome caused by the organism.

| Penicillins | | | | | | | | |
| Antipseudomonal Penicillins | | Macrolides | | Tetracyclines | | Glycylcycline | Misc | |
ticarcillin/ clavulanate	piperacillin/ tazobactam	erythromycin	clarithromycin, azithromycin	tetracycline, doxycycline	minocycline	tigecycline	colistin	cotrimoxazole (TMP-SMX)
1-2	1-2	0	0	0	0	1-2[f]	1-2	1-2
0-1	1-2	0	0	2		2c		2
1-2	1-2	0	0	0	0	1-2	0-2d	1-2
0	1	0	0	0	1	1-2	1	0
2	2	0	0	1		2	2	1
2	2	1	1-2	1-2	1-2	2	2	1-2
2	2	0	0	1		2	2	2
0	0	1-2	2	1	1	1-2c		1
2	2	0	2	0	0	2	2	
2	2	0	1	1[f]	1[f]	1	0	0
2	2	*	*	*	*	*		1
2	2	0	0	1	1	0-1	2	2
2	2	0	0	0	0	0-1	0	1
1	1-2	0	0	0	0	0	2	0
2	2	0	1	0-1	0-1	1		1
1	1		1	0-1	0-1	1		1-2
1-2	1	0	0		1-2	1-2	0	1-2

Table 23 Aerobic Gram-Positive Bacteria: Aminoglycosides, Carbapenems, Cephalosporins, and Penicillins

Aerobes	gentamicin, streptomycin	ertapenem	imipenem, meropenem	cefazolin, cephalexin	cefotetan, cefoxitin	cefuroxime	cefotaxime, ceftriaxone	ceftazidime
	Aminogly-cosides	Carba-penems		1st Gen	2nd Gen		3rd Gen	
					Cephalosporins[a]			
Corynebacterium jeikeium	0	0	0	0	0	0	0	0
Enterococcus								
E faecalis	syn[b]	0	1	0	0	0	0	0
E faecium	syn[b]	0	1	0	0	0	0	0
VRE	syn[b]	0	0	0	0	0	0	0
Listeria monocytogenes	syn[b]		1-2	0	0	0	0	0
Nocardia	syn[b]	2	1	0	0	0	1	1
Staphylococcus								
MRSA, MRSE	syn[b]	0	0	0	0	0	0	0
MSSA, MSSE	syn[b]	1-2	1-2	2	0-1	1	1	0
Streptococcus								
Group A, B, C	0-syn[b]	2	2	2	1	1	2	1
S pneumoniae (pen susceptible)	0	2	2	1	0-1	1	2	1
S pneumoniae (pen intermediate)	0	2	2	0	0	1	1-2	0
S pneumoniae (pen resistant)	0	2	2	0	0	0	1	0
Viridans group	0	2	2	1	0-1	0-1	2	1

[a] Representative agents; not all-inclusive.

[b] Synergistic activity when combined with appropriate agent; do not use as monotherapy.

[c] Activity for susceptible isolates.

[d] More than 80% of staphylococci are resistant to penicillin or ampicillin.

0 = Little or no activity; 1 = moderate activity, with some resistance noted; 2 = good activity; blank box = inadequate data to rank.

[f] High or increasing rates of resistance reported. Do not use empirically without susceptibility data.

| Cephalosporins[a] | | Penicillins[a] | | | | | |
| 4th Gen | Other | Natural Penicillins | Antistaph Penicillins | Amino-penicillins | | Anti-pseudomonal Penicillins | |
cefepime	ceftaroline	penicillin	nafcillin, dicloxacillin	ampicillin, amoxicillin	amoxicillin/clavulanate, ampicillin/sulbactam	ticarcillin/clavulanate	piperacillin/tazobactam
0	0	0	0	0	0	0	0
0	0-1	2[c]	0	2[c]	2[c]	0	1-2[c]
0	0	1[c]	0	1[c]	1[c]	0	1[c]
0	0	1[c]	0	1[c]	1[c]	0	0
0		1-2	0	2	2		1
1		0	0	0	1		
0	2	0	0	0	0	0	0
1	2	0-2[d(f)]	2	0-2[d(f)]	1-2	1-2	1-2
2	2	2	2	2	2	2	2
2	2	2		2	2	2	2
2	2	1		1	1	1	1
1	2	0-1	0	0-1	0-1	0-1	0-1
2	2	2	1	2	2	2	2

Table 24 Aerobic Gram-Positive Bacteria: Macrolides, Fluoroquinolones, Tetracyclines, Tigecycline, and Antibacterial Classes

Aerobes	Macrolides		Fluoroquinolones			Tetracyclines	
	erythromycin	clarithromycin, azithromycin	ciprofloxacin	levofloxacin	moxifloxacin, gemifloxacin	tetracycline, doxycycline	minocycline
Corynebacterium jeikeium	0	0	0	0	0	0	0
Enterococcus							
E faecalis	0	0	0-1	1[b]	1[b]	0	0-1
E faecium (non-VRE)	0	0	0-1	1[b]	1[b]	0	1
VRE	0	0	0	0	0	0	1
Listeria monocytogenes	*	*				*	*
Nocardia	0-1	0-1	0-1	1	1	1	1
Staphylococcus							
MRSA, MRSE	1[d]	1[d]	0-1	1[d]	1[d]	1	1
MSSA, MSSE	1	1	0-1	1	1	1	1-2
Streptococcus							
Group A, B, C	1	1	0-1	1	1-2	1	1
S pneumoniae (pen susceptible)	1	1	0	1-2	2	1	1
S pneumoniae (pen intermediate)	1	1	0	1-2	2	1	1
S pneumoniae (pen resistant)	0-1	0-1	0	1-2	2	0-1	0-1
Viridans group	1	1		1-2	1-2	1	1

[a] In vitro or animal models; limited clinical experience.

[b] More active agents are available for systemic infections.

[c] For severe enterococcal infections, tigecycline and daptomycin have not been studied extensively.

[d] May be more active against community-acquired MRSA.

0 = Little or no activity; 1 = moderate activity, with some resistance noted; 2 = good activity; blank box = inadequate data to rank.

* Concern exists about antimicrobial tissue penetration related to the most common infectious syndrome caused by the organism.

Glycylcycline	Misc					
tigecycline	clindamycin	TMP-SMX	daptomycin	linezolid	metronidazole	vancomycin
	0	0	1-2[a]	2[a]	0	2
1-2[c]	0	0	1-2[c]	2	0	2
1-2[c]	0	0	1-2[c]	2	0	2
1-2[c]	0	0	1-2[c]	1-2	0	0
*	*	1-2	*	1-2	0	1
1	0	2		1-2	0	0
2	1[d]	1[d]	2	2	0	2
2	1-2	1-2	2	2	0	2
2	1	0-1	2	2	0	2
2	1	1	*	2	0	2
2		1	*	2	0	2
2[a]	0	0	*	2[a]	0	2
1-2	1	0-1	2[a]	2[a]	0	2

Table 25 Anaerobic Bacteria: Aminoglycosides, Carbapenems, Cephalosporins, and Penicillins

| Anaerobes | Aminogly-cosides | Carba-penems | | Cephalosporins[a] | | | | |
| | | | | 1st Gen | 2nd Gen | | 3rd Gen | |
	gentamicin, streptomycin	ertapenem	imipenem, meropenem	cefazolin, cephalexin	cefotetan, cefoxitin	cefuroxime	cefotaxime, ceftriaxone	ceftazidime
Actinomyces	0	2	2				1-2[b]	
Bacteroides	0	2	2	0	1		1	0
Clostridium difficile (enteric)								
C perfringens	0	2	2		1	1	1	
Fusobacterium	0	2	2		1		1	
Peptostreptococcus	0	2	2	2	2	2	2	1
Porphyromonas, Prevotella	0	2	2	0	1	1	1	

[a] Representative agents; not all-inclusive.

[b] In vitro or animal models; limited clinical experience.

0 = Little or no activity; 1 = moderate activity, with some resistance noted; 2 = good activity; blank box = inadequate data to rank.

| Cephalosporins[a] | | Penicillins[a] | | | | | |
| 4th Gen | Other | Natural Penicillins | Antistaph Penicillins | Amino-penicillins | | Anti-pseudomonal Penicillins | |
cefepime	ceftaroline	penicillin	nafcillin, dicloxacillin	ampicillin, amoxicillin	amoxicillin/clavulanate, ampicillin/sulbactam	ticarcillin/clavulanate	piperacillin/tazobactam
1-2[b]		2	0	2	2[b]	2[b]	2[b]
	0	0-1	0	0-1	1-2	2	2
1	1	2	0	1	2	2	2
1		1-2		1	2	2	2
2	2	2	0	1-2	2	2	2
	0	1	0	1	2	2	2

Table 26 Anaerobic Bacteria: Macrolides, Fluoroquinolones, Tetracyclines, Tigecycline, and Other Medication Classes

Anaerobes	Macrolides			Fluoroquinolones			Tetracyclines	
	erythromycin	fidaxomicin	clarithromycin, azithromycin	ciprofloxacin	levofloxacin	moxifloxacin, gemifloxacin	tetracycline, doxycycline	minocycline
Actinomyces	1-2		1-2	1[a]	1[a]	1[a]	1-2	1-2
Bacteroides	0		0	0	0	1-2	0-1	0-1
Clostridium difficile (enteric)		2						
C perfringens	1		1			1	1	1
Fusobacterium						1-2	1	1
Peptostreptococcus	1		1		1	1-2	1	1
Prevotella, Porphyromonas						1-2		

[a] In vitro or animal models; limited clinical experience.

[b] Use oral or intracolonic vancomycin for *C difficile*.

0 = Little or no activity; 1 = moderate activity, with some resistance noted; 2 = good activity; blank box = inadequate data to rank.

[(l)] High or increasing rates of resistance reported. Do not use empirically without susceptibility data.

Glycylcycline	Misc						
tigecycline	clindamycin	TMP-SMX	daptomycin	linezolid	metronidazole	dalfopristin/ quinupristin	vancomycin
1-2	1-2		1[a]	1-2[a]	0	1[a]	1-2[a]
1-2	1[l]	0	0	1[a]	2	0	0
					2		2[b]
2	2		2[a]	2[a]	2	2[a]	1
1-2[a]	2	0	0		2		0
2	2	0	2[a]	1-2[a]	2	2[a]	2
2	2			2[a]	2		

Table 27 Select Fungal Organisms

Medication	Aspergillus	Blastomyces dermatitidis	Candida albicans, C tropicalis, C parapsilosis	C glabrata	C krusei
amphotericin B product	2[a]	2	2	1-2	1-2
caspofungin, micafungin, anidulafungin	1-2[a]	0-1[b]	2[c]	2	2
fluconazole	0	1	2	1[d]	0
flucytosine	0	0	2[e]	2[e]	0
itraconazole	2	1-2	2	1[d]	0
posaconazole	2[b]	1-2[b]	2	1-2[f]	2
voriconazole	2[a]	1[b]	2	1-2[f]	2

[a] Combination therapy with an echinocandin plus voriconazole or an amphotericin B product is sometimes used for severe infections (no randomized controlled trials but retrospective cohort studies suggest improved outcomes). *Aspergillus terreus* is less susceptible to amphotericin.

[b] Limited clinical data.

[c] Higher minimum inhibitory concentrations noted against *C parapsilosis* and some failures reported. Clinical significance not entirely clear.

[d] Susceptibilities often in the susceptible, dose-dependent range (requires more aggressive dosing).

[e] Not typically used alone. Flucytosine should be used in combination therapy to treat candidal infections and in combination induction therapy to treat cryptococcal meningitis.

[f] Some azole cross-resistance observed. Not preferred in patients with recent azole therapy without susceptibility testing.

0 = Little or no activity; 1 = moderate activity, with some resistance noted; 2 = good activity; blank box = inadequate data to rank.

[i] High or increasing rates of resistance reported. Do not use empirically without susceptibility data.

C lusitaniae, C guilliermondii	Coccidioides	Cryptococcus	Fusarium	Histoplasma	Pseudallescheria boydii (Scedosporium apiospermum)	Zygomycetes
(f)	2	2	1	2	1	2
1-2	0	0	0	1[b]	0	0
1-2	1-2	2	0	1		0
1[e]	1[e]	1-2[e]	0	0	0	0
1	1-2	1	0	2	1	0-1
1-2	1-2[b]	1-2[b]	1[b]	1-2[b]	1-2[b]	1-2[b]
1-2	1-2[b]	1-2[b]	1	1[b]	1-2	0

Table 28 Select Viral Organisms (Excluding Human Immunodeficiency Virus)

Medication	HSV	VZV	CMV	HBV	HCV	Influenza A	Influenza B
acyclovir	2	2	0	0	0	0	0
adefovir	1	0	0	1	0	0	0
amantadine	0	0	0	0	0	1[a]	0
boceprevir	0	0	0	0	2	0	0
cidofovir	2[b]	2[c]	2	0	0	0	0
entecavir	0	0	0	2	0	0	0
famciclovir (penciclovir)	2	2	0	0-1	0	0	0
foscarnet	2[b]	2[c]	2[d]	0	0	0	0
ganciclovir	2[c]	2[c]	2	0	0	0	0
interferon alpha	0	0	0	2	2[e]	0	0
lamivudine	0	0	0	1	0	0	0
oseltamivir	0	0	0	0	0	2	2
ribavirin	0	0	0	0	2[e]	0	0
rimantadine	0	0	0	0	0	1[a]	0
telaprevir	0	0	0	0	2	0	0
tenofovir	0	0	0	1-2	0	0	0
valacyclovir	2	2	0	0	0	0	0
valganciclovir	2[c]	2[c]	2	0	0	0	0
zanamivir	0	0	0	0	0	2	2

[a] High rates of resistance have been reported for amantadine or rimantadine in patients with influenza A, so neither is currently recommended by the Centers for Disease Control and Prevention for treatment or prophylaxis.

[b] Active against many acyclovir-resistant strains of herpes simplex virus; not used as a first-line treatment for sensitive strains due to enhanced toxicity compared with that of alternate drugs.

[c] Not used as a first-line treatment due to enhanced toxicity compared with that of alternate drugs.

[d] Foscarnet is active against many ganciclovir-resistant strains.

[e] Interferon (pegylated) is used in combination with ribavirin.

0 = Little or no activity; 1 = moderate activity, with some resistance noted; 2 = good activity.

Bacteria: Preferred and Alternate Treatment Options

Table 29 Specific Treatment of Bacterial Organisms

Organisms	First-Line Treatment[a]	Alternate Treatment[a]
Acinetobacter	A carbapenem[b] (except ertapenem)	tigecycline, piperacillin/ tazobactam, ampicillin/ sulbactam, ceftazidime, cefepime, a fluoroquinolone, an aminoglycoside, colistin (as colistimethate), minocycline, doxycycline, sulbactam
Actinomyces	penicillin	ampicillin, amoxicillin, doxycycline, a cephalosporin, clindamycin, erythromycin
Aeromonas	A fluoroquinolone	A carbapenem,[b] TMP-SMX, gentamicin, a 3rd-gen cephalosporin
Alcaligenes xylosoxidans (also known as *Achromobacter xylosoxidans*)	A carbapenem,[b] piperacillin/tazobactam	ceftazidime, cefepime, TMP-SMX
Bacillus	vancomycin	clindamycin, a carbapenem,[b] a fluoroquinolone
B anthracis (anthrax)	ciprofloxacin, doxycycline	amoxicillin, penicillin, levofloxacin, imipenem
Bacteroides fragilis	metronidazole	A carbapenem,[b] a β-lactam/ β-lactamase inhibitor,[c] clindamycin, moxifloxacin, cefotetan, cefoxitin, tigecycline
Bartonella		
B henselae	A macrolide,[d] doxycycline	A fluoroquinolone, rifampin
B quintana	A macrolide,[d] doxycycline	
Bordetella pertussis	A macrolide[d]	TMP-SMX
Borrelia burgdorferi (Lyme disease)	doxycycline, amoxicillin	penicillin, cefuroxime, cefotaxime, ceftriaxone, azithromycin, clarithromycin

(Continues)

Table 29 Specific Treatment of Bacterial Organisms (*Cont'd.*)

Organisms	First-Line Treatment[a]	Alternate Treatment[a]
Brucella	doxycycline plus 1 of the following: gentamicin, streptomycin, or rifampin	TMP-SMX, ciprofloxacin, chloramphenicol; each with or without 1 of the following: gentamicin, streptomycin, or rifampin
Burkholderia cepacia	Often a colonizer not requiring treatment; TMP-SMX	ceftazidime, cefepime, a carbapenem,[b] a fluoroquinolone, minocycline, tigecycline
Campylobacter		
C fetus	ampicillin, imipenem, gentamicin	chloramphenicol
C jejuni	A macrolide[d]	doxycycline, a fluoroquinolone
Capnocytophaga	clindamycin, amoxicillin/ clavulanate	A carbapenem,[b] doxycycline, a β-lactam/β-lactamase inhibitor,[c] erythromycin, a fluoroquinolone
Chlamydophila pneumoniae	doxycycline, a macrolide[d]	A fluoroquinolone, another tetracycline, tigecycline
Citrobacter freundii	A carbapenem[b]	A fluoroquinolone, an aminoglycoside, TMP-SMX, cefepime, piperacillin/ tazobactam, tigecycline, aztreonam
Clostridium		
C difficile	metronidazole, vancomycin (oral)	nitazoxanide, rifaximin, fidaxomicin
C perfringens	penicillin with or without clindamycin	metronidazole, clindamycin, a β-lactam/β-lactamase inhibitor,[c] a carbapenem[b]
C tetani	metronidazole plus tetanus immune globulin and tetanus toxoid	doxycycline plus tetanus immune globulin and tetanus toxoid; or penicillin plus tetanus immune globulin and tetanus toxoid
Corynebacterium		
C diphtheriae	erythromycin plus antitoxin	clindamycin plus antitoxin; or penicillin plus antitoxin
C jeikeium (group JK)	vancomycin	Base treatment on susceptibility results; consider linezolid, daptomycin, dalfopristin/ quinupristin

Table 29 Specific Treatment of Bacterial Organisms (Cont'd.)

Organisms	First-Line Treatment[a]	Alternate Treatment[a]
Coxiella burnetii (Q fever)	Acute: doxycycline	Acute: A fluoroquinolone, a macrolide[d]
	Chronic (eg, endocarditis): doxycycline plus hydroxychloroquine; or doxycycline plus a fluoroquinolone	Chronic: doxycycline plus a fluoroquinolone; or doxycycline plus rifampin
Ehrlichia	doxycycline	tetracycline, rifampin
Eikenella corrodens	ampicillin, amoxicillin, a 3rd-gen cephalosporin	doxycycline, a β-lactam/β-lactamase inhibitor,[c] a fluoroquinolone
Enterobacter	A carbapenem[b]	A fluoroquinolone, TMP-SMX, piperacillin/tazobactam, an aminoglycoside, cefepime, tigecycline, aztreonam, colistin (as colistimethate), tigecycline
Enterococcus[e]		
ampicillin-sensitive	ampicillin,[f] amoxicillin,[f] penicillin[f]	vancomycin,[f] linezolid, a β-lactam/β-lactamase inhibitor,[c] dalfopristin/quinupristin (active for E faecium only), daptomycin, tigecycline, telavancin
ampicillin-resistant, vancomycin-sensitive	vancomycin[f]	linezolid, daptomycin,[e] dalfopristin/quinupristin (E faecium only), tigecycline, telavancin
VRE	linezolid	daptomycin,[e] dalfopristin/quinupristin (E faecium only), tigecycline
Erysipelothrix rhusiopathiae	penicillin	A cephalosporin, a fluoroquinolone, clindamycin, a carbapenem[b]
Escherichia coli	ceftriaxone, cefotaxime, cefepime ESBL-producing strain: A carbapenem[b]	A fluoroquinolone (with increasing resistance), an aminoglycoside, another cephalosporin, piperacillin/tazobactam, ticarcillin/clavulanate, TMP-SMX, tigecycline, aztreonam, a carbapenem,[b] colistin (as colistimethate)

(Continues)

Table 29 Specific Treatment of Bacterial Organisms (*Cont'd.*)

Organisms	First-Line Treatment[a]	Alternate Treatment[a]
Francisella tularensis (tularemia)	streptomycin, gentamicin CNS infection: doxycycline plus either gentamicin or streptomycin	doxycycline, a fluoroquinolone, chloramphenicol
Fusobacterium	penicillin	metronidazole, clindamycin, a β-lactam/β-lactamase inhibitor,[c] a carbapenem[b]
Gardnerella vaginalis (bacterial vaginosis)	metronidazole	metronidazole (vaginal), clindamycin (vaginal or oral), or furazolidone
Haemophilus influenzae	ceftriaxone, cefotaxime	A fluoroquinolone, TMP-SMX, azithromycin, clarithromycin, a β-lactam/β-lactamase inhibitor,[c] doxycycline, a 2nd-, 3rd-, or 4th-gen cephalosporin, a carbapenem[b]
Klebsiella pneumoniae	ceftriaxone, cefotaxime, cefepime ESBL-producing strain: A carbapenem[b] Carbapenemase-producing strain: Consult an infectious diseases expert	A fluoroquinolone, an aminoglycoside, TMP-SMX, a β-lactam/β-lactamase inhibitor,[c] a carbapenem,[b] tigecycline, colistin (as colistimethate)
Legionella	A newer fluoroquinolone[g] azithromycin with or without rifampin	Another macrolide,[d] doxycycline, TMP-SMX
Leuconostoc	ampicillin, amoxicillin, penicillin	clindamycin, doxycycline, a macrolide[d]
Listeria monocytogenes	ampicillin with or without gentamicin or penicillin with or without gentamicin	TMP-SMX, meropenem
Moraxella catarrhalis	A 2nd- or 3rd-gen cephalosporin	A fluoroquinolone, azithromycin, clarithromycin, TMP-SMX, cefepime, a carbapenem,[b] tetracycline, tigecycline, a β-lactam/β-lactamase inhibitor[c]
Morganella morganii	cefepime, a fluoroquinolone	A carbapenem,[b] piperacillin/ tazobactam, an aminoglycoside, TMP-SMX, aztreonam

Table 29 Specific Treatment of Bacterial Organisms (*Cont'd.*)

Organisms	First-Line Treatment[a]	Alternate Treatment[a]
Mycobacterium	See treatment sections for tuberculosis (Table 72) and nontuberculosis mycobacterial infections (text chapter following Table 72)	
Mycoplasma pneumoniae	A macrolide[d]	doxycycline, a fluoroquinolone, tigecycline
Neisseria		
N gonorrhoeae	ceftriaxone, cefixime	cefotaxime, a fluoroquinolone (variable resistance), spectinomycin
N meningitidis	penicillin, ceftriaxone, cefotaxime	ampicillin, a fluoroquinolone, TMP-SMX
Nocardia asteroides	TMP-SMX	minocycline, imipenem with or without amikacin, another sulfonamide, ceftriaxone with or without amikacin, amoxicillin/ clavulanate, linezolid
Pasteurella multocida	penicillin, ampicillin, amoxicillin	doxycycline, a 2nd- or 3rd-gen cephalosporin, TMP-SMX, a β-lactam/β-lactamase inhibitor,[c] a carbapenem[b]
Peptostreptococcus	penicillin, ampicillin, amoxicillin	clindamycin, a cephalosporin, a newer fluoroquinolone,[g] a carbapenem,[b] vancomycin, a β-lactam/β-lactamase inhibitor[c]
Propionibacterium acnes (systemic infection)	penicillin	clindamycin, doxycycline, a carbapenem[b]
Proteus		
P mirabilis/	ampicillin, amoxicillin	A cephalosporin, a fluoro-quinolone, an aminoglycoside, TMP-SMX, a β-lactam/β-lactamase inhibitor,[c] a carbapenem[b]
P vulgaris	A carbapenem[b]	A fluoroquinolone, an aminoglycoside, TMP-SMX, a β-lactam/β-lactamase inhibitor,[c] a 3rd- or 4th-gen cephalosporin, aztreonam, colistin (as colistimethate)
Providencia	A carbapenem[b]	A fluoroquinolone, an aminoglycoside, TMP-SMX, a β-lactam/β-lactamase inhibitor,[c] a 3rd- or 4th-gen cephalosporin, aztreonam, colistin (as colistimethate)

(*Continues*)

Table 29 Specific Treatment of Bacterial Organisms (Cont'd.)

Organisms	First-Line Treatment[a]	Alternate Treatment[a]
Pseudomonas aeruginosa	cefepime, ceftazidime, a carbapenem[b] (except ertapenem); consider addition of an aminoglycoside or ciprofloxacin for severe infection or until susceptibilities are known	ciprofloxacin, levofloxacin, piperacillin/tazobactam, colistin (as colistimethate), aztreonam
Rickettsia	doxycycline	A fluoroquinolone, chloramphenicol
Salmonella	A fluoroquinolone, ceftriaxone	amoxicillin, ampicillin, chloramphenicol, TMP-SMX, a 3rd- or 4th-gen cephalosporin, furazolidone
Serratia	A carbapenem[b]	A fluoroquinolone, an aminoglycoside, cefepime, TMP-SMX, piperacillin/tazobactam, aztreonam
Shigella	A fluoroquinolone	TMP-SMX, azithromycin, furazolidone, a 3rd- or 4th-gen cephalosporin
Staphylococcus[h]		
oxacillin/methicillin-sensitive	nafcillin, oxacillin, a 1st-gen cephalosporin, dicloxacillin	clindamycin (if double-disk diffusion test is negative), TMP-SMX, minocycline
		Broad-spectrum agents with activity against methicillin-sensitive staphylococci include cefepime, ceftriaxone, β-lactam/β-lactamase inhibitors,[c] carbapenems,[b] newer fluoroquinolones[g]
oxacillin-resistant (MRSA, MRSE)	vancomycin, linezolid, daptomycin[e]	tigecycline; or, depending on susceptibility of mild to moderate infections or step-down therapy: TMP-SMX, minocycline, a newer fluoroquinolone,[g] dalfopristin/quinupristin, telavancin, ceftaroline
vancomycin-intermediate or vancomycin-resistant (VISA, VRSA)	Notify infection control immediately; obtain infectious diseases consultation	

Table 29 Specific Treatment of Bacterial Organisms (*Cont'd.*)

Organisms	First-Line Treatment[a]	Alternate Treatment[a]
Stenotrophomonas maltophilia	TMP-SMX (consider adding ticarcillin/ clavulanate for severe infection)	ticarcillin/clavulanate, tigecycline, a fluoroquinolone, minocycline
Streptococcus		
S pneumoniae	See new CLSI breakpoints for meningeal and nonmeningeal infections	
penicillin susceptible	penicillin, ampicillin	A cephalosporin, a macrolide,[d] clindamycin, doxycycline, a newer fluoroquinolone,[g] TMP-SMX, or any of the agents listed below for penicillin-intermediate or penicillin resistant under first-line or alternate treatment
penicillin intermediate	ceftriaxone, cefotaxime, a newer fluoroquinolone[g]; high-dose penicillin, ampicillin, or amoxicillin	cefepime, vancomycin, linezolid, tigecycline, a carbapenem,[b] clindamycin, TMP-SMX, ceftaroline Variable resistance may be seen with macrolides[d]
penicillin resistant	vancomycin	linezolid, dalfopristin/ quinupristin, tigecycline, a newer fluoroquinolone,[g] ceftaroline
S pneumoniae meningitis	vancomycin plus either ceftriaxone with or without rifampin or cefotaxime with or without rifampin	cefepime or meropenem
Group A, B, C, or G	penicillin, cephalosporin	Another penicillin, a macrolide[d] or clindamycin (variable resistance), vancomycin, linezolid, daptomycin, tigecycline, telavancin, ertapenem
Viridans group	penicillin, a cephalosporin For endocarditis and infection in immunocompromised patients: Base treatment on susceptibility testing	vancomycin, a newer fluoroquinolone,[g] a β-lactam/ β-lactamase inhibitor,[c] ertapenem

(*Continues*)

Table 29 Specific Treatment of Bacterial Organisms (*Cont'd.*)

Organisms	First-Line Treatment[a]	Alternate Treatment[a]
Treponema pallidum (syphilis)	penicillin	doxycycline, ceftriaxone
Ureaplasma	A macrolide,[d] doxycycline	levofloxacin or moxifloxacin
Vibrio		
V cholerae	doxycycline	A fluoroquinolone, TMP-SMX
V vulnificus	doxycycline	ceftriaxone, cefotaxime, ciprofloxacin
Yersinia		
Y enterocolitica	A fluoroquinolone, gentamicin, TMP-SMX, doxycycline	chloramphenicol, ceftriaxone, cefotaxime
Y pestis (plague)	streptomycin	TMP-SMX, gentamicin, doxycycline, chloramphenicol, ciprofloxacin

[a] Depending on susceptibility.

[b] Carbapenems: meropenem, imipenem, doripenem, and ertapenem; ertapenem has minimal activity against *Pseudomonas*, *Acinetobacter*, and *Enterococcus*.

[c] β-Lactam/β-lactamase inhibitors: piperacillin/tazobactam, ampicillin/sulbactam, amoxicillin/clavulanate, and ticarcillin/clavulanate.

[d] Macrolides: erythromycin, clarithromycin, and azithromycin.

[e] Insufficient data exist for use of daptomycin for serious enterococcal infections; do **NOT** use for pneumonia (high failure rates, inactivated by surfactant).

[f] Add gentamicin or streptomycin when cidal activity is required (eg, for infective endocarditis) and agents are susceptible for synergy.

[g] Newer (respiratory) fluoroquinolones: moxifloxacin, levofloxacin, and gemifloxacin.

[h] Consider addition of rifampin for deep-seated staphylococcal infections (eg, infective endocarditis) that do not respond well or are in the presence of prosthetic material. *S coagulase*–negative bacteria is a common contaminant that can also cause serious infection.

Adapted from Drugs for bacterial infections. Treat Guidel Med Lett. 2010 Jun;8(94):43-52. Used with permission.

Bacterial Drug Resistance

Table 30   Select Bacterial Resistance Issues

Pertinent Organisms	Resistance Issue	Treatment
EXTENDED-SPECTRUM β-LACTAMASE–PRODUCING (ESBL) GRAM-NEGATIVE BACILLI (Some labs no longer specifically test for this because of the 2010 CLSI breakpoint changes and recommendations)		
Escherichia coli, Klebsiella **Less common:** *Proteus mirabilis, Enterobacter*	Generally resistant to penicillins and cephalosporins[a]; may appear susceptible to piperacillin/tazobactam but with a potentially higher failure rate than with a carbapenem	First-line: A carbapenem (Note: Some regions have seen considerable carbapenem resistance by a different mechanism in *Klebsiella*) Alternates: A fluoroquinolone or tigecycline, but there is less clinical experience with these
ampC-MEDIATED RESISTANCE IN GRAM-NEGATIVE BACILLI		
Enterobacter and *Citrobacter* (also may be seen in *Morganella morganii, Providencia, Serratia,* and indole-positive *Proteus*)	2nd- and 3rd-gen cephalosporins should generally be avoided even if organism is reported to be susceptible, because of potential for induction or selection of *ampC*-mediated β-lactamase (derepressed β-lactamase production), which can lead to development of resistance during treatment	First-line: A carbapenem Alternates (depending on susceptibility testing): A fluoroquinolone, TMP-SMX, tigecycline, piperacillin/tazobactam, an aminoglycoside, cefepime (better activity than 3rd-gen cephalosporins[b]) If *ampC*-mediated resistance occurs, a carbapenem is typically the only active β-lactam
CARBAPENEMASE-PRODUCING GRAM-NEGATIVES (eg, KPC or NDM-1) (Many labs no longer specifically test for this because of the 2010 CLSI breakpoint changes and recommendations)		
K pneumoniae, less common in other Enterobacteriaceae and *Pseudomonas aeruginosa*	Resistance to carbapenems and other β-lactams; also often has concomitant resistance to other classes of drugs	Per susceptibility testing; colistin (as colistimethate), polymyxin, and tigecycline often have in vitro activity

(Continues)

Table 30 Select Bacterial Resistance Issues (*Cont'd.*)

Pertinent Organisms	Resistance Issue	Treatment
METHICILLIN-RESISTANT *Staphylococcus aureus* (MRSA)		
S aureus	Oxacillin-resistant (methicillin-resistant) staphylococci are resistant to all currently available β-lactams except ceftaroline; both nosocomial and community-acquired strains are seen	First-line: vancomycin, linezolid, daptomycin[c]
		Alternates (depending on susceptibility testing): doxycycline, minocycline, TMP-SMX, clindamycin (test for inducible resistance), dalfopristin/quinupristin, tigecycline, ceftaroline, newer fluoroquinolones[d]
	CA-MRSA isolates tend to be more susceptible than nosocomial isolates to non–β-lactams (eg, TMP-SMX, clindamycin, tetracycline, fluoroquinolones)	
VANCOMYCIN- INTERMEDIATE OR VANCOMYCIN-RESISTANT STAPHYLOCOCCI (VISA OR VRSA)		
S aureus with **vancomycin MIC ≥4**	Organisms with reduced susceptibility or complete resistance to vancomycin have been reported	Contact infection control immediately and obtain infectious diseases consultation
VANCOMYCIN-RESISTANT ENTEROCOCCI (VRE)		
Enterococcus	Enterococci with resistance to vancomycin	First-line: linezolid
		Alternates: daptomycin,[c] dalfopristin/quinupristin (only for *E faecium*), tigecycline; may be susceptible to penicillin and ampicillin

[a] May show in vivo susceptibility to cephamycins (eg, cefotetan, cefoxitin), but failures have been reported and other mechanisms can confer resistance.

[b] Resistance to cefepime is less likely than that with 3rd-gen agents, but has been reported. If inducible β-lactamase production occurs, organisms should be considered resistant to penicillins and cephalosporins.

[c] Do not use daptomycin for pneumonia because it is inactivated by surfactant. It has in vitro activity against enterococci, but studies on serious enterococcal infections are limited.

[d] Newer fluoroquinolones include moxifloxacin, levofloxacin, and gemifloxacin. Staphylococcal resistance to fluoroquinolones has been reported to develop while patients are receiving therapy.

Fungi: Preferred and Alternate Treatment Options

Table 31 Fungal Organism–Specific Treatment

Organism	First-Line Treatment	Alternate Treatment (Depending on Susceptibility)
Aspergillus	voriconazole	An amphotericin B product[a] (less active for A flavus and A terreus), itraconazole, an echinocandin,[b] posaconazole
Blastomyces	An amphotericin B product[a] (initial therapy for severe pulmonary or disseminated infections, for CNS disease, and for immunocompromised or pregnant patients); itraconazole (for mild-to-moderate disease)	voriconazole, posaconazole, fluconazole (less active)
Candidal infection (systemic)		
Candida unspeciated[c]	An echinocandin[b] (for life-threatening disease, azole preexposure, candidemia, or unstable patient; consider in neutropenic patient); fluconazole (for stable patient with no azole preexposure)	voriconazole, an amphotericin B product,[a] itraconazole, posaconazole (not for candidemia)
C albicans, C parapsilosis, or C tropicalis	fluconazole, an echinocandin[b] (for life-threatening disease or unstable patient)	An amphotericin B product,[a] voriconazole, itraconazole, posaconazole (not for candidemia)
C glabrata	An echinocandin,[b] voriconazole (for patient with no azole preexposure or with documented susceptibility)	An amphotericin B product,[a,d] itraconazole,[e] higher-dose fluconazole[e] (for patient with no preexposure or with documented susceptibility), posaconazole (not for candidemia)
C guilliermondii or C lusitaniae	voriconazole, fluconazole	An echinocandin,[b] an amphotericin B product,[a,d] posaconazole (not for candidemia)

(Continues)

Table 31 Fungal Organism–Specific Treatment (*Cont'd.*)

Organism	First-Line Treatment	Alternate Treatment (Depending on Susceptibility)
C krusei	An echinocandin,[b] voriconazole	An amphotericin B product,[a,d] posaconazole (not for candidemia)
Candidal infection (localized)		
Candidal oropharyngeal or thrush	nystatin (topical), clotrimazole, fluconazole	voriconazole, an amphotericin B product (oral liquid), itraconazole, an echinocandin,[b] posaconazole
Candidal esophagitis[f]	fluconazole	itraconazole, voriconazole, an echinocandin, posaconazole, an amphotericin B product[a]
Candidal urinary tract infection (*Candida* in urine often represents colonization, especially in catheterized patients)	fluconazole	An amphotericin B product,[a] flucytosine
Candidal vulvovaginal infection	An azole (intravaginal), oral fluconazole	itraconazole, intravaginal boric acid (refractory cases)
Coccidioides	fluconazole, itraconazole, an amphotericin B product[a] (initial therapy for pregnant patients or patients with respiratory failure or rapidly progressive disease)	voriconazole
Cryptococcus	fluconazole, an amphotericin B product[a] (often with flucytosine for induction therapy for CNS disease)	voriconazole, itraconazole, posaconazole (not for CNS disease)
Fusarium	voriconazole, an amphotericin B product[a]	posaconazole
Histoplasma (symptomatic)	itraconazole, an amphotericin B product[a] (initial therapy for patients with severe infection or CNS disease)	voriconazole, fluconazole (both have less activity than itraconazole)

Table 31 Fungal Organism–Specific Treatment (*Cont'd.*)

Organism	First-Line Treatment	Alternate Treatment (Depending on Susceptibility)
Mucormycosis (eg, *Mucor, Rhizopus*)	An amphotericin B product[a,d]	posaconazole
Paracoccidioides	itraconazole, an amphotericin B product[a] (with maintenance sulfonamide or an azole)	voriconazole, sulfonamide, ketoconazole
Pneumocystis jiroveci (**PCP**)	TMP-SMX; add corticosteroids for severe disease	pentamidine IV, TMP plus dapsone, atovaquone, clindamycin plus primaquine
Scedosporium (*Pseudalles-cheria*)	voriconazole	posaconazole, itraconazole, terbinafine (in combination with an azole)
Sporothrix	itraconazole, an amphotericin B product[a]	potassium iodide, terbinafine
Tinea pedis	terbinafine (topical), an azole (topical)	oral fluconazole, griseofulvin, itraconazole

[a] Includes amphotericin B deoxycholate, liposomal amphotericin B, and amphotericin B lipid complex.

[b] The echinocandins include caspofungin, micafungin, and anidulafungin. Echinocandins may display a higher minimum inhibitory concentration (MIC) for *C guilliermondii* and *C parapsilosis*, but their clinical implication is unclear.

[c] Speciation and susceptibility testing for serious infections is recommended. Review institution- and population-specific rates of non-*albicans* species of *Candida*. De-escalate to fluconazole if appropriate, on the basis of speciation and susceptibility tests.

[d] May exhibit a higher MIC with amphotericin. Some resistance seen.

[e] Both fluconazole MIC and itraconazole MIC for *C glabrata* are often in the susceptible but dose-dependent category. If either drug is used, higher than usual doses are suggested. If susceptibility results show susceptible isolate (MIC ≤8 for fluconazole or ≤0.125 for itraconazole), use usual doses. When there is no susceptibility information with azole preexposure, either an echinocandin or an amphotericin B product is preferable due to the possibility of azole cross-resistance.

[f] Do **NOT** use topical therapy (eg, nystatin, clotrimazole, or amphotericin oral suspension) for esophageal disease. Systemic therapy is needed.

Viruses: Preferred and Alternate Treatment Options

Table 32 Antiviral Organism-Specific Treatment (Non-HIV Infections)

Organism	First-Line Treatment	Alternate Treatment
CMV	ganciclovir, valganciclovir	foscarnet, cidofovir, ganciclovir ocular implant,[a] fomivirsen[a] intravitreal injection
HSV	acyclovir,[b] famciclovir, valacyclovir	foscarnet (for acyclovir-resistant strains), trifluridine eye drops (for keratoconjunctivitis), ganciclovir,[c] valganciclovir[c]
HBV[d]	pegylated interferon, entecavir, tenofovir[e]	lamivudine,[e] adefovir, telbivudine, emtricitabine[e]
HCV	pegylated interferon plus ribavirin plus one of the following: boceprevir or telaprevir	
Influenza virus (treatment or prophylaxis)	oseltamivir, zanamivir	peramivir (IV only), amantadine or rimantadine for select seasonal strains, see CDC Web site for yearly recommendations (http://www.cdc.gov/flu/)
Varicella-zoster virus	acyclovir,[b] famciclovir, valacyclovir	foscarnet (for acyclovir-resistant strains)

[a] Ocular implants and intravitreal injections for CMV retinitis should generally be used in combination with systemic therapy to prevent spread to the contralateral eye and other organs.

[b] Intravenous acyclovir should be used for HSV CNS disease and for sight-threatening disease or severe varicella-zoster virus in immunocompromised patients.

[c] Active against acyclovir-susceptible strains of HSV, but not the preferred treatment due to toxicity and cost.

[d] HBV vaccine should be administered as a preventive strategy to persons at risk (including health care workers).

[e] Also has anti-HIV activity and thus is commonly used in HIV patients with HCV coinfection (tenofovir, lamivudine, and emtricitabine).

Infectious Syndromes in Adults

Clinical Approach to Patients With Infection

Four-Step Approach to Successful Management of Infectious Diseases

- **Define the host:** Identify factors that influence the type of infection, disease progression, and prognosis, which include:
  - Host factors such as patient age, immune status (eg, immunosuppression or the absence of a spleen), the presence of foreign bodies (eg, central venous catheter, permanent pacemaker, intracardiac defibrillator, prosthetic heart valves, prosthetic joints), or other comorbid conditions, **AND**
  - The environmental setting (community-acquired vs hospital-acquired or nursing home–acquired infection) or recent antibiotic use (increased risk for multidrug-resistant infections and *Clostridium difficile* colitis)
- **Define the infection syndrome:** Determine the anatomical location of infection and the extent of inflammation (eg, the "-itis": meningitis, pyelonephritis, peritonitis, pneumonitis, endocarditis), the rate of progression, and the severity of infection (eg, localized vs multiorgan involvement or hemodynamic instability).
- **Define the microbiology:** Determine the suspected pathogen(s) on the basis of the host and syndrome information or identify the confirmed pathogen(s) from available laboratory test results (eg, cultures, stains, serologies, antigens). Appropriate cultures should be obtained before initiating antimicrobial therapy: Consider 2 separate blood cultures and, as clinically indicated, the culture of other sites (eg, urine, cerebrospinal fluid, deep wounds, respiratory secretions, other body fluids).
- **Determine the optimal antimicrobial therapy:** Base decisions about antimicrobial therapy on an integration of the information about host, syndrome, and suspected or confirmed microbiology. When appropriate, target antimicrobial therapy against confirmed or suspected pathogens. Ensure that the selected antimicrobial therapy is dosed correctly and can adequately penetrate the anatomical site of infection.

Additional Considerations

Source Control

- Identify infection that is amenable to source control measures, specifically the drainage of an abscess or local focus of infection, the debridement of infected necrotic tissue, or the removal of a potentially infected device. Examples include:

- **Drainage:** Intra-abdominal abscess, thoracic empyema, and cholangitis
- **Debridement:** Necrotizing fasciitis, intestinal infarction, osteomyelitis, septic arthritis, and mediastinitis
- **Device removal:** Infected permanent pacemaker or intracardiac defibrillator, vascular catheter, urinary catheter, and intrauterine device
- **Definitive control:** Sigmoid resection for recurrent diverticulitis and cholecystectomy for gangrenous cholecystitis
- Recognize sepsis, severe sepsis, and septic shock (see definitions listed below).

Emergent Antimicrobial Intervention

- Identify syndromes requiring urgent antimicrobial intervention (eg, neutropenia with gram-negative bacteriemia, bacterial meningitis, thoracic or subdural empyema, severe sepsis, septic shock, infective endocarditis with heart failure).
- Pay particular attention to Gram stain results (which are rapidly available), cultures, molecular diagnostic results, and drug susceptibility information to further direct therapy.
- Review each patient's drug allergies and organ function (eg, renal, hepatic) for optimal selection and dosing of antimicrobial therapy.
- Ensure selected antibiotic adequately penetrates site of infection (eg, cerebrospinal fluid).

Severe Sepsis or Septic Shock

- Accomplish aggressive resuscitation with fluids, vasopressors, and/or blood products as indicated within the first 6 hours of resuscitation, with targets of central venous pressure 8-12 mm Hg, mean arterial pressure ≥65 mm Hg, urine output ≥0.5 mL/kg/h, and central venous or mixed venous oxygen saturation ≥70%.
- Initiate antibiotic therapy within the first hour after recognition of severe sepsis or septic shock by appropriate cultures.
- Obtain an infectious diseases consultation for all serious and complex infections.
- Correctly define clinical syndrome:
  - **Sepsis:** Hyperthermia or hypothermia, tachypnea, and tachycardia in the presence of infection
  - **Severe sepsis:** Sepsis associated with acute organ dysfunction:
    - **Respiratory dysfunction:** Bilateral pulmonary infiltrates with a ratio of Pao_2 to Fio_2 <300 mm Hg
    - **Renal dysfunction:** Urine output <0.5 mL/kg/h for at least 2 hours or serum creatinine >2.0 mg/dL
    - **Coagulation abnormalities:** International normalized ratio >1.5 or an activated partial thromboplastin time >60 seconds
    - **Thrombocytopenia:** Platelet count <100,000/mcL)
    - **Hypoperfusion:** Serum lactate level >2.0 mmol/L)
    - **Hyperbilirubinemia:** Total plasma bilirubin level >2.0 mg/dL

- **Hypotension:** Systolic blood pressure <90 mm Hg, mean arterial pressure <65 mm Hg, or a reduction in systolic blood pressure >40 mm Hg from baseline).
- **Septic shock:** Severe sepsis (despite adequate volume resuscitation) associated with acute circulatory failure (systolic blood pressure <90 mm Hg, mean arterial pressure <65 mm Hg, or a reduction in systolic blood pressure >40 mm Hg from baseline).[a]

[a] Dellinger RP, et al. Crit Care Med. 2008 Jan;36(1):296-327. Erratum in: Crit Care Med. 2008 Apr;36(4):1394-6.

Respiratory Tract Infections

Clinical Syndromes and Common Pathogens

Acute Bronchitis

Diagnostic criteria include productive cough, symptoms of upper respiratory infection, and negative findings on chest radiographs. Viral agents are the most common cause; antibiotics are therefore not beneficial.

- **Viral causes:** Influenza, parainfluenza, and other respiratory viruses affect >70% of patients
- **Less common but potentially antibiotic-responsive infectious agents:** *Mycoplasma pneumoniae*, *Chlamydophila pneumoniae*, *Bordetella pertussis*

Community-Acquired Pneumonia

Diagnostic criteria for community-acquired pneumonia (CAP) include acute or subacute onset of fever, cough, dyspnea, or pleuritic chest pain that develops in previously healthy persons.

- **Common bacteria:** *Streptococcus pneumoniae*, *M pneumoniae*, *C pneumoniae*, *Legionella pneumophila*, *Haemophilus influenzae*, and occasionally community-acquired methicillin-resistant *Staphylococcus aureus* (CA-MRSA)
- **Viral causes:** Influenza (seasonal), parainfluenza, varicella, respiratory syncytial virus (seasonal; more significant in infants and immunocompromised adults)
- **More chronic symptoms in specific epidemiologic conditions:** Mycobacteria (tuberculosis and nontuberculosis mycobacteria [eg, MAC {*Mycobacterium avium-intracellulare* complex}, *Mycobacterium kansasii*]), fungi (*Histoplasma*, *Blastomyces*, *Coccidioides*), and zoonoses (*Coxiella burnetii* [Q fever], *Francisella tularensis*)

Aspiration Pneumonia

Diagnostic criteria include fever, cough, or pulmonary infiltrate in a lower lung field after a single or recurrent aspiration event. Acute aspiration may cause chemical lung injury, which does not require antibiotic therapy. Not all aspiration results in bacterial pneumonia.

- **Common bacteria:** Mixed oral or upper intestinal bacterial flora; may include anaerobes

Hospital-Acquired or Health Care–Associated Pneumonia

Hospitalized patients or those in a nursing home or a skilled care facility for >2 days are at risk of hospital-acquired or health care–associated pneumonia; the diagnosis excludes patients in whom the organism was incubating at admission. This type of infection is most common in patients who are intubated for >2-3 days. Diagnostic criteria include fever, new pulmonary infiltrate, and respiratory distress. Clinical diagnosis is difficult in intubated patients.

- **Early-onset common bacteria:** Within 4 days after admission to a health care facility, with no risk factors for multidrug-resistant (MDR) organisms (see Table 33 on "Risk Factors for MDR Pathogens Causing Hospital-Acquired Pneumonia, Health Care–Associated Pneumonia, and Ventilator-Associated Pneumonia"): *S pneumoniae*, *H influenzae*, *S aureus*, *Escherichia coli*, *Klebsiella pneumoniae*, *Proteus*, *Serratia marcescens*
- **Late-onset common bacteria:** Onset occurs >5 days after admission to a health care facility or risk factors for MDR pathogens (see Table 33): Organisms as delineated above, for early onset, plus *Pseudomonas aeruginosa*, *Enterobacter*, *K pneumoniae* (including ESBL), *Acinetobacter*, and MRSA

  Data from Mandell LA, et al. Clin Infect Dis. 2007 Mar 1;44 Suppl 2:S27-72.

Table 33 Risk Factors for MDR Pathogens Causing Hospital-Acquired Pneumonia, Health Care–Associated Pneumonia, and Ventilator-Associated Pneumonia

Antimicrobial therapy in preceding 90 days
Current hospitalization of ≥5 days
High frequency of antibiotic resistance in community or in specific hospital unit
Presence of risk factors for health care–associated pneumonia
Hospitalization for ≥2 days in preceding 90 days
Residence in nursing home or extended-care facility
Home infusion therapy (including antibiotics)
Chronic dialysis in preceding 30 days
Home wound care
Family member with MDR pathogen
Immunosuppressive disease or therapy

Adapted from American Thoracic Society; Infectious Diseases Society of America. Am J Respir Crit Care Med. 2005 Feb 15;171(4):388-416. Used with permission.

Pneumonia in Immunocompromised Hosts

Diagnostic criteria include fever, cough, dyspnea, and pleuritic chest pain. Dyspnea may be more pronounced than indicated by findings on chest radiographs. Management often requires invasive procedures (bronchoscopy or open-lung biopsy) for diagnosis of opportunistic infections.

- Cell-mediated (T-cell) immune dysfunction (patients with HIV [human immunodeficiency virus]; organ transplant recipients; patients on chronic corticosteroids)
  - Usual CAP pathogens

- *Legionella*, *Nocardia*, *Pneumocystis jiroveci* (PCP), *Cryptococcus neoformans*, *Histoplasma capsulatum*, cytomegalovirus, *Toxoplasma gondii*
- Neutropenia
  - Usual CAP pathogens
  - *P aeruginosa*, *Aspergillus* (eg, *A fumigatus*), agents of mucormycosis (eg, *Mucor*, *Rhizopus*)

Novel Characteristics of Respiratory Pathogens

- **S pneumoniae:** Acute high fever, productive cough, shortness of breath; rapid progression; air-space consolidation commonly seen on chest radiographs; bacteremia and pleural space infections also common
- **M pneumoniae:** Sore throat, dry cough, headache; occasional pleural effusion; chest radiograph and examination findings often discordant with mild symptoms; extrapulmonary findings include erythema multiforme and Stevens-Johnson syndrome, hemolytic anemia, changes in cardiac conduction, myocarditis or pericarditis, aseptic meningitis or encephalitis, Guillain-Barré syndrome, Raynaud phenomenon, glomerulonephritis, bullous myringitis
- **C pneumoniae:** Sore throat and prolonged dry cough; biphasic symptoms; variable findings on chest radiographs; less common extrapulmonary findings include endocarditis, meningoradiculitis, encephalitis
- **L pneumophila and other species:** Typically high fever; nonproductive or minimally productive cough; variable presentation with sometimes severe symptoms; rapidly progressive and often fatal; findings on chest radiographs include segmental to lobar infiltrate; hyponatremia, hypophosphatemia, and diarrhea
- **H influenzae**
  - Type B more common in children 4 months to 4 years of age (decreased incidence with *H influenzae* type B vaccine); also associated with pediatric meningitis, epiglottis, otitis, and cellulitis
  - Non–type B *H influenzae* pneumonia common in elderly patients and patients with chronic obstructive pulmonary disease; also associated with sinusitis and otitis
  - **CA-MRSA:** Infrequent cause of pneumonia but can be rapidly progressive or necrotizing
- **Respiratory Zoonoses**
  - *Chlamydophila psittaci* (psittacosis): Exposure to birds
  - *Coxiella burnetii* (Q fever): Exposure to cattle, goats, sheep
  - *Brucella*: Risk for abattoir workers
  - *Bacillus anthracis* (respiratory anthrax): "Woolsorter's disease" (less common)
  - *Francisella tularensis* (tularemia): Exposure to rabbits
  - *Rhodococcus equi*: Exposure to horses, cattle, pigs, sheep
  - *Yersinia pestis* (pneumonic plague): Exposure to another human with plague or exposure to rodents or fleas

Data from Mandell LA, et al. Clin Infect Dis. 2007 Mar 1;44 Suppl 2:S27-72.

Table 34 Empiric Therapy[a]

Condition	Treatment Options
Acute bronchitis	Supportive measures only; antibiotic therapy not indicated in most cases
Community-acquired pneumonia (CAP)	
Outpatient, no previous antibiotic therapy	**One of the following:**
	azithromycin or clarithromycin (if high-level resistance in region is uncommon[b]); **OR**
	doxycycline; **OR**
	A respiratory fluoroquinolone[c] (levofloxacin, moxifloxacin, or gemifloxacin)
Outpatient, recent antibiotic therapy, presence of comorbid conditions[d] or other risk factors for drug-resistant *S pneumoniae*	After recent antibiotic therapy, use alternate antimicrobial class:
	A newer fluoroquinolone (levofloxacin, moxifloxacin, or gemifloxacin); **OR**
	A combination of either azithromycin or clarithromycin plus 1 of the following: high-dose amoxicillin, amoxicillin/clavulanate, or an alternate β-lactam (ceftriaxone, cefuroxime, or cefpodoxime)
Hospitalized patient (non-ICU)	A fluoroquinolone (levofloxacin or moxifloxacin); **OR**
	A combination of a select β-lactam (ceftriaxone, cefotaxime, ertapenem, or ampicillin) plus a select macrolide (azithromycin or clarithromycin)
ICU admission	Combination therapy with a select β-lactam (ceftriaxone, cefotaxime, or ampicillin/sulbactam) plus either a fluoroquinolone (levofloxacin or moxifloxacin) or azithromycin
	If *P aeruginosa* is a concern:
	An antipseudomonal β-lactam[e] plus either ciprofloxacin or levofloxacin; **OR**
	An antipseudomonal β-lactam[e] plus an aminoglycoside and azithromycin
Possible CA-MRSA	Add vancomycin or linezolid to a CAP regimen; avoid daptomycin because it is inactivated by surfactant
Aspiration pneumonia	
Outpatient management	**EITHER**
	amoxicillin/clavulanate
	OR
	clindamycin

Table 34 Empiric Therapy[a] *(Cont'd.)*

Condition	Treatment Options
Hospitalized patient	**One of the following:**
	A β-lactam/β-lactamase inhibitor (ampicillin/sulbactam, piperacillin/tazobactam, or ticarcillin/clavulanate); **OR**
	A 3rd- or 4th-gen cephalosporin combined with either metronidazole or clindamycin; **OR**
	A fluoroquinolone combined with either metronidazole or clindamycin; **OR**
	meropenem, ertapenem, doripenem, or imipenem
Hospital-acquired or health-care–associated pneumonia[f]	
Early onset and no risk factors for MDR organisms	ceftriaxone, cefotaxime, a respiratory fluoroquinolone, ampicillin/sulbactam, piperacillin/tazobactam, ticarcillin/clavulanate, or ertapenem
Late onset or risk factors for MDR organisms	A select β-lactam (cefepime, ceftazidime, imipenem, meropenem, doripenem, or piperacillin/tazobactam) plus ciprofloxacin, levofloxacin, or an aminoglycoside
	With suspected MRSA: Add vancomycin or linezolid

[a] Initiate therapy after cultures are obtained. For pathogen-directed therapy, see Section IV: on "Treatment of Specific Organisms."

[b] In regions with high-level macrolide-resistant *S pneumoniae* rates >25%, consider alternate treatments.

[c] Treat with levofloxacin 750 mg for 5 days or 500 mg for 10 days. A fluoroquinolone should generally not be used as first-line treatment for outpatient therapy in previously healthy patients with no risk factors for drug-resistant *S pneumoniae* because of possible overuse that can lead to increased resistance.

[d] Comorbid conditions include chronic heart, lung, liver, and renal disease; diabetes mellitus; alcoholism; malignancies; asplenia; immunosuppressing conditions or use of immunosuppressing drugs; use of antimicrobials within the past 3 months (in which case, an alternate drug from a different class should be selected); and other risks for drug-resistant *S pneumoniae* infection.

[e] Antipseudomonal β-lactams include piperacillin/tazobactam, cefepime, ceftazidime, imipenem, doripenem, and meropenem.

[f] De-escalate antimicrobials on the basis of culture results. For hospital-acquired or health care–associated pneumonia, shorten the traditional duration of therapy to 7-8 days when patients respond and the etiologic agent is not *Pseudomonas* (similar success rates, less super-resistance, fewer adverse effects).

Data from Mandell LA, et al. Clin Infect Dis. 2007 Mar 1;44 Suppl 2:S27-72 and American Thoracic Society; Infectious Diseases Society of America. Am J Respir Crit Care Med. 2005 Feb 15;171(4):388-416.

Other Considerations

- With persistent fever despite apparently appropriate therapy, consider empyema
- With CAP, early transition to oral therapy is not associated with adverse outcomes; it decreases costs and adverse effects, and it may lead to shorter lengths of stay
- With CAP, administer antibiotics as soon as feasible for hospitalized patients; draw blood cultures (if any) before administration of antibiotics
- Vaccination for S pneumoniae and influenza virus decreases incidence and severity of CAP (now a core measure of the Centers for Medicare and Medicaid Services and the Joint Commission, which accredits and certifies health care organizations and programs)

Infective Endocarditis: Diagnosis and Treatment

Common Infective Endocarditis Pathogens

Native Valves
- Viridans streptococci
- *Staphylococcus aureus*
- Enterococci
- HACEK organisms

Prosthetic Valves
- Same as native valves, plus
  - Coagulase-negative staphylococci
  - Fungi
  - Gram-negative rods (early postoperative period)

Elements of Diagnosis

The diagnosis of infective endocarditis (IE) rests on demonstrated evidence of cardiac involvement and persistent bacteremia due to microorganisms that typically cause endocarditis. Establishing a microbiologic diagnosis is critical to therapeutic decisions. Every effort should be made to identify the causative organism.

Table 35 Definition of Infective Endocarditis by the Modified Duke Criteria

Definite IE
- Pathologic criteria
  - Microorganisms: Demonstrated by culture or histologic examination of a vegetation, a vegetation that has embolized, or an intracardiac abscess specimen; or
  - Pathologic lesions: Vegetation or intracardiac abscess confirmed by histologic findings that show active endocarditis
- Clinical criteria
  - 2 Major criteria; or
  - 1 Major criterion and 3 minor criteria; or
  - 5 Minor criteria

Possible IE
- 1 Major criterion and 1 minor criterion; or
- 3 Minor criteria

Rejected
- Firm alternate diagnosis explaining evidence of IE; or
- Resolution of IE syndrome with antibiotic therapy for ≤4 days; or
- No pathologic evidence of IE at surgery or autopsy, with antibiotic therapy for ≤4 days; or
- Does not meet the above criteria for possible IE

Adapted from Li JS, et al. Clin Infect Dis. 2000 Apr;30(4):633-8. Used with permission.

Table 36 Definition of Terms Used in the Modified Duke Criteria for the Diagnosis of Infective Endocarditis

Major criteria

- Blood culture positive for IE
    - Typical microorganisms consistent with IE from 2 separate blood cultures:
        - Viridans streptococci, *Streptococcus bovis*, HACEK group, *S aureus*; or
        - Community-acquired enterococci, in the absence of a primary focus; or
    - Microorganisms consistent with IE from persistently positive blood cultures, defined as follows:
        - At least 2 positive cultures of blood samples drawn >12 hours apart; or
        - All of 3 or a majority of ≥4 separate cultures of blood (with first and last samples drawn at least 1 hour apart)
    - Single positive blood culture for *Coxiella burnetii* or antiphase 1 IgG antibody titer >1:800
- Evidence of endocardial involvement
- Echocardiogram positive for IE (TEE recommended in patients with prosthetic valves, rated at least "possible IE" by clinical criteria, or complicated IE [paravalvular abscess]; TTE as first test in other patients), defined as follows:
    - Oscillating intracardiac mass on valve or supporting structures, in the path of regurgitant jets, or on implanted material in the absence of an alternative anatomical explanation; or
    - Abscess; or
    - New partial dehiscence of prosthetic valve
- New valvular regurgitation (worsening or changing of preexisting murmur not sufficient)

Minor criteria

- Predisposition: Predisposing heart condition or injection drug use
- Fever: Temperature >38°C
- Vascular phenomena: Major arterial emboli, septic pulmonary infarcts, mycotic aneurysm, intracranial hemorrhage, conjunctival hemorrhages, and Janeway lesions
- Immunologic phenomena: Glomerulonephritis, Osler nodes, Roth spots, and rheumatoid factor
- Microbiologic evidence: Positive blood culture but does not meet a major criterion as noted above[a] or serologic evidence of active infection with organism consistent with IE

[a] Excludes single positive cultures for coagulase-negative staphylococci and organisms that do not cause endocarditis.

Adapted from Li JS, et al. Clin Infect Dis. 2000 Apr;30(4):633-8. Used with permission.

Table 37 Use of Echocardiography During Diagnosis and Treatment

Initial echocardiography
- Perform as soon as possible (<12 hours after initial evaluation)
- Use TEE primarily; obtain TTE views of any abnormal findings for later comparison
- Perform TTE if TEE is not immediately available
- Use TTE in small children, as it may be sufficient

Repeat echocardiography
- Perform TEE as soon as possible after positive TTE in patients at high risk of complications for potential impact on prognosis and management
- Repeat TEE 7-10 days after initial TEE if suspicion exists without diagnosis of IE or with worrisome clinical course during early treatment of IE

Adapted from Baddour LM, et al. Circulation. 2005 Jun 14;111(23):e394-434. Errata in: Circulation. 2005 Oct 11;112(15):2373. Circulation. 2007 Apr 17;115(15):e408. Circulation. 2007 Nov 20;116(21):e547. Circulation. 2008 Sep 16;118(12):e497. Used with permission.

Table 38 Echocardiographic Features That Suggest Potential Need for Surgical Intervention

Vegetation
- Persistent vegetation after systemic embolization
- Anterior mitral leaflet vegetation, particularly if >10 mm[a]
- Embolic events (≥1) during first 2 weeks of antimicrobial therapy[a]
- Increased vegetation size despite appropriate antimicrobial therapy[a,b]

Valvular dysfunction
- Acute aortic or mitral insufficiency with signs of ventricular failure[b]
- Heart failure unresponsive to medical therapy[b]
- Valve perforation or rupture[b]

Perivalvular extension
- Valvular dehiscence, rupture, or fistula[c]
- New heart block[b,c]
- Large abscess or extension of abscess despite appropriate antimicrobial therapy

[a] Surgery may be required because of risk of embolization.

[b] Surgery may be required because of heart failure or failure of medical therapy.

[c] Echocardiography should not be the primary modality used to detect or monitor heart block.

Adapted from Baddour LM, et al. Circulation. 2005 Jun 14;111(23):e394-434. Errata in: Circulation. 2005 Oct 11;112(15):2373. Circulation. 2007 Apr 17;115(15):e408. Circulation. 2007 Nov 20;116(21):e547. Circulation. 2008 Sep 16;118(12):e497. Used with permission.

Treatment of Endocarditis: Pathogen-Directed Therapy

Table 39 Therapy of Native Valve Endocarditis Caused by Highly Penicillin-Susceptible Viridans Group Streptococci and *S bovis* (MIC ≤0.12 mcg/mL)

Regimen	Dosage[a] and Route	Duration	Comments
EITHER			
penicillin G	12-18 million units per day IV, either continuously or in 4-6 equally divided doses	4 wk	Preferred options in most patients >65 y or with impaired 8th cranial nerve function or impaired renal function
OR			
ceftriaxone	2 g per day IV or IM	4 wk	
EITHER			
penicillin G	12-18 million units per day IV, either continuously or in 6 equally divided doses	2 wk	The 2-week regimen is not intended for patients with a known cardiac abscess or extracardiac infection or for those with Cl_{cr} <20 mL/min, impaired 8th cranial nerve function, or infection with *Abiotrophia*, *Granulicatella*, or *Gemella*
PLUS			
gentamicin	3 mg/kg per day IV or IM	2 wk	
OR			
ceftriaxone	2 g per day IV or IM	2 wk	
PLUS			
gentamicin[b]	3 mg/kg per day IV or IM	2 wk	
vancomycin[c]	30 mg/kg per day IV in 2 equally divided doses not to exceed 2 g per day unless serum levels are inappropriately low	4 wk	Use vancomycin for patients unable to tolerate penicillin or ceftriaxone Adjust dosage to obtain a trough level of 10-15 mcg/mL

[a] Recommended dosages are for adult patients with normal renal function.

[b] Other potentially nephrotoxic drugs (eg, NSAIDs) should be used with caution in patients receiving gentamicin therapy.

[c] Infuse vancomycin over at least 1 hour to reduce the risk of histamine release (red man syndrome).

Adapted from Baddour LM, et al. Circulation. 2005 Jun 14;111(23):e394-434. Errata in: Circulation. 2005 Oct 11;112(15):2373. Circulation. 2007 Apr 17;115(15):e408. Circulation. 2007 Nov 20;116(21):e547. Circulation. 2008 Sep 16;118(12):e497. Used with permission.

Table 40 Therapy of Native Valve Endocarditis Caused by Relatively Penicillin-Resistant Strains of Viridans Group Streptococci and *S bovis* (MIC >0.12 mcg/mL to ≤0.5 mcg/mL)

Regimen	Dosage[a] and Route	Duration	Comments
EITHER			
penicillin G	24 million units per day IV, either continuously or in 4-6 equally divided doses	4 wk	Use an enterococcal endocarditis regimen for patients with endocarditis caused by penicillin-resistant strains (MIC >0.5 mcg/mL)
PLUS			
gentamicin	3 mg/kg per day IV or IM	2 wk	
OR			
ceftriaxone	2 g per day IV or IM	4 wk	
PLUS			
gentamicin	3 mg/kg per day IV or IM	2 wk	
vancomycin[b]	30 mg/kg per day IV in 2 equally divided doses not to exceed 2 g per day unless serum levels are inappropriately low	4 wk	Use vancomycin only for patients unable to tolerate penicillin or ceftriaxone

[a] Recommended dosages are for adult patients with normal renal function.

[b] Adjust vancomycin dosage to obtain a trough level of 10-15 mcg/mL.

Adapted from Baddour LM, et al. Circulation. 2005 Jun 14;111(23):e394-434. Errata in: Circulation. 2005 Oct 11;112(15):2373. Circulation. 2007 Apr 17;115(15):e408. Circulation. 2007 Nov 20;116(21):e547. Circulation. 2008 Sep 16;118(12):e497. Used with permission.

Table 41 Therapy for Endocarditis of Prosthetic Valves or Other Prosthetic Material Caused by Viridans Group Streptococci and *S bovis*

Regimen	Dosage[a] and Route	Duration	Comments
PENICILLIN-SUSCEPTIBLE STRAIN (MIC ≤0.12 mcg/mL) EITHER			
penicillin G	24 million units per day IV, either continuously or in 4-6 equally divided doses	6 wk	Use of either penicillin G with gentamicin or ceftriaxone with gentamicin has **NOT** demonstrated superior cure rates compared with penicillin or ceftriaxone monotherapy for patients with a highly susceptible strain

(Continues)

Table 41 Therapy for Endocarditis of Prosthetic Valves or Other Prosthetic Material Caused by Viridans Group Streptococci and *S bovis* (Cont'd.)

Regimen	Dosage[a] and Route	Duration	Comments
PENICILLIN-SUSCEPTIBLE STRAIN (MIC ≤0.12 mcg/mL) (Continued)			
PLUS (optional)			
gentamicin	3 mg/kg per day IV or IM	2 wk	Do **NOT** use gentamicin in patients with Cl$_{cr}$ <30 mL/min
OR			
ceftriaxone	2 g per day IV or IM	6 wk	
PLUS (optional)			
gentamicin	3 mg/kg per day IV or IM	2 wk	Do **NOT** use gentamicin in patients with Cl$_{cr}$ <30 mL/min
vancomycin[b]	30 mg/kg per day IV in 2 equally divided doses	6 wk	Use vancomycin only for patients unable to tolerate penicillin or ceftriaxone
PENICILLIN RELATIVELY OR FULLY RESISTANT STRAIN (MIC >0.12 mcg/mL)			
EITHER			
penicillin G	24 million units per day IV, either continuously or in 4-6 equally divided doses	6 wk	
PLUS			
gentamicin	3 mg/kg per day IV or IM	6 wk	
OR			
ceftriaxone	2 g per day IV or IM	6 wk	
PLUS			
gentamicin	3 mg/kg per day IV or IM	6 wk	
vancomycin[b]	30 mg/kg per day IV in 2 equally divided doses	6 wk	Use vancomycin only for patients unable to tolerate penicillin or ceftriaxone

[a] Recommended dosages are for adult patients with normal renal function.

[b] Adjust vancomycin dosage to obtain a trough level of 10-15 mcg/mL.

Adapted from Baddour LM, et al. Circulation. 2005 Jun 14;111(23):e394-434. Errata in: Circulation. 2005 Oct 11;112(15):2373. Circulation. 2007 Apr 17;115(15):e408. Circulation. 2007 Nov 20;116(21):e547. Circulation. 2008 Sep 16;118(12):e497. Used with permission.

Table 42 Therapy for Endocarditis Caused by Staphylococci in the Absence of Prosthetic Materials

Regimen	Dosage[a] and Route	Duration	Comments
OXACILLIN-SUSCEPTIBLE STRAINS			
EITHER			
nafcillin[b]	12 g per day IV in 4-6 equally divided doses	6 wk	Use 6 weeks for complicated right-sided IE and for left-sided IE; or use 2 weeks for uncomplicated right-sided IE
PLUS (optional)			
gentamicin[c]	3 mg/kg per day IV or IM in 2-3 equally divided doses	3-5 days	Clinical benefit of aminoglycosides has **NOT** been established
			Consider skin testing for oxacillin-susceptible staphylococci and when there is a questionable history of immediate-type hypersensitivity to penicillin
OR			
oxacillin[b]	12 g per day IV in 4-6 equally divided doses	6 wk	
PLUS (optional)			
gentamicin[c]	3 mg/kg per day IV or IM in 2-3 equally divided doses	3-5 days	Clinical benefit of aminoglycosides has **NOT** been established
			Consider skin testing for oxacillin-susceptible staphylococci and when there is a questionable history of immediate-type hypersensitivity to penicillin

(*Continues*)

Table 42 Therapy for Endocarditis Caused by Staphylococci in the Absence of Prosthetic Materials (*Cont'd.*)

Regimen	Dosage[a] and Route	Duration	Comments
OXACILLIN-SUSCEPTIBLE STRAINS (Continued)			
For penicillin-allergic (non-anaphylactoid type) patients:			
cefazolin	6 g per day IV in 3 equally divided doses	6 wk	Avoid cephalosporins in patients with anaphylactoid-type hypersensitivity to β-lactams; use vancomycin instead
PLUS (optional)			
gentamicin[c]	3 mg/kg per day IV or IM in 2-3 equally divided doses	3-5 days	Clinical benefit of aminoglycosides has **NOT** been established
OXACILLIN-RESISTANT STRAINS			
vancomycin	30 mg/kg per day IV in 2 equally divided doses	6 wk	Adjust to achieve a trough level of 10-15 mcg/mL (some experts recommend a higher trough range of 15-20 mcg/mL)

[a] Recommended dosages are for adult patients with normal renal function.

[b] May use penicillin G 24 million units per day in place of nafcillin or oxacillin for penicillin-susceptible strain (MIC ≤0.1 mcg/mL).

[c] Administer gentamicin in close temporal proximity to vancomycin, nafcillin, or oxacillin.

Adapted from Baddour LM, et al. Circulation. 2005 Jun 14;111(23):e394-434. Errata in: Circulation. 2005 Oct 11;112(15):2373. Circulation. 2007 Apr 17;115(15):e408. Circulation. 2007 Nov 20;116(21):e547. Circulation. 2008 Sep 16;118(12):e497. Used with permission.

Table 43 Therapy for Prosthetic Valve Endocarditis Caused by Staphylococci

Regimen	Dosage[a] and Route	Duration	Comments
OXACILLIN-SUSCEPTIBLE STRAINS			
EITHER			
nafcillin	12 g per day IV in 6 equally divided doses	≥6 wk	Use penicillin G 24 million units per day instead of nafcillin or oxacillin if strain is penicillin-susceptible (MIC ≤0.1 mcg/mL) and does not produce β-lactamase
PLUS			
rifampin	900 mg per day IV or oral in 3 equally divided doses	≥6 wk	
AND PLUS			
gentamicin	3 mg/kg per day IV or IM in 2-3 equally divided doses	2 wk	Use vancomycin in patients with immediate-type hypersensitivity reactions to β-lactam antibiotics
OR			
oxacillin	12 g per day IV in 6 equally divided doses	≥6 wk	Substitute cefazolin for nafcillin or oxacillin in patients with nonimmediate-type hypersensitivity reaction to penicillin
PLUS			
rifampin	900 mg per day IV or oral in 3 equally divided doses	≥6 wk	
AND PLUS			
gentamicin[b]	3 mg/kg per day IV or IM in 2-3 equally divided doses	2 wk	
OXACILLIN-RESISTANT STRAINS			
vancomycin	30 mg/kg per day IV in 2 equally divided doses	≥6 wk	Adjust vancomycin to achieve a trough level of 10-15 mcg/mL (some experts recommend a higher trough range of 15-20 mcg/mL)
PLUS			
rifampin	900 mg per day IV or oral in 3 equally divided doses	≥6 wk	
AND PLUS			
gentamicin[b]	3 mg/kg per day IV or IM in 2-3 equally divided doses	2 wk	

[a] Recommended dosages are for adult patients with normal renal function.

[b] Adjust gentamicin dosage to achieve a peak serum level of 3-4 mcg/mL and a trough level of <1 mcg/mL.

Adapted from Baddour LM, et al. Circulation. 2005 Jun 14;111(23):e394-434. Errata in: Circulation. 2005 Oct 11;112(15):2373. Circulation. 2007 Apr 17;115(15):e408. Circulation. 2007 Nov 20;116(21):e547. Circulation. 2008 Sep 16;118(12):e497. Used with permission.

Table 44 Therapy for Native Valve or Prosthetic Valve Enterococcal Endocarditis Caused by Strains Susceptible to Penicillin, Gentamicin,[a] or Vancomycin

Regimen	Dosage[b] and Route	Duration	Comments
EITHER			
ampicillin	12 g per day IV in 6 equally divided doses	4-6 wk	Native valve: Use 4-week therapy for symptoms lasting ≤3 months and 6-week therapy for symptoms lasting >3 months
PLUS			
gentamicin[c]	3 mg/kg per day IV or IM in 3 equally divided doses	4-6 wk	
OR			
penicillin G	18-30 million units per day IV either continuously or in 6 equally divided doses	4-6 wk	Prosthetic valve or other prosthetic cardiac material: Use 6-week minimum therapy
PLUS			
gentamicin[c]	3 mg/kg per day IV or IM in 3 equally divided doses	4-6 wk	
vancomycin[d]	30 mg/kg per day IV in 2 equally divided doses	6 wk	Use vancomycin only for patients unable to tolerate penicillin or ampicillin
PLUS			
gentamicin[c]	3 mg/kg per day IV or IM in 3 equally divided doses	6 wk	Use 6 weeks of vancomycin therapy because of decreased activity against enterococci

[a] For strains resistant to gentamicin and susceptible to streptomycin, substitute streptomycin 15 mg/kg per day IV or IM in 2 divided doses. See full-text article of Baddour et al (see below) for management of enterococcal IE strains that are penicillin resistant and for management of strains resistant to penicillin, aminoglycosides, or vancomycin.

[b] Recommended dosages are for adult patients with normal renal function.

[c] Adjust gentamicin dosage to achieve a peak serum level of 3-4 mcg/mL and a trough level of <1 mcg/mL. Patients with Cl_{Cr} <50 mL/min should be treated in consultation with an infectious diseases specialist.

[d] Adjust vancomycin dosage to obtain a trough level of 10-15 mcg/mL.

Adapted from Baddour LM, et al. Circulation. 2005 Jun 14;111(23):e394-434. Errata in: Circulation. 2005 Oct 11;112(15):2373. Circulation. 2007 Apr 17;115(15):e408. Circulation. 2007 Nov 20;116(21):e547. Circulation. 2008 Sep 16;118(12):e497. Used with permission.

Table 45 Therapy for Both Native Valve and Prosthetic Valve Endocarditis Caused by HACEK[a] Microorganisms

Regimen	Dosage[b] and Route	Duration	Comments
ceftriaxone **OR**	2 g per day IV or IM	Native valve: 4 wk Prosthetic valve: 6 wk	Can substitute cefotaxime or another 3rd- or 4th-gen cephalosporin for ceftriaxone
ampicillin-sulbactam **OR**	12 g per day IV in 4 equally divided doses	Native valve: 4 wk Prosthetic valve: 6 wk	
ciprofloxacin[c]	1,000 mg per day oral or 800 mg per day IV in 2 equally divided doses	Native valve: 4 wk Prosthetic valve: 6 wk	Use fluoroquinolones only for patients unable to tolerate a cephalosporin or ampicillin; levofloxacin or moxifloxacin may be substituted; fluoroquinolones are not generally recommended for patients <18 y

[a] HACEK stands for the group of slow-growing gram-negative bacteria than can cause endocarditis: *Haemophilus parainfluenzae, H aphrophilus, H paraphrophilus, H influenzae, Actinobacillus actinomycetemcomitans, Cardiobacterium hominis, Eikenella corrodens,* and *Kingella kingae.*

[b] Recommended dosages are for adult patients with normal renal function.

[c] The fluoroquinolones are highly active in vitro against HACEK microorganisms. Few published data exist on the use of fluoroquinolone therapy for endocarditis caused by HACEK.

Adapted from Baddour LM, et al. Circulation. 2005 Jun 14;111(23):e394-434. Errata in: Circulation. 2005 Oct 11;112(15):2373. Circulation. 2007 Apr 17;115(15):e408. Circulation. 2007 Nov 20;116(21):e547. Circulation. 2008 Sep 16;118(12):e497. Used with permission.

Other Treatment Considerations

Role of Surgery

Obtain prompt surgical evaluation of patients with congestive heart failure, fungal IE, multiresistant organisms, gram-negative IE, or endocarditis of prosthetic valves, and of patients with echocardiographic features suggesting the need for surgical intervention (see preceding section above on "Elements of Diagnosis").

Care During and After Completion of Antimicrobial Treatment

- Initiate before or at completion of antimicrobial therapy:
  - Transthoracic echocardiogram to establish new baseline
  - Drug rehabilitation referral for patients who use illicit injection drugs
  - Patient education about the signs of endocarditis and the need for antibiotic prophylaxis before certain dental, surgical, or invasive procedures
  - Thorough dental evaluation and treatment, if not performed earlier in the evaluation
  - Prompt removal of intravenous catheter after administration of antimicrobial therapy
- Short-term follow-up:
  - Obtain at least 3 sets of blood cultures from separate sites for any febrile illness and before initiation of antibiotic therapy
  - Conduct a physical examination for evidence of congestive heart failure
  - Evaluate for toxicity due to current or prior antimicrobial therapy
- Long-term follow-up:
  - Obtain at least 3 sets of blood cultures from separate sites for any febrile illness and before initiation of antibiotic therapy
  - Evaluate valvular and ventricular function (eg, echocardiography)
  - Encourage scrupulous oral hygiene and frequent professional office visits

Adapted from Baddour LM, et al. Circulation. 2005 Jun 14;111(23):e394-434. Errata in: Circulation. 2005 Oct 11;112(15):2373. Circulation. 2007 Apr 17;115(15):e408. Circulation. 2007 Nov 20;116(21):e547. Circulation. 2008 Sep 16;118(12):e497. Used with permission.

Infective Endocarditis Prophylaxis

Prevention of Endocarditis

The guidelines for the prevention of infective endocarditis (IE) issued by the American Heart Association underwent a major revision in 2007. Key changes include the following:

- Dental procedures have been found to be associated with a small number of cases of IE. Thus, even if prophylaxis was 100% effective, it would prevent only an extremely small number of cases.
- The emphasis has shifted from antibiotic prophylaxis to good oral health and to increased access to dental care.
- Prophylactic antibiotics based on a patient's lifetime risk for acquiring IE are no longer recommended. Instead, prophylaxis focuses on patients at highest risk for adverse outcomes from IE.

Candidates for Prophylaxis

Only those patients with conditions that expose them to the highest risk for adverse outcomes from IE should receive prophylaxis. These high-risk conditions include:

- Prosthetic cardiac valve
- A history of IE
- Congenital heart disease (CHD) **ONLY** for the following specific conditions:
  - Unrepaired cyanotic CHD, including palliative shunts and conduits
  - Completely repaired congenital heart defect with prosthetic material or a prosthetic device placed either during surgery or by catheter intervention during the first 6 months after the procedure
  - CHD repair with residual defects at, or adjacent to, the site of a prosthetic patch or prosthetic device
- Development of cardiac valvulopathy after cardiac transplantation

(Adapted from Wilson W, et al. Circulation. 2007 Oct 9;116[15]:1736-54. Epub 2007 Apr 19. Erratum in: Circulation. 2007 Oct 9;116[15]:e376-7. Used with permission.)

Infective Endocarditis Prophylaxis for Specific Procedures

Prophylactic antibiotics should be administered **ONLY** to patients with the high-risk conditions listed above.

Dental Procedures

Prophylaxis is directed against viridans group streptococci.

- Procedures for which dental prophylaxis should be given to appropriate candidates include any procedures that involve manipulation of gingival tissue or the periapical region of the teeth or that involve perforation of the oral mucosa.
- Procedures that do **NOT** require prophylaxis include routine anesthetic injections through noninfected tissue, dental radiographs, placement of removable prosthodontic or orthodontic appliances, adjustment of orthodontic appliances, and placement of orthodontic brackets.
- Prophylaxis is not necessary after the shedding of deciduous teeth or for bleeding from trauma to the lips or oral mucosa.

Table 46 Prophylactic Regimens for Infective Endocarditis Before Dental Procedures[a,b]

Clinical Situation	Adult Prophylaxis (Use Only 1 Drug per Clinical Situation)	Pediatric Prophylaxis (Use Only 1 Drug per Clinical Situation)
Oral regimen	amoxicillin 2 g oral	amoxicillin 50 mg/kg oral
Unable to take oral medication	ampicillin 2 g IM or IV **OR** cefazolin 1 g IM or IV **OR** ceftriaxone 1 g IM or IV	ampicillin 50 mg/kg IM or IV **OR** cefazolin 50 mg/kg IM or IV **OR** ceftriaxone 50 mg/kg IM or IV
Allergy to penicillin or ampicillin (oral regimen)	cephalexin[c,d] 2 g oral **OR** clindamycin 600 mg oral **OR** azithromycin 500 mg oral **OR** clarithromycin 500 mg oral	cephalexin[c,d] 50 mg/kg oral **OR** clindamycin 20 mg/kg oral **OR** azithromycin 15 mg/kg oral **OR** clarithromycin 15 mg/kg oral

Table 46 Prophylactic Regimens for Infective Endocarditis Before Dental Procedures[a,b] (*Cont'd.*)

Clinical Situation	Adult Prophylaxis (Use Only 1 Drug per Clinical Situation)	Pediatric Prophylaxis (Use Only 1 Drug per Clinical Situation)
Allergy to penicillin or ampicillin (unable to take oral medication)	cefazolin[d] 1 g IM or IV **OR** ceftriaxone[d] 1 g IM or IV **OR** clindamycin 600 mg IM or IV	cefazolin[d] 50 mg/kg IM or IV **OR** ceftriaxone[d] 50 mg/kg IM or IV **OR** clindamycin 20 mg/kg IM or IV

[a] Give a single dose 30-60 minutes before the procedure.

[b] If the antibiotic is inadvertently not administered before the procedure, it may be administered up to 2 hours after the procedure.

[c] Or substitute another 1st- or 2nd-generation cephalosporin in an equivalent dose.

[d] Do not use a cephalosporin in patients with a history of anaphylaxis, angioedema, or urticaria after treatment with penicillin or ampicillin.

Adapted from Wilson W, et al. Circulation. 2007 Oct 9;116(15):1736-54. Epub 2007 Apr 19. Erratum in: Circulation. 2007 Oct 9;116(15):e376-7. Used with permission.

Respiratory Procedures

For candidates for prophylaxis as listed above:

- It may be reasonable to give one of the prophylactic regimens recommended above for dental procedures (see Table 46 on "Prophylactic Regimens for Infective Endocarditis Before Dental Procedures") before an invasive procedure (eg, tonsillectomy, adenoidectomy) involving the respiratory tract that necessitates incision or biopsy of the respiratory mucosa.
- Prophylaxis is **NOT** recommended for bronchoscopy unless the procedure involves incision of the respiratory tract mucosa.

Gastrointestinal or Genitourinary Procedures

For candidates for prophylaxis as listed above:

- Prophylaxis solely to prevent IE is **NO** longer recommended.
- For patients scheduled for an elective urinary tract manipulation who also have an enterococcal urinary tract infection or colonization, it may be reasonable to administer antibiotic therapy to eradicate enterococci from the urine before the procedure.
- If the urinary tract procedure is not elective, it may be reasonable to administer an antimicrobial regimen that contains an agent active against enterococci.
- Amoxicillin or ampicillin is the preferred agent for enterococcal coverage; vancomycin may be administered to patients who are unable to tolerate ampicillin.

Procedures Involving Infected Skin, Skin Structure, or Musculoskeletal Tissue

For candidates for prophylaxis as listed above:

- It is reasonable for the regimen administered to treat the infection to contain an agent active against staphylococci and β-hemolytic streptococci.
- An antistaphylococcal penicillin or a cephalosporin is preferable; vancomycin or clindamycin may be administered to patients who are unable to tolerate a β-lactam or who are known or suspected to have an infection caused by methicillin-resistant *Staphylococcus aureus*.

Other Prophylactic Considerations

- The presence of fever or other manifestations of systemic infection indicates the possibility of IE. In these cases, it is important to obtain blood cultures and other relevant tests before administration of a prophylactic antibiotic. Failure to do so may result in a delay in the diagnosis and treatment of a concomitant case of IE.
- If a patient is already receiving long-term antibiotic therapy with an antibiotic that is also recommended for IE prophylaxis for a dental procedure, an antibiotic from a different class should be used.
- If a patient requires a dental procedure while receiving parenteral antibiotic therapy for treatment of IE, the antibiotic therapy should be continued and the timing should be adjusted so that a dose is administered 30-60 minutes before the dental procedure.
- Patients who undergo surgery for placement of prosthetic heart valves or prosthetic intravascular or intracardiac material should be given surgical prophylaxis directed primarily against *Staphylococcus*.
- Antibiotic prophylaxis for dental procedures is not recommended for patients who have coronary artery bypass grafts or coronary artery stents.

(Adapted from Wilson W, et al. Circulation. 2007 Oct 9;116[15]:1736-54. Epub 2007 Apr 19. Erratum in: Circulation. 2007 Oct 9;116[15]:e376-7. Used with permission.)

Intravascular Catheter-Related Infections

Elements of Diagnosis

- Catheter cultures should be performed only if a catheter-related bloodstream infection (CRBSI) is suspected. Do **NOT** obtain routine or surveillance blood cultures through catheters.
- Always draw peripheral and blood cultures through the catheter lumen before starting empiric antimicrobial therapy.

A definite diagnosis of CRBSI requires one of the following:

- Growth of >15 CFU (colony-forming units) from the catheter tip, plus positive peripheral blood cultures; **OR**
- Microbial growth from blood cultures drawn through the catheter hub at least 2 hours before microbial growth from peripherally obtained blood cultures (differential time to positivity)

Table 47 Commonly Encountered Pathogens in Catheter-Related Bloodstream Infections

Clinical Situation	Common Organisms
All CRBSIs	*Staphylococcus*, including coagulase-negative staphylococci (most common) and *S aureus*, and select gram-positive bacilli (eg, *Corynebacterium*, *Bacillus*)
Prolonged hospitalization, critically ill (ICU) patients, femoral catheters, and immunosuppressed patients, including those with neutropenia	*Staphylococcus* and gram-negative bacilli (GNB), including *Pseudomonas aeruginosa*
Any of the above risk factors and total parenteral nutrition, prolonged use of antibacterial agents, and known *Candida* colonization	*Staphylococcus*, GNB, and *Candida*

- Once culture results are known, therapy should be de-escalated on the basis of the susceptibility profile of the responsible pathogen.
- For pathogen-specific therapy, see Section IV, Table 29 ("Specific Treatment of Bacterial Organisms") and Table 31 ("Fungal Organism–Specific Treatment").

Table 48 Complicated and Uncomplicated Central Venous Catheter (CVC) Infections

CVC-related infection is considered uncomplicated if:
- Fever and blood cultures resolve in ≤72 hours
- Patient has no foreign or prosthetic intravascular devices
- There is no evidence of endocarditis, suppurative thrombophlebitis, or osteomyelitis
- There is no active malignancy or immunosuppression (in cases of S aureus infection)

CVC-related infection is considered complicated with:
- Tunnel infection or port abscess
- Septic thrombosis, endocarditis, or osteomyelitis
- Bacteremia lasting >72 hours despite appropriate antimicrobial therapy

Catheter Removal vs Retention, and Duration of Treatment

- See Figure 3 and Figure 4 for a decision algorithm regarding catheter removal vs retention and duration of antimicrobial treatment.
- CVC should be removed in cases of complicated infection (see definitions above), regardless of causative pathogen.
- Infected short-term CVC should generally be removed.
- Infected long-term CVC (surgically implanted catheters such as the Hickman, Broviac, and Groshong catheters, as well as totally implantable catheters with subcutaneous ports) with fungi, mycobacteria, P aeruginosa, drug-resistant bacteria (including VRE, ESBL-producing, and other multidrug resistant GNB) should be removed. With S aureus, consider removal of infected catheter and provide prolonged antimicrobial therapy except in select situations as noted below.
- Patients with CRBSI due to S aureus may be treated with a shorter course (≥14 days) of systemic antibiotics if they are not diabetic, have no active malignancy, are not receiving immunosuppression, are not neutropenic, have no prosthetic intravascular device (eg, pacemaker, prosthetic valve, vascular graft), have negative transesophageal echocardiography, or have bacteremia and fever that resolve within 72 hours of catheter removal and initiation of appropriate antimicrobial therapy.
- When denoting duration of antimicrobial therapy, **day 1 is the first day of negative blood cultures**.

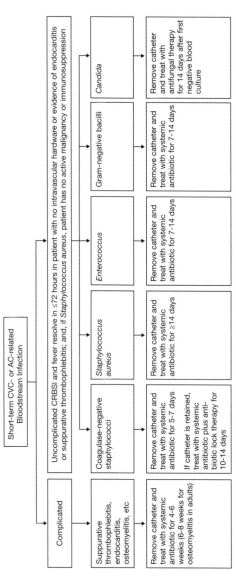

Figure 3 Management of Short-term Central Venous Catheter–Related Bloodstream Infections. AC indicates arterial catheter; CRBSI, catheter-related blood-stream infection; CVC, central venous catheter. (Adapted from Mermel LA, et al. Clin Infect Dis. 2009 Jul 1;49[1]:1-45. Used with permission.)

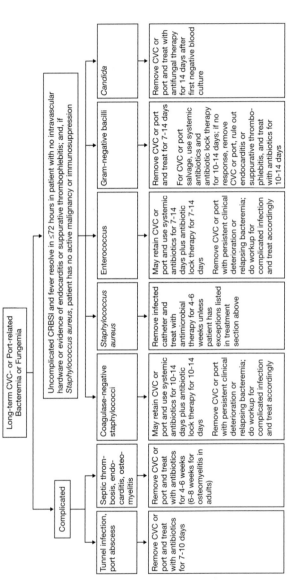

Figure 4 Management of Long-term Central Venous Catheter–Related Bloodstream Infections. CRBSI indicates catheter-related bloodstream infection; CVC, central venous catheter (Adapted from Mermel LA, et al. Clin Infect Dis. 2009 Jul 1;49[1]:1–45. Used with permission.)

Antibiotic Lock Therapy

- Antibiotic lock therapy is indicated for patients with uncomplicated long-term CVC and totally implantable catheters infected by select susceptible bacteria when catheter retention is the goal. The highest success rates have been found with coagulase-negative staphylococcus. For additional information on antibiotic lock solution options, see Mermel LA, et al. Clin Infect Dis. 2009 Jul 1;49(1):1-45.
- For CRBSIs, antibiotic lock therapy should be used in conjunction with systemic antibiotic therapy.
- If antimicrobial lock therapy cannot be used and CVC retention is the goal, systemic antibiotics should be infused through the colonized catheter lumen.

Other Considerations

- Repeat blood cultures should be obtained if CVC retention is attempted. If blood cultures remain positive after 72 hours of appropriate antibiotics, remove the CVC.
- There is no need to perform routine blood cultures after completing antimicrobial therapy for CRBSI.
- Linezolid should not be used for empiric therapy.

Central Nervous System Infections

Empiric Therapy for Acute Bacterial Meningitis

Elements of Diagnosis and Treatment

- **Clinical:** The diagnosis of meningitis is suggested by the constellation of headache, fever, and neck stiffness. Some patients may also experience changes in mental status.
- **Radiology:** Computed tomograms or magnetic resonance imaging of the brain may be indicated for immunocompromised patients and patients with papilledema or focal neurologic deficits. However, neuroimaging should not delay initiation of antimicrobial therapy.
- **Laboratory:** Cerebrospinal fluid (CSF) typically shows neutrophilic pleocytosis, high protein, and low glucose. Gram stain may provide rapid initial clues to the causative agent while awaiting results of CSF and blood cultures.
- **Treatment**
  - Acute bacterial meningitis is a medical emergency. Institute empiric antimicrobial therapy promptly and adjust it after isolating the etiologic agent. The duration of pathogen-directed therapy depends on the causative organism (see Table 50 on "Pathogen-Directed Therapy")
  - Use adjunctive dexamethasone 0.15 mg/kg q6h for 2-4 days for neonates or children with *Haemophilus influenzae* meningitis and for adults with proven or suspected *Streptococcus pneumoniae* meningitis. Administer the first dose of dexamethasone before or concurrent with the first dose of antimicrobial therapy.
  - Consider adding rifampin for suspected *S pneumoniae*, pending susceptibilities if dexamethasone is used. If *S pneumoniae* is β-lactam susceptible, rifampin can be discontinued.

Table 49 Empiric Therapy

Patient Variable	Suspected Pathogens	First-Line Treatment
Age		
<1 mo	S agalactiae Escherichia coli Listeria monocytogenes Klebsiella	ampicillin plus either cefotaxime or an aminoglycoside
1-23 mo	S pneumoniae Neisseria meningitidis E coli S agalactiae H influenzae	vancomycin[a] plus either ceftriaxone or cefotaxime
2-50 y	N meningitidis S pneumoniae	vancomycin[a] plus either ceftriaxone or cefotaxime
>50 y	S pneumoniae N meningitidis L monocytogenes Aerobic gram-negative bacilli	vancomycin[a] plus ampicillin and plus 1 of the following: ceftriaxone, cefotaxime, or cefepime
Head trauma		
Basilar skull fracture	S pneumoniae H influenzae Group A (β-hemolytic) streptococci	vancomycin[a] plus either ceftriaxone or cefotaxime
Penetrating trauma	S aureus Coagulase-negative staphylococci Aerobic gram-negative bacilli, including Pseudomonas aeruginosa	vancomycin[a] plus 1 of the following: cefepime, ceftazidime, or meropenem
Postneurosurgery	S aureus Coagulase-negative staphylococci Aerobic gram-negative bacilli, including P aeruginosa	vancomycin[a] plus 1 of the following: cefepime, ceftazidime, or meropenem
CSF shunt-related	Coagulase-negative staphylococci S aureus Aerobic gram-negative bacilli, including P aeruginosa Propionibacterium acnes	vancomycin[a] plus 1 of the following: cefepime, ceftazidime, or meropenem

[a] Monitor serum levels. Maintain vancomycin trough concentration at 15-20 mcg/mL.

Adapted from Tunkel AR, et al. Clin Infect Dis. 2004 Nov 1;39(9):1267-84. Epub 2004 Oct 6. Used with permission.

Pathogen-Directed Therapy for Acute Bacterial Meningitis

Elements of Diagnosis and Treatment

- **Clinical:** Adjust antimicrobial therapy on the basis of the results of Gram stain, bacterial cultures, and antimicrobial susceptibility pattern.
- **Laboratory:** Use results of antimicrobial susceptibilities to guide the choice of pathogen-directed therapy.
- **Treatment:** Continue adjunctive dexamethasone 0.15 mg/kg q6h for 2-4 days in neonates or children with *H influenzae* meningitis and in adults with proven or suspected *S pneumoniae* meningitis.

Table 50 Pathogen-Directed Therapy

Pathogens	First-Line Treatment
Enterococcus	
ampicillin-susceptible	ampicillin plus gentamicin
ampicillin-resistant	vancomycin plus gentamicin
ampicillin- and vancomycin-resistant	linezolid
E coli and other Enterobacteriaceae	A 3rd- or 4th-gen cephalosporin (eg, ceftriaxone, cefotaxime, ceftazidime, cefepime)
H influenzae	
β-Lactamase negative	ampicillin, cefotaxime, or ceftriaxone
β-Lactamase positive	ceftriaxone or cefotaxime
L monocytogenes	ampicillin with or without an aminoglycoside **OR** penicillin G with or without an aminoglycoside
N meningitidis penicillin MIC	
<0.1 mcg/mL	penicillin, ampicillin, ceftriaxone, or cefotaxime
0.1-1.0 mcg/mL	ceftriaxone or cefotaxime
P aeruginosa	cefepime or ceftazidime
S aureus	
MRSA	vancomycin
MSSA	nafcillin or oxacillin

Alternate Treatment	Duration
linezolid	Individualize[a]
meropenem, aztreonam, TMP-SMX, or a fluoroquinolone[b]	21 days[a]
cefepime or a fluoroquinolone[b]	7 days[a]
cefepime or a fluoroquinolone[b]	
TMP-SMX or meropenem	21 days[a]
meropenem or a fluoroquinolone[b]	7 days[a]
meropenem or a fluoroquinolone[b]	
meropenem, ciprofloxacin, levofloxacin, or aztreonam	Individualize[a]
TMP-SMX or linezolid	
vancomycin or meropenem	Individualize[a]

(Continues)

Table 50 Pathogen-Directed Therapy (*Cont'd.*)

Pathogens	First-Line Treatment
S epidermidis (MRSE)	vancomycin
S agalactiae	penicillin or ampicillin
S pneumoniae	
penicillin susceptible	penicillin G, ampicillin, ceftriaxone, or cefotaxime
penicillin intermediate	ceftriaxone or cefotaxime
penicillin resistant	vancomycin plus either cefotaxime or ceftriaxone
cefotaxime or ceftriaxone MIC ≥0.5 mcg/mL	vancomycin plus either cefotaxime or ceftriaxone

[a] Duration of therapy may have to be individualized on the basis of the patient's clinical response.

[b] CSF levels vary by agent.

Adapted from Tunkel AR, et al. Clin Infect Dis. 2004 Nov 1;39(9):1267-84. Epub 2004 Oct 6. Used with permission.

Alternate Treatment	Duration
linezolid	Individualize[a]
ceftriaxone or cefotaxime	14-21 days[a]
cefepime	10-14 days[a]
cefepime or meropenem	
fluoroquinolone	
fluoroquinolone	

Table 51 Recommended Doses of Select Antimicrobial Agents for Treatment of Meningitis in Children and Adults With Normal Renal and Hepatic Function

Antimicrobial Agents	Children (After Neonatal Period)		Adults	
	Dose	Total Max Daily Dose	Dose	Total Daily Dose
ampicillin	300 mg/kg/24h divided q6h	12 g	2 g q4h	12 g
cefepime	150 mg/kg/24h divided q8h	6 g	2 g q8h	6 g
cefotaxime	225-300 mg/kg/24h divided q6h	12 g	2 g q4h (or 3 g q6h)	12 g
ceftazidime	150 mg/kg/24h divided q8h	6 g	2 g q8h	6 g
ceftriaxone	80-100 mg/kg/24h divided q12h	4 g	2 g q12h	4 g
ciprofloxacin	NA	NA	400 mg q8h (or 600 mg q12h)	800-1,200 mg

(*Continues*)

Table 51 Recommended Doses of Select Antimicrobial Agents for Treatment of Meningitis in Children and Adults With Normal Renal and Hepatic Function (*Cont'd.*)

| Antimicrobial Agents | Children (After Neonatal Period) | | Adults | |
	Dose	Total Max Daily Dose	Dose	Total Daily Dose
meropenem	120 mg/kg/ 24h divided q8h	6 g	2 g q8h	6 g
moxifloxacin	NA	NA	400 mg q24h	400 mg
nafcillin	200 mg/kg/ 24h divided q6h	12 g	2 g q4h	12 g
oxacillin	200 mg/kg/ 24h divided q6h	12 g	2 g q4h	12 g
penicillin G	300,000 units/ kg/24h divided q4-6h	24 million units	20-24 million units per day or 4 million units q4h, as continuous IV infusion (load with 4-5 million units)	20-24 million units
rifampin	10-20 mg/kg/24h divided q12-24h	600 mg	600 mg q24h	600 mg
TMP-SMX	10-20 mg/kg/24h divided q6-12h	20 mg/kg	15-20 mg/ kg/24h divided q6-12h	15-20 mg/kg
vancomycin[a]	60 mg/kg/24h divided q6h	60 mg/kg	40-45 mg/ kg/24h divided q8-12h[a]	Individualize[a]

[a] Monitor serum levels and maintain trough concentration of 15-20 mcg/mL.

Adapted from Tunkel AR, et al. Clin Infect Dis. 2004 Nov 1;39(9):1267-84. Epub 2004 Oct 6. Used with permission.

Cryptococcal and Tubercular Meningitis

Elements of Diagnosis and Treatment

- **Clinical:** The constellation of headache, fever, and neck stiffness is frequently associated with cryptococcal or tubercular meningitis. Changes in mental status may occur in many cases. Certain risk factors (eg, immunocompromised state or exposure history) may be apparent.
- **Radiology:** Neuroimaging may be indicated for immunocompromised patients and for patients with papilledema or focal neurologic deficits.
- **Laboratory:** Conduct CSF examination with Gram stain and culture, in addition to blood cultures. Cryptococcal antigen may be detected in CSF and blood.
- **Adjunctive treatment of tubercular meningitis:** Administer adjunctive dexamethasone 0.15 mg/kg q6h for 2-4 days
- **Treatment of cryptococcal meningitis:** See Tables 73-78 on "Fungal Infections"

Table 52 Treatment of Tubercular Meningitis

Empiric Therapy	First-Line Treatment	Alternate Treatment
Mycobacterium tuberculosis	isoniazid 300 mg/24h plus all 3 of the following for 2 mo: rifampin 600 mg/24h, pyrazinamide 15-30 mg/kg/24h, and ethambutol 15-20 mg/kg/24h; then isoniazid 300 mg/24h and rifampin 600 mg/24h for 7-10 mo	Management of drug-resistant TB should be guided by susceptibility testing and patients should be referred to a TB management expert

Urinary Tract Infections

Elements of Diagnosis

Table 53 Elements of Diagnosis of Urinary Tract Infections

Clinical Syndromes	Diagnostic Considerations
Asymptomatic bacteriuria	**Clinical diagnosis:** Urine culture >10^5 CFU/mL in absence of symptoms; common in elderly and in patients with chronic catheterization, spinal cord injuries, and neurogenic bladder; typically requires no treatment **EXCEPT** during pregnancy and in young children
Cystitis in women (uncomplicated)	**Clinical diagnosis:** Cultures typically not needed; urine dipstick esterase-positive urine culture should show >10^2 CFU/mL; symptoms include dysuria and frequency
	Common pathogens: 75-95% *Escherichia coli* and other gram-negative bacteria; 5-20% *Staphylococcus saprophyticus* and *Enterococcus*
Pyelonephritis (community acquired)	**Clinical diagnosis:** Symptoms same as for cystitis (see above) plus low back or flank pain and fever; urinalysis for pyuria and bacteriuria; urine culture recommended
	Common pathogens: *E coli* and other gram-negative bacteria (eg, *Klebsiella*, *Enterobacter*, *Proteus mirabilis*); most common gram-positive pathogens are *S saprophyticus* and *Enterococcus*
UTI in men (community acquired)	**Clinical diagnosis:** Dysuria, urinary frequency; evaluate for anatomical obstructive anomaly (ie, by postvoiding urinary tract ultrasound) in noncatheterized men
	Common pathogens: 80% *E coli*; in elderly, *Enterococcus*
Bacterial prostatitis	
Acute	**Clinical diagnosis:** Fever, dysuria, urinary frequency, pelvic pain, rectal examination reveals tender prostate, possibly elevated PSA; urinalysis (pyuria and bacteriuria); culture of expressed prostate secretions for pathogen
	Common pathogens: *E coli*; less frequent pathogens include *Klebsiella*, *Enterobacter*, *P mirabilis*, and *Staphylococcus aureus*

Table 53 Elements of Diagnosis of Urinary Tract Infections (*Cont'd.*)

Clinical Syndromes	Diagnostic Considerations
Chronic	**Clinical diagnosis:** Low-grade fever, recurrent bacteriuria, pyuria; possibly elevated PSA; rectal examination reveals nontender prostate; culture of expressed prostate secretions for pathogen
	Common pathogens: *E coli* (80%), *Klebsiella*, *Enterobacter*, *P mirabilis*, *Enterococcus*, and *S aureus*
Catheter-associated UTI	**Clinical diagnosis:** Symptoms of dysuria, frequency, urgency, suprapubic pain, fever, costovertebral tenderness, plus the presence of an indwelling urinary catheter for at least 48 hours; urine culture >10^2 CFU/mL; pyuria
	Common pathogens: *E coli* and *Proteus*, *Enterobacter*, *Pseudomonas*, and *Serratia*; usually no treatment needed unless symptomatic
Candiduria	**Clinical diagnosis:** Urinalysis with yeast (ie, *Candida*); urine culture >10^3 CFU/mL with or without pyuria; urine dipstick not contributory
	Frequently represents colonization, common with urinary catheters and poor collection procedures; depending on presentation, may not require treatment
Ileal conduit or urinary diversion	**Clinical diagnosis:** Nonsterile source for urine collection; urine cultures are often polymicrobial and noninterpretable

Empiric Antimicrobial Selection

Table 54 Empiric Therapy for Acute Uncomplicated Cystitis

Host Considerations	Empiric Antimicrobial Selection
Healthy women	First-line Treatment • TMP-SMX 160/800 mg bid for 3 days[a] • nitrofurantoin monohydrate macrocrystals 100 mg bid for 5 days[b]
	Alternate Treatment (if first-line agents cannot be used) • ciprofloxacin 250 mg bid for 3 days[a] • ciprofloxacin XR 500 mg daily for 3 days[a] • levofloxacin 250 mg daily for 3 days[a] • fosfomycin 3 g once[c] • amoxacillin/clavulanate 500/125 mg bid for 3 days[d] • cefdinir 100 mg bid for 3 days • cefpodoxime proxetil 100 mg bid for 3 days
Men; symptoms for >1 week; recent antimicrobial use; diabetes; age >65 y	Consider 7-day treatment: • TMP-SMX 160/800 mg bid[a] • TMP 100 mg bid[a] • ciprofloxacin 250 mg bid[a] • ciprofloxacin XR 500 mg daily[a] • levofloxacin 250 mg daily[a] • amoxicillin/clavulanate 500/125 mg bid[d]
Pregnancy	3-Day treatment preferred: • amoxicillin/clavulanate 500/125 bid[d] • nitrofurantoin monohydrate macrocrystals 100 mg bid[b] • cefpodoxime 100 mg bid • cefdinir 100 mg bid
	Note: • Avoid use of TMP-SMX (pregnancy category C) in 1st and 3rd trimesters of pregnancy • Avoid use of fluoroquinolones in pregnancy

[a] Empiric use of TMP-SMX or TMP alone is acceptable only if there is <20% TMP-SMX resistance in the community. Some geographic areas are also seeing increasing rates of resistance to fluoroquinolones. Check local susceptibility data. Fluoroquinolones should be reserved for patients not able to take first-line agents or for patients with pyelonephritis.

[b] Avoid nitrofurantoin in patients with Cl_{cr}<60 mL/min.

[c] Listed as alternate due to cost and potential usefulness for more resistant organisms.

[d] Can consider amoxicillin alone for streptococcal or enterococcal organisms on Gram stain; otherwise, use empiric amoxicillin with caution, because many common urinary pathogens are resistant; patients should be followed closely.

Data from Gupta K, et al. Clin Infect Dis. 2011 Mar 1;52(5):e103-120. Used with permission.

Table 55 Empiric Therapy for Acute Pyelonephritis

Host Considerations	Empiric Antimicrobial Selection[a]
Outpatient (uncomplicated)	Treat with 1 of the following: • ciprofloxacin 500 mg bid for 7 days[b] or ciprofloxacin XR 1 g daily for 7 days[b] • levofloxacin 750 mg daily for 5 days[b] • TMP-SMX 160/800 mg bid for 14 days[b] If *Enterococcus* is suspected by Gram stain, options include: • amoxicillin 500 mg tid or 875 mg bid for 14 days • amoxicillin/clavulanate 875 mg/125 mg bid for 14 days
Inpatient (uncomplicated): Initial therapy (pending urine culture results): 14 days total (IV and oral)	Treat with 1 of the following: • ciprofloxacin 400 mg IV q12h[b] • levofloxacin 500 mg IV q24h[b] • ceftriaxone 1 g IV q24h • cefotaxime 1 g IV q8h • cefepime 1 g IV q12h • aztreonam 1 g IV q8h If *Enterococcus* is suspected by Gram stain, options include: • ampicillin 1-2 g IV q6h • ampicillin/sulbactam 1.5-3.0 g IV q6h • vancomycin (if recent penicillin use) 15 mg/kg IV q12h

Inpatient (complicated[c]): Uroseptic or hemodynamically unstable	Empiric coverage against more common organisms, including Enterobacteriaceae, *Enterococcus*, and S *saprophyticus*
	• Community-acquired UTI
	  • ampicillin 1-2 g IV q6h plus either ciprofloxacin 400 mg q8-12h or levofloxacin 500-750 mg q24h
	  • ampicillin/sulbactam 1.5-3.0 g IV q6h
	  • piperacillin/tazobactam 3.375 g IV q6h
	  • For patients with penicillin allergy:
	    • vancomycin 15 mg/kg IV q12h plus one of the following:
	      • ceftriaxone 1-2 g IV q24h
	      • cefotaxime 1-2 g IV q8h
	      • ciprofloxacin 400 mg q8-12h
	      • levofloxacin 500-750 mg q24h

(*Continues*)

Table 55 Empiric Therapy for Acute Pyelonephritis (*Cont'd.*)

Host Considerations	Empiric Antimicrobial Selection[a]
Inpatient (complicated[c]): Uroseptic or hemodynamically unstable (Continued)	<ul><li>Catheter-associated and health care facility–acquired UTI (also includes activity against *Pseudomonas aeruginosa*)<ul><li>ampicillin 1-2 g q6h IV plus either ciprofloxacin 400 mg q8-12h or levofloxacin 500-750 mg q24h</li><li>piperacillin/tazobactam 3.375-4.25 g q6h</li><li>cefepime 1-2 g q12h plus ampicillin 1-2 g q6h</li><li>meropenem 1 g IV q8h</li><li>imipenem 500 mg IV q6h</li><li>doripenem 500 mg IV q8h</li><li>Consider adding vancomycin for possible penicillin- or ampicillin-resistant *Enterococcus*[a]</li></ul></li></ul>

[a] Urine culture is recommended for directing targeted effective therapy; urine Gram stain can assist in the initial selection of an antimicrobial agent.

[b] If local susceptibility is <90% for *E coli*, give an initial dose of ceftriaxone 1 g.

[c] Complicated UTI (nosocomial or concomitant with structural or functional abnormalities or nursing home exposure).

Table 56 Empiric Therapy for Special Conditions

Syndrome	Empiric Antimicrobial Selection[a]
Acute bacterial prostatitis	Treat with 1 of the following:<ul><li>ciprofloxacin 500 mg bid for 4 weeks</li><li>levofloxacin 500 mg daily for 4 weeks</li><li>TMP-SMX DS bid for 4 weeks[b]</li></ul>
Chronic bacterial prostatitis	Treat with 1 of the following:<ul><li>ciprofloxacin 500 mg bid for 6-12 weeks</li><li>levofloxacin 500 mg daily for 6-12 weeks</li><li>TMP-SMX DS bid for 6-12 weeks[b]</li><li>Relapse: Treat for 12 weeks</li><li>Failures: Consider suppression with TMP-SMX SS daily or nitrofurantoin 50 mg daily</li></ul>
Candiduria	Treat with 1 of the following:<ul><li>Removal of Foley catheter resolves infection in 40% of patients</li><li>Treat with fluconazole 200-400 mg daily for 7-14 days only if patient is symptomatic, is neutropenic, or has renal allograft or urologic instrumentation</li><li>For patients with fluconazole-resistant *Candida*:<ul><li>Consider amphotericin with or without 5-flucytosine</li></ul></li></ul>

Table 56 Empiric Therapy for Special Conditions (*Cont'd.*)

Syndrome	Empiric Antimicrobial Selection[a]
Candida pyelonephritis	Treat with 1 of the following: • fluconazole 400 mg (6 mg/kg) daily for 14 days • For patients with fluconazole-resistant *Candida*: • Consider amphotericin with or without 5-flucytosine

[a] Urine or prostate fluid cultures are recommended for directing targeted effective therapy; urine Gram stain can assist in the initial selection of an antimicrobial agent.
[b] Empiric use of TMP-SMX or TMP alone is acceptable only if there is <20% TMP-SMX resistance in the community.

Pathogen-Directed Therapy

Table 57 Pathogen-Directed Therapy of Urinary Tract Infections

Common Pathogens	Preferred Antimicrobial Therapy[a]	
	First-Line Treatment	**Alternate Treatment**
Enterobacteriaceae (E coli; Klebsiella, Proteus, Enterobacter, Citrobacter, Serratia, Salmonella, and Providencia)	Treat with 1 of the following: • a fluoroquinolone[b,c] • a 2nd- or 3rd-gen cephalosporin (except for *Enterobacter, Citrobacter*, and some *Serratia*; may have inducible β-lactamase production) • cefepime • TMP-SMX[c]	Treat with 1 of the following: • aztreonam • β-lactam/β-lactamase inhibitor combinations[d] • a carbapenem[e]
Enterococcus		
penicillin- or ampicillin-susceptible	Treat with 1 of the following: • penicillin • amoxicillin • ampicillin	Treat with 1 of the following: • β-lactam/β-lactamase inhibitor combinations[d] (except ticarcillin/clavulanate) • a carbapenem[e] (except ertapenem)
penicillin- or ampicillin-resistant	vancomycin	Treat with 1 of the following: • daptomycin • nitrofurantoin[f]

(*Continues*)

Table 57 Pathogen-Directed Therapy of Urinary Tract Infections (Cont'd.)

| Common Pathogens | Preferred Antimicrobial Therapy[a] | |
	First-Line Treatment	Alternate Treatment
VRE	Treat with 1 of the following: • daptomycin • nitrofurantoin[f]	linezolid
S saprophyticus	Treat with 1 of the following: • a 1st-, 2nd-, 3rd-, or 4th-gen cephalosporin • TMP-SMX[c] • a fluoroquinolone[b]	Treat with 1 of the following: • β-lactam/β-lactamase inhibitor combinations[d] • a carbapenem[e]
P aeruginosa	Treat with 1 of the following: • ciprofloxacin • levofloxacin • cefepime • ceftazidime • aztreonam	Treat with 1 of the following: • a carbapenem[e] (except ertapenem) • piperacillin/tazobactam
S aureus[g]		
MSSA	Treat with 1 of the following: • cefazolin, cephalexin, or other 1st-gen cephalosporin • TMP-SMX	Treat with 1 of the following: • β-lactam/β-lactamase inhibitor combinations[d] • a carbapenem
MRSA	Treat with 1 of the following: • vancomycin • TMP-SMX	Treat with 1 of the following: • daptomycin • linezolid
Candida albicans	fluconazole	amphotericin with or without 5-flucytosine

[a] Urine or prostate fluid cultures are recommended for directing effective therapy; urine Gram stain can assist in the initial selection of an antimicrobial agent.

[b] Acceptable fluoroquinolones are levofloxacin and ciprofloxacin but **NOT** moxifloxacin, as it does not penetrate the urinary tract well.

[c] Most communities have >20% TMP-SMX resistance; in these circumstances, particularly with upper UTI, a fluoroquinolone is preferable. For lower UTI, a 7-day course of nitrofurantoin may help stem fluoroquinolone resistance and overuse.

[d] β-Lactam/β-Lactamase inhibitors: piperacillin/tazobactam, ticarcillin/clavulanate, ampicillin/sulbactam, or amoxicillin/clavulanate.

[e] Acceptable carbapenems are imipenem, meropenem, doripenem, or ertapenem.

[f] Use nitrofurantoin only for lower UTI.

[g] Remove catheter in cases of catheter-associated infection. In noncatheter-associated cases, evaluate patients for hematogenous S aureus dissemination.

Soft Tissue Infections: Nontoxigenic

(See also section on Soft Tissue Infections: Necrotizing or Toxigenic, pages 206-209.)

Elements of Diagnosis

Clinical Diagnosis

- Diagnosis is largely based on history and physical examination.
- Recurrent cellulitis is common (≥20% of patients).
- Leukocytosis may or may not be found.
- Blood cultures have low yields (about 2-4%).
- Radiologic procedures are not generally needed, except to evaluate patients for osteomyelitis (eg, chronic infections, postsurgical infections, diabetic foot, plantar puncture wounds with prolonged symptoms), deep-tissue abscess, or necrotizing process.
- Epidemiologic findings may influence causative pathogens and thus the choice of antibiotic therapy.
- For cellulitis, elevate involved area, if feasible, to reduce induration.

Table 58 Treatment of Nontoxigenic Soft Tissue Infections

Syndrome and Common Pathogens	First-Line Treatment	Alternate Treatment
CELLULITIS OR ERYSIPELAS		
Uncomplicated cellulitis; no known exposures (eg, to β-hemolytic streptococci or *Staphylococcus aureus*)	cefazolin, nafcillin, oxacillin, dicloxacillin, cephalexin, or cefadroxil	clindamycin, vancomycin, or doxycycline
CA-MRSA likely (eg, spider bite–like lesions, abscesses, exposure to persons with CA-MRSA, or nonresponding or recurrent furuncles or impetigo)	minocycline, doxycycline, TMP-SMX, or (with negative inducible-resistance test) clindamycin Moderate to severe infection: vancomycin Incision and drainage important for purulent lesions	Moderate to severe infection: linezolid, daptomycin, tigecycline, ceftaroline, or telavancin

(Continues)

Table 58 Treatment of Nontoxigenic Soft Tissue Infections (*Cont'd.*)

Syndrome and Common Pathogens	First-Line Treatment	Alternate Treatment
CELLULITIS OR ERYSIPELAS (Continued)		
Erysipelas (β-hemolytic streptococci, usually group A)	penicillin	cefazolin, cephalexin, cefadroxil, nafcillin, oxacillin, dicloxacillin, clindamycin, or vancomycin
Immunocompromised (β-hemolytic streptococci, S aureus, Pseudomonas aeruginosa and other gram-negative bacteria, fungi, viruses)	Empiric therapy depends on clinical presentation; modify on basis of established etiology, cultures, and sensitivities	
IMPETIGO		
S aureus, group A streptococci	cefazolin, nafcillin, oxacillin, dicloxacillin, cephalexin, cefadroxil, minocycline, or topical mupirocin	β-lactam allergic or MRSA: vancomycin, linezolid, clindamycin (with negative inducible-resistance test), daptomycin, or telavancin
WOUND INFECTION		
Bite wounds (often polymicrobial: Pasteurella, Capnocytophaga, anaerobes, viridans group streptococci, Eikenella, Haemophilus)	ampicillin/sulbactam or amoxicillin/clavulanate Wound cleaning is important Tetanus vaccination (if not up to date)	One of the following: piperacillin/tazobactam, ticarcillin/clavulanate, a carbapenem[a], or moxifloxacin; **OR** combination therapy with one of the following: levofloxacin, ciprofloxacin, TMP-SMX, a 3rd- or 4th-gen cephalosporin, or doxycycline **PLUS** one of the following: metronidazole or clindamycin
Surgical site: Clean procedures: Staphylococcus and Streptococcus	Debridement plus antimicrobials based on surgical site and culture results (see Stevens DL et al[c])	

Table 58 Treatment of Nontoxigenic Soft Tissue Infections (*Cont'd.*)

Syndrome and Common Pathogens	First-Line Treatment	Alternate Treatment
WOUND INFECTION (Continued)		
GI procedures: Intestinal flora	Debridement plus antimicrobials based on surgical site and culture results (see Stevens DL et al[c])	
Rapidly progressive infection in first 48 hours after surgery: *Clostridium* and *Streptococcus pyogenes*		
Plantar puncture (*S aureus*, group A streptococci, gram-negative bacteria such as *P aeruginosa*)	Antibiotics should optimally be based on culture results Empiric therapy: cefepime, levofloxacin, or ciprofloxacin Tetanus vaccination (if not up to date)	moxifloxacin (if *Pseudomonas* is not found or suspected)
DIABETIC FOOT OR PRESSURE ULCER		
Diabetic foot (often mixed aerobic and anaerobic infection)	β-lactam/β-lactamase inhibitor[b] plus glucose control	A carbapenem[a] or tigecycline; **OR** a combination of metronidazole plus one of the following: moxifloxacin, levofloxacin, or cefepime
Pressure ulcers (often mixed aerobic and anaerobic infection; may include MRSA or VRE)	β-lactam/β-lactamase inhibitor[b] or a carbapenem	A fluoroquinolone plus metronidazole; **OR** cefepime plus metronidazole; **OR** tigecycline MRSA: vancomycin, linezolid, daptomycin, ceftaroline, or telavancin VRE: linezolid, daptomycin, or tigecycline

[a] The carbapenems include meropenem, imipenem, doripenem, and ertapenem.

[b] The β-lactam/β-lactamase inhibitors include piperacillin/tazobactam, ticarcillin/clavulanate, ampicillin/sulbactam, and amoxicillin/clavulanate.

[c] Stevens DL, et al. Clin Infect Dis. 2005 Nov 15;41(10):1373-406. Epub 2005 Oct 14. Erratum in: Clin Infect Dis. 2006 Apr 15;42(8):1219. Dosage error in article text. Clin Infect Dis. 2005 Dec 15;41(12):1830.

Marine or Water Exposure

β-Hemolytic streptococci and staphylococci are possible pathogens or copathogens of nontoxigenic soft tissue infections related to marine or water exposure. Base treatment on exposure history and culture data.

- **Salt water or brackish water:** *Vibrio vulnificus*
- **Freshwater:** *Aeromonas, Pseudomonas* (also common with hot tubs), *Plesiomonas, Edwardsiella,* and *Erysipelothrix*
- **Fish tank or saltwater fish–related injury:** *Mycobacterium marinum*

Table 59 Treatment of Nontoxigenic Soft Tissue Infections Due to Marine or Water Exposure

Type of Therapy	First-Line Treatment	Alternate Treatment
Empiric therapy	A newer fluoroquinolone (moxifloxacin or gemifloxacin) or a 3rd- or 4th-gen cephalosporin	A carbapenem,[a] β-lactam/β-lactamase inhibitor,[b] or (for *Aeromonas, Plesiomonas,* or *Edwardsiella*) TMP-SMX
	Salt water exposure: Add a tetracycline	
	Fish tank exposure: Consider rifampin plus ethambutol, with or without a fluoroquinolone	Fish tank exposure: doxycycline, minocycline, TMP-SMX, or clarithromycin (with or without rifampin)
	Sewage exposure: Add metronidazole	
Pathogen-directed therapy	See Table 29 on "Specific Treatment of Bacterial Organisms" and section on "Nontuberculosis Mycobacterial Infections" (pages 255-265)	

[a] The carbapenems include meropenem, imipenem, doripenem, and ertapenem.

[b] The β-lactam/β-lactamase inhibitors include piperacillin/tazobactam, ticarcillin/clavulanate, ampicillin/sulbactam, and amoxicillin/clavulanate.

Other Considerations

- **Use of macrolides:** Not as useful today as empiric therapy in penicillin-allergic patients, because resistance to these drugs is found in some strains of β-hemolytic streptococci
- **CA-MRSA:** Should be considered if the patient does not respond to oral β-lactam therapy or if other close contacts have been infected with this organism, or if the patient presents with purulence
- **Referral for management:** Lymphedema, refractory tinea pedis, chronic dermopathies, or venous insufficiency
- **Additional measures:** May be required in cases of frequent recurrence, including possible chronic daily suppressive therapy with antibiotics; elimination or prevention of interdigital tinea is important
- **Osteomyelitis:** Consider evaluation for osteomyelitis in cases of chronic infections, postsurgical infections, pressure ulcers, and plantar puncture wounds that are highly contaminated
- **Plantar puncture wounds:** Clean thoroughly, remove foreign bodies, and administer a tetanus vaccination (if not up to date); surgical drainage or debridement may also be needed

Soft Tissue Infections: Necrotizing or Toxigenic

Necrotizing or Toxigenic Soft Tissue Infections

Elements of Diagnosis

- A high index of suspicion is critical in the diagnosis of necrotizing or toxigenic soft tissue infections.
- Minor or major trauma can predispose patients to necrotizing soft tissue infections, which are more common in obese patients, patients with diabetes mellitus, and immunocompromised patients.[a]
- Necrotizing or toxigenic soft tissue infections should be considered in the differential diagnosis of patients with presumed cellulitis and extreme pain disproportionate to localized skin and soft tissue findings.
- Symptoms include swelling, erythema, and pain. These may progress to tense edema, blisters, necrosis, crepitus, or subcutaneous gas.[a]
- Systemic symptoms include tachycardia, fever, and hypotension progressing to shock.[a] Ultrasonography, computed tomography, and magnetic resonance imaging can be helpful in making a diagnosis, but **immediate surgical consultation** should be obtained when necrotizing fasciitis is suspected.
- Laboratory abnormalities sometimes include increased creatine phosphokinase, creatinine, peripheral white blood cell count, C-reactive protein, erythrocyte sedimentation rate, and decreased albumin.

[a] Anaya DA, Dellinger EP. Clin Infect Dis. 2007 Mar 1;44(5):705-10. Epub 2007 Jan 22.

Table 60 Treatment of Soft Tissue Infections

Syndrome and Common Pathogens	First-Line Treatment	Alternate Treatment
TOXIC SHOCK SYNDROME		
Staphylococcus aureus, β-hemolytic streptococci, viridans group streptococci	**EITHER** nafcillin plus clindamycin **OR** cefazolin plus clindamycin	Combination therapy with one of the following (especially for suspected MRSA): vancomycin, linezolid, daptomycin, telavancin, or tigecycline **PLUS** clindamycin
NECROTIZING FASCIITIS		
EMPIRIC THERAPY		
Mixed flora (various anaerobic and aerobic bacteria), β-hemolytic streptococci (groups A, B, C, F, G), and CA-MRSA	Broad-spectrum empiric coverage until the pathogen is identified should include clindamycin plus one of the following: ampicillin/sulbactam, piperacillin/tazobactam, ticarcillin/clavulanate, or a carbapenem[a] For patients allergic to penicillin: **EITHER** tigecycline plus a fluoroquinolone or clindamycin and plus a fluoroquinolone **OR** cefepime plus metronidazole[b] and plus clindamycin If CA-MRSA is prevalent in local community: add vancomycin	CA-MRSA: linezolid, daptomycin, telavancin, or tigecycline
PATHOGEN-DIRECTED THERAPY		
Type 1		
Mixed aerobic and anaerobic infection; often seen in patients with severe trauma or diabetes mellitus (eg, Fournier gangrene)	**One of the following:** piperacillin/tazobactam, ticarcillin/clavulanate, or a carbapenem[a]	tigecycline

(*Continues*)

Table 60 Treatment of Soft Tissue Infections (Cont'd.)

Syndrome and Common Pathogens	First-Line Treatment	Alternate Treatment
NECROTIZING FASCIITIS (Continued)		
PATHOGEN-DIRECTED THERAPY (Continued)		
	For patients allergic to penicillin: **EITHER** A newer fluoroquinolone plus metronidazole **OR** cefepime[b] plus metronidazole Add clindamycin for its toxin-inhibiting properties	
Type 2 β-Hemolytic streptococci (usually *Streptococcus pyogenes*)	penicillin G plus clindamycin Patients allergic to penicillin: vancomycin plus clindamycin	cefazolin can be used when penicillin allergy does not produce an immediate reaction (eg, anaphylaxis, hives) plus clindamycin
Type 3 Clostridial myonecrosis due to *Clostridium*, especially *C perfringens*	penicillin plus clindamycin	**EITHER** penicillin plus tetracycline **OR** A carbapenem[a]
Type 4 CA-MRSA	vancomycin	**EITHER** linezolid, daptomycin, telavancin, tigecycline **OR** (If negative inducible resistance test) clindamycin

[a] The carbapenems include meropenem, imipenem, doripenem, and ertapenem.

[b] Only for patients without life-threatening (immunoglobulin E–mediated) allergic reaction to penicillin.

Other Considerations

- Necrotizing fasciitis and clostridial myonecrosis often require immediate and serial surgical debridement.
- Complications include multiple organ failure or metastatic foci of infection.
- Intraoperative findings of necrotizing fasciitis include gray necrotic tissue, lack of bleeding, thrombosed vessels, dishwater pus, and lack of resistance to blunt finger dissection.[a]
- Initial histopathologic findings of surgically resected tissues may be of prognostic importance. A poor neutrophilic response with numerous organisms seen on routine stains suggests a poor prognosis.
- Despite aggressive treatment, as many as 15-30% (or more) of patients affected by necrotizing fasciitis and clostridial myonecrosis may die.
- Hyperbaric oxygen as a treatment has not been fully defined and is not routinely recommended.
- Case cohort studies and case reports have suggested some benefit to treatment with intravenous immunoglobulin in specific circumstances (eg, streptococcal toxic shock). However, due to the lack of randomized controlled trials, intravenous immunoglobulin should probably be reserved for select patients.
- Viridans group streptococci can cause toxic shock syndrome in severely immunocompromised patients (eg, bone marrow transplant patients with prolonged neutropenia).
- Surgical exploration of the incision is needed when toxic shock syndrome occurs.

[a] Anaya DA, Dellinger EP. Clin Infect Dis. 2007 Mar 1;44(5):705-10. Epub 2007 Jan 22.

Surgical Prophylaxis

Common Pathogens Targeted By Prophylaxis Regimens

Surgical prophylaxis should be directed toward the microorganism likely to cause infection after the operation.

Table 61 Antimicrobial Prophylaxis for Surgery

Nature of Operation	Common Pathogens	Recommended Antimicrobials	Adult Dosage Before Surgery[a]
Cardiac	*Staphylococcus aureus*, *S epidermidis*	cefazolin **OR** vancomycin[b]	1-2 g IV[c,d] 15 mg/kg IV
Gastrointestinal			
Esophageal, gastroduodenal	Enteric gram-negative bacilli, gram-positive cocci	**High risk[e] only:** cefazolin[f]	1-2 g IV[d]
Biliary tract	Enteric gram-negative bacilli, enterococci, clostridia	**High risk[g] only:** cefazolin[f]	1-2 g IV[d]
Colorectal	Enteric gram-negative bacilli, anaerobes, enterococci	**Oral options:** neomycin plus erythromycin base	1 g×3 doses[h] 1 g×3 doses[h]
		OR neomycin plus metronidazole	2 g×2 doses[h] 2 g×2 doses[h]
		Parenteral options: cefoxitin[f] or cefotetan[f]	1-2 g IV
		OR cefazolin plus metronidazole	1-2 g IV[d] 0.5 g IV
		OR ampicillin/sulbactam[f]	3 g IV

Table 61 Antimicrobial Prophylaxis for Surgery (*Cont'd.*)

Nature of Operation	Common Pathogens	Recommended Antimicrobials	Adult Dosage Before Surgery[a]
Appendectomy, nonperforated[i]	Same as for colorectal	cefoxitin[f] or cefotetan[f]	1-2 g IV
		OR	
		cefazolin plus metronidazole	1-2 g IV[d] 0.5 g IV
		OR	
		ampicillin/ sulbactam[f]	3 g IV
Genitourinary			
Cystoscopy alone	Enteric gram-negative bacilli, enterococci	**High risk[j] only:** ciprofloxacin **OR** TMP-SMX	500 mg oral or 400 mg IV 1 DS tablet
Cystoscopy with manipulation or upper tract instrumentation[k]	Enteric gram-negative bacilli, enterococci	ciprofloxacin **OR** TMP-SMX	500 mg oral or 400 mg IV 1 DS tablet
Open or laparoscopic surgery[l]	Enteric gram-negative bacilli, enterococci	cefazolin[f]	1-2 g IV[d]
Gynecologic and obstetric			
Vaginal, abdominal, or laparoscopic hysterectomy	Enteric gram-negative bacilli, anaerobes, group B streptococci, enterococci	cefoxitin,[f] cefotetan,[f] or cefazolin[f] **OR** ampicillin/ sulbactam[f]	1-2 g IV 1-2 g IV[d] 3 g IV
Cesarean section	Same as for hysterectomy	cefazolin[f]	1-2 g IV
Abortion	Same as for hysterectomy	doxycycline	300 mg oral[m]

(*Continues*)

Table 61 Antimicrobial Prophylaxis for Surgery (*Cont'd.*)

Nature of Operation	Common Pathogens	Recommended Antimicrobials	Adult Dosage Before Surgery[a]
Head and neck surgery			
Incisions through oral or pharyngeal mucosa	Anaerobes, enteric gram-negative bacilli, *S aureus*	clindamycin **OR** cefazolin plus metronidazole	600-900 mg IV 1-2 g IV[d] 0.5 g IV
Neurosurgery	*S aureus*, *S epidermidis*	cefazolin **OR** vancomycin[b]	1-2 g IV[d] 15 mg/kg IV
Orthopedic	*S aureus*, *S epidermidis*	cefazolin[n] or cefuroxime[n] **OR** vancomycin[b,n]	1-2 g IV[d] 1.5 g IV 15 mg/kg IV
Thoracic (noncardiac)	*S epidermidis*, streptococci, enteric gram-negative bacilli	cefazolin or cefuroxime **OR** vancomycin[b]	1-2 g IV[d] 1.5 g IV 15 mg/kg IV
Vascular			
Arterial surgery involving a prosthesis, the abdominal aorta, or a groin incision	*S aureus*, *S epidermidis*, enteric gram-negative bacilli	cefazolin **OR** vancomycin[b]	1-2 g IV[d] 15 mg/kg IV
Lower extremity amputation for ischemia	*S aureus*, *S epidermidis*, enteric gram-negative bacilli, clostridia	cefazolin **OR** vancomycin[b]	1-2 g IV[d] 15 mg/kg IV

[a] Parenteral prophylactic antimicrobials can be given as a single IV dose begun ≤60 minutes before the operation. For patients undergoing prolonged operations (>4 hours) or who have major blood loss, additional intraoperative doses should be given at intervals 1-2 times the half-life of the drug for the duration of the procedure in patients with normal renal function. If vancomycin or a fluoroquinolone is used, the infusion should be started 60-120 minutes before the initial incision to minimize the possibility of an infusion reaction close to the time of anesthesia induction and to have adequate tissue levels at the time of incision. (Bratzler DW, et al. Clin Infect Dis. 2004 Jun 15;38[12]:1706-15. Epub 2004 May 26.)

[b] Vancomycin can be used in hospitals in which MRSA and *S epidermidis* are frequent causes of postoperative wound infection, in patients previously colonized with MRSA, or in patients who are allergic to penicillin or cephalosporin. For operations in which enteric gram-negative bacilli are common pathogens, use another drug such as an aminoglycoside (eg, gentamicin, tobramycin, or amikacin).

Table 61 Antimicrobial Prophylaxis for Surgery (*Cont'd.*)

^c Some consultants recommend an additional dose when patients are removed from bypass during open-heart surgery.

^d Consider 3 g for patients weighing >120 kg, with a 2-g intraoperative repeat dose as needed.

^e Morbid obesity, esophageal obstruction, decreased gastric acidity, or decreased gastrointestinal motility.

^f For patients allergic to penicillin and cephalosporin, a reasonable alternative is clindamycin with one of the following: gentamicin, ciprofloxacin, levofloxacin, or aztreonam.

^g Age >70 years, acute cholecystitis, nonfunctioning gallbladder, obstructive jaundice, or common duct stones.

^h On the day before an 8 AM operation, administer neomycin 1 g plus erythromycin 1 g at 1 PM, 2 PM, and 11 PM, or administer neomycin 2 g plus metronidazole 2 g at 7 PM and 11 PM.

ⁱ For a ruptured viscus, therapy is often continued for about 5 days.

^j Urine culture positive or unavailable, preoperative catheter, transrectal prostatic biopsy, or placement of prosthetic material.

^k Shockwave lithotripsy or ureteroscopy.

^l Including percutaneous renal surgery, procedures with entry into the urinary tract, and those involving implantation of a prosthesis. If manipulation of bowel is involved, give prophylaxis according to colorectal guidelines.

^m Divided into 100 mg 1 hour before the abortion and 200 mg one-half hour after it.

ⁿ If a tourniquet is to be used in the procedure, the entire dose of antibiotic must be infused prior to its inflation.

Adapted from Antimicrobial prophylaxis for surgery. Treat Guidel Med Lett. 2009 Jun;7(82):47-52. Used with permission.

Other Considerations

- Infusion just before incision is critical to success but continuation beyond a 24-hour maximum (48-hour maximum for cardiac surgery) is not necessary; resistance and complications may result from prolonged use of prophylaxis
- Surgical prophylaxis guidelines and quality indicators specify starting antibiotics within 1 hour of incision; prophylactic agents that require a longer infusion time (eg, vancomycin and fluoroquinolones) should be started within 1-2 hours of surgery, and infusions should optimally be completed before incision
- Most patients with mild penicillin allergy can receive cephalosporin prophylaxis, depending on allergy history or skin test results
- Cardiac, orthopedic, craniotomy, and vascular surgeries in institutions with a high rate of MRSA infection may require vancomycin as the primary agent (although increased efficacy is unproven)
- Recommendations to improve adherence to guidelines and core measures include:
  - Stocking only the appropriate doses in the operating room

- Assigning responsibility for administration of medications to nurses in the preoperative holding area or in the anesthesia area (rather than administering medications before patients transfer to the operating room)
- Using preprinted order sets
- Involving staff in infection control, infectious diseases, and pharmacy as resources
- Using visible reminders such as checklists and stickers

See also Bratzler et al.[a]

[a] Bratzler DW, et al. Clin Infect Dis. 2004 Jun 15;38(12):1706-15. Epub 2004 May 26.

Osteomyelitis

Elements of Diagnosis

- **Clinical:** Localized pain and tenderness of involved bone; systemic signs and symptoms of acute hematogenous osteomyelitis
- **Radiology:** Bone destruction or sequestrum in chronic cases; use of nuclear scanning, magnetic resonance imaging, or computed tomography may aid diagnosis and staging
- **Laboratory:** White blood cell count is often normal; erythrocyte sedimentation rate and C-reactive protein are usually elevated

Table 62 Treatment of Osteomyelitis in Adults With Normal Organ Function

Clinical Feature	First-Line Treatment	Alternate Treatment
EMPIRIC THERAPY		
Acute pain, swelling with fever, leukocytosis	cefazolin 1-2 g IV q8h[a,b]	vancomycin 15 mg/kg IV q12h[b]
Wound drainage, painful surgical site, prior surgery	vancomycin 15 mg/kg IV q12h[b]	daptomycin 6 mg/kg IV q24h[b]; **OR**
		linezolid 600 mg IV or oral q12h[b]
Chronic pain, ulceration, or swelling without systemic symptoms (eg, foot ulceration in patients with diabetes mellitus)	Establish diagnosis; define microbiology before determining treatment options	
PATHOGEN-DIRECTED THERAPY		
Staphylococcus		
oxacillin-sensitive	nafcillin or oxacillin 1.5-2.0 g IV q4-6h for 4-6 weeks; **OR**	vancomycin 15 mg/kg IV q12h for 4-6 weeks
	cefazolin 1-2 g IV q8h for 4-6 weeks	
oxacillin-resistant	vancomycin 15 mg/kg IV q12h for 4-6 weeks	linezolid 600 mg oral or IV q12h for 4-6 weeks; **OR**
		daptomycin 6 mg/kg IV q24h for 4-6 weeks

(Continues)

Table 62 Treatment of Osteomyelitis in Adults With Normal Organ Function (*Cont'd.*)

Clinical Feature	First-Line Treatment	Alternate Treatment
PATHOGEN-DIRECTED THERAPY (Continued)		
β-Hemolytic *Streptococcus* or penicillin-sensitive *S pneumoniae*	penicillin G 20×10⁶ units IV per day either continuously or in 6 equally divided doses for 4-6 weeks; **OR** ceftriaxone 2 g IV or IM q24h for 4-6 weeks; **OR** cefazolin 1-2 g IV q8h for 4-6 weeks	vancomycin 15 mg/kg IV q12h for 4-6 weeks
Enterobacteriaceae	ceftriaxone[c] 2 g IV q24h for 4-6 weeks; **OR** ciprofloxacin 500-750 mg oral q12h for 4-6 weeks	imipenem 500 mg IV q6h for 4-6 weeks; **OR** meropenem 1 g IV q8h (or 500 mg IV q6h) for 4-6 weeks; **OR** ertapenem 1 g IV q24h for 4-6 weeks; **OR** aztreonam 1 g IV q8h for 4-6 weeks
Pseudomonas, Enterobacter	meropenem 1 g IV q8h or 500 mg IV q6h for 4-6 weeks; **OR** imipenem 500 IV q6h for 4-6 weeks; **OR** cefepime 2 g IV q8-12h for 4-6 weeks	ciprofloxacin 750 mg oral q12h for 4-6 weeks; **OR** ceftazidime[c] 2 g IV q8h for 4-6 weeks; **OR** aztreonam 1-2 g IV q8h for 4-6 weeks
Polymicrobial infection (eg, diabetic foot)	Treatment depends on type and severity; refer to published guidelines in Lipsky et al[d]	

[a] Consider using vancomycin in clinical situations with a high risk of methicillin-resistant *S aureus* or if patient is hemodynamically unstable.

[b] Consider addition of gram-negative coverage in ill-appearing, hemodynamically unstable, or immunocompromised patients.

[c] Avoid use for organisms that produce extended-spectrum β-lactamases or for organisms that may have inducible β-lactamases (eg, *Enterobacter*).

[d] Lipsky BA, et al. Clin Infect Dis. 2004 Oct 1;39(7):885-910. Epub 2004 Sep 10.

Other Considerations

Surgery

Chronic osteomyelitis typically requires surgical debridement. To medically manage acute and chronic osteomyelitis when triaging, consult with a surgeon who manages bone and joint infections.

Therapy for Specific Scenarios

- **Hardware retained:** Consider chronic suppression until fusion
- **Vertebral osteomyelitis:** Medical management alone may be sufficient
- **Sternal osteomyelitis (eg, poststernotomy):** Surgical debridement is often required

Management of Complications

- **No clinical or laboratory improvement:** Reassess diagnosis and adequacy of surgical debridement
- **Recurrence of infectious syndrome:** Consider the possibility that the patient has received suboptimal medical treatment; reassess adequacy of surgical debridement; and consider removal of any hardware

Acute Native Joint Infections

Elements of Diagnosis

- **Clinical:** Acute monoarticular swelling, typically of a large joint, with fever and pain
- **Radiology:** Normal osseus structures (early) with soft-tissue swelling
- **Laboratory:** Elevated leukocytes, erythrocyte sedimentation rate, and C-reactive protein
- **Arthrocentesis:** >50,000-100,000 leukocytes (predominantly neutrophils), absence of crystals, Gram stain often negative

Table 63 Treatment of Acute Joint Infections

Clinical Feature or Pathogen	First-Line Treatment	Alternate Treatment
EMPIRIC THERAPY[a]		
Acute joint swelling with fever, leukocytosis, and joint pain; no prior surgery	vancomycin 15 mg/kg IV q12h[b]	daptomycin 6 mg/kg IV q24h
Wound drainage, painful joint, prior surgery	vancomycin 15 mg/kg IV q12h[b]	daptomycin 6 mg/kg IV q24h[c] or linezolid 600 mg IV or oral q12h[c]
Polyarticular synovitis with rash in young, sexually active patient (suspect disseminated *Neisseria gonorrhoeae*)	ceftriaxone 2 g IV q24h	ciprofloxacin (note increasing quinolone resistance to *N gonorrhoeae*) 500 mg oral q12h[c] or 400 mg IV q12h[c]; or cefotaxime 1-2 g IV q8h
Chronic monoarticular swelling without systemic symptoms	Establish diagnosis before determining treatment	
Gram stain positive	Treat as for *Staphylococcus* if gram-positive cocci	
	Treat as for *Pseudomonas* if gram-negative bacilli	
PATHOGEN-DIRECTED THERAPY[a]		
Staphylococcus aureus		
oxacillin-sensitive	**EITHER**	
	nafcillin or oxacillin 1.5-2.0 g IV q4-6h for 3-4 wk	vancomycin 15 mg/kg IV q12h for 3-4 wk
	OR	
	cefazolin 1-2 g IV q8h for 3-4 wk	

Table 63 Treatment of Acute Joint Infections (*Cont'd.*)

Clinical Feature or Pathogen	First-Line Treatment	Alternate Treatment
PATHOGEN-DIRECTED THERAPY[a] (Continued)		
oxacillin-resistant	vancomycin 15 mg/kg IV q12h for 3-4 wk	**EITHER** linezolid 600 mg oral or IV q12h for 3-4 wk **OR** daptomycin 6 mg/kg IV q24h for 3-4 wk
β-Hemolytic streptococci or penicillin-sensitive pneumococci	Any 1 of the following: penicillin G 20,000 units per day IV either continuously or in 6 equally divided doses for 2-3 wk **OR** ceftriaxone 2 g IV q24h for 2-3 wk **OR** cefazolin 1-2 g IV q8h for 2-3 wk	vancomycin 15 mg/kg IV q12h for 2-3 wk
Enterobacteriaceae	**EITHER** ceftriaxone[d] 2 g IV q24h for 3-4 wk **OR** ciprofloxacin 500-750 mg oral q12h for 3-4 wk	**EITHER** ertapenem 1 g IV q24h for 3-4 wk **OR** aztreonam 1-2 g IV q8h for 3-4 wk
Pseudomonas	**EITHER** cefepime 2 g IV q12h for 3-4 wk **OR** meropenem 1 g IV q8h for 3-4 wk	**EITHER** ciprofloxacin 750 mg oral q12h for 3-4 wk **OR** ceftazidime[d] 2 g IV q8h for 3-4 wk

[a] Adult doses for normal organ function and antimicrobial selection should be based on drug susceptibility testing.

[b] Consider the addition of gram-negative coverage in ill-appearing, hemodynamically unstable, or immunocompromised patients.

[c] Resistance in *N gonorrhoeae* is increasing in several regions and among men who have sex with other men; susceptibility testing is suggested.

[d] Avoid use for organisms that produce extended-spectrum β-lactamases or for organisms that may have inducible β-lactamases (eg, *Enterobacter, Citrobacter, Serratia*).

Table 64 Management of Complications

Complicating Factors	Management
No clinical or laboratory improvement	Reassess diagnosis, consider noninfectious etiology, rule out concomitant crystal arthritis, consider atypical organisms
Periarticular osteomyelitis	Consider surgical debridement
Recurrence of infectious syndrome	Consider suboptimal medical treatment, reassess adequacy of surgical debridement, rule out periarticular osteomyelitis
Long-term postseptic degenerative arthritis	Consider total joint arthroplasty

Table 65 Therapy for Specific Scenarios

Scenario	Management
Presence of prosthetic joint	Typically caused by oxacillin-resistant staphylococci; consider vancomycin therapy
Septic arthritis after an animal bite	Consider 1 of the following: piperacillin/tazobactam 3.375 IV q6h, ampicillin/sulbactam 3 g IV q6h, or a carbapenem[a]
Immunocompromised host or standard bacterial cultures that are negative	Consider evaluating for fungal or mycobacterial organisms and treating for them as necessary

[a] The carbapenems include meropenem, imipenem, ertapenem, or doripenem.

Gastrointestinal Infections

Orofacial Infections, Esophagitis, and Gastritis

Elements of Diagnosis

Orofacial Infections

- **Ludwig angina:** Acute soft tissue infection usually of dental origin; spreads rapidly and is bilateral; involves submandibular and sublingual spaces and can spread to the neck; may include respiratory obstruction from edema
- **Acute necrotizing ulcerative gingivitis (eg, Vincent angina, trench mouth):** Mixed bacterial infection with gingival ulcerations and gingival breakdown, usually due to poor dental hygiene
- **Lemierre syndrome:** Suppurative jugulovenous thrombophlebitis, pharyngitis, and bacteremia, with potential for abscess formation and extension to mediastinum or septic pulmonary emboli; caused most commonly by *Fusobacterium necrophorum*
- **Peritonsillar abscess (quinsy):** Usually due to group A streptococci, often with anaerobic bacteria; often results in enlarged displaced tonsils, severe pharyngeal pain, dysphagia

Esophagitis

- **More common in immunocompromised patients:** Human immunodeficiency virus (HIV) infection, hematologic malignancy, postchemotherapy, organ transplantation
- **Most common pathogens:** *Candida* (especially *C albicans*), herpes simplex virus (HSV), cytomegalovirus (CMV)
- **Less common pathogens:** *Histoplasma capsulatum, Blastomyces dermatitidis, Mycobacterium tuberculosis* and other *Mycobacterium, Actinomyces*
- **Noninfectious causes:** Gastroesophageal reflux disease, radiotherapy, antineoplastic chemotherapy, aphthous ulcers (in 5% of AIDS patients and also in some patients with acute HIV infection)
- **Symptoms:** Odynophagia, dysphagia, and substernal chest pain; oral thrush common with HIV-associated candidal esophagitis; pain common with HSV and CMV esophagitis

Helicobacter pylori *Gastric and Peptic Ulcer Disease*

- *H pylori* colonization and infection are more common with increasing age and in developing countries
- *H pylori* gastric colonization is associated with a 3- to 4-fold increase in the risk for development of either gastric or duodenal ulceration; more than 90% of duodenal ulcerations are associated with *H pylori* infection (in the absence of drug-associated causes)
- *H pylori*–associated chronic gastritis is considered a risk factor for development of gastric carcinoma and gastric mucosa-associated lymphoid tissue (MALT)

- Diagnosis of *H pylori* infection can be made by endoscopy and biopsy or by noninvasive techniques such as serologic analysis, breath test, or fecal antigen analysis

Table 66 Treatment of Gastrointestinal Infections: I. Oropharyngeal Infections, Esophagitis, and Gastritis

Syndrome or Common Pathogen	First-Line Treatment	Alternate Treatment
TREATMENT OF OROPHARYNGEAL INFECTIONS		
Ludwig angina Viridans group streptococci or other streptococci, *Fusobacterium*, *Bacteroides*, *Actinomyces*	ampicillin/sulbactam, amoxicillin/clavulanate, piperacillin/tazobactam, or a carbapenem	**EITHER** penicillin G plus metronidazole **OR** clindamycin
Acute ulcerative or necrotizing gingivitis *Bacteroides*, *Fusobacterium*, spirochetes, viridans group streptococci or other streptococci	See above	See above
Lemierre syndrome *F necrophorum*, *Bacteroides*	See above	See above
Peritonsillar abscess Group A streptococci, anaerobes	See above	See above
TREATMENT OF ESOPHAGITIS*		
***Candida*[a]**	fluconazole	itraconazole, an echinocandin,[b] voriconazole, amphotericin B product, or amphotericin B lipid complex
HSV[a]	acyclovir, valacyclovir, famciclovir	foscarnet (for acyclovir-resistant strains)
CMV	IV ganciclovir, valganciclovir	foscarnet
Aphthous ulcers	prednisone	thalidomide

Table 66 Treatment of Gastrointestinal Infections: I. Oropharyngeal Infections, Esophagitis, and Gastritis (Cont'd.)

Syndrome or Common Pathogen	First-Line Treatment	Alternate Treatment
TREATMENT OF GASTRITIS		
H pylori	A PPI plus amoxicillin and clarithromycin	**One of the following combinations:**
	For patients with penicillin allergy: A PPI plus metronidazole and clarithromycin	bismuth, metronidazole, tetracycline, and a PPI; **OR**
	For patients with macrolide allergy: A PPI plus amoxicillin and metronidazole	A PPI plus levofloxacin and amoxicillin; **OR**
		A PPI plus rifabutin and amoxicillin

[a] Suppressive therapy may be needed after treatment in AIDS patients and in markedly immunosuppressed patients.

[b] The echinocandins include caspofungin, micafungin, and anidulafungin.

* Mandell, Douglas, and Bennett's principles and practice of infectious diseases. Vol 1. 7th ed. Elsevier Churchill Livingstone; c2010. pp. 1335-7.

Diarrhea

Elements of Diagnosis

Noninflammatory Diarrhea
- **Site:** Predominantly in the small intestine
- **Stool volume:** Large, watery diarrhea
- **Fecal leukocytes:** No
- **Common organisms**
  - **Bacteria:** *Vibrio cholerae*, enterotoxigenic *Escherichia coli* (ETEC), *Bacillus cereus*, *Staphylococcus aureus*, *Clostridium perfringens* (type A enterotoxin)
  - **Viruses:** *Rotavirus*, *Calicivirus*, Norwalk-like viruses, adenovirus, *Astrovirus*
  - **Parasites:** *Giardia lamblia*, *Cryptosporidium*

Inflammatory Diarrhea
- **Site:** Predominantly in the colon
- **Stool volume:** Small
- **Fecal leukocytes:** Yes
- **Common organisms**
  - **Bacteria:** *Shigella*, *Salmonella*, *Campylobacter jejuni*, *Vibrio parahaemolyticus*, enteroinvasive *E coli* (EIEC), *E coli* O157:H7 (enterohemorrhagic), *Clostridium difficile* (cytotoxin), *M tuberculosis*
  - **Viruses:** CMV
  - **Parasites:** *Entamoeba histolytica*, *Schistosoma japonicum*, *S mansoni*

Invasive Enteric Infections With Secondary Dissemination
- **Sites:** Ileum, colon
- **Stool volume:** Small
- **Fecal leukocytes:** Yes
- **Common organisms**
  - **Bacteria:** *S typhi, Yersinia enterocolitica, Vibrio vulnificus, Listeria monocytogenes, Brucella, Tropheryma whippelii* (small-bowel predominance with *T whippelii*)
  - **Parasites:** *E histolytica, Strongyloides stercoralis, Trichinella spiralis*

Evaluation of Food-Borne Diarrhea[*]
- **Vomiting:** Primary symptom, possibly with diarrhea
  - **Viral gastroenteritis:** *Rotavirus, Norovirus,* and other caliciviruses
  - **Preformed bacterial toxins (short incubation period of <6 hours):** *S aureus* toxin, *Bacillus* toxin
- **Noninflammatory diarrhea:** Acute watery diarrhea without fever or dysentery; sometimes accompanied by fever
  - **Viral gastroenteritis:** *Astrovirus, Norovirus,* other caliciviruses, enteric adenovirus, *Rotavirus*
  - **Bacteria:** ETEC and *V cholerae*
  - **Parasites:** *G lamblia, Cryptosporidium, Cyclospora cayetanensis*
- **Inflammatory diarrhea:** Invasive disease; possibly fever and (on gross examination) bloody stools
  - **Bacteria:** *Campylobacter, Shigella, Salmonella,* EIEC, *V parahaemolyticus, E coli* O157:H7, *Y enterocolitica*
  - **Parasites:** *E histolytica*
- **Seafood ingestion:** *Vibrio, Anisakis,* and other genera
- **Persistent (≥14 days) diarrhea:** Especially common in travelers to mountainous regions or areas with untreated water
  - **Parasites:** *C cayetanensis, E histolytica, Cryptosporidium, G lamblia*
- **Neurologic manifestations:** Paresthesia, respiratory depression, bronchospasm, cranial nerve palsy
  - **Bacteria:** *Clostridium botulinum* toxin, *Campylobacter*-associated Guillain-Barré syndrome
  - **Other:** Organophosphate pesticides, thallium poisoning, fish poisoning
- **Systemic illness:** Fever, weakness, arthritis, jaundice
  - **Bacteria:** *L monocytogenes, S typhi* and *S paratyphi, Brucella, V vulnificus*
  - **Viral:** HAV and HEV
  - **Parasites:** *T spiralis, Toxoplasma gondii, E histolytica* with extraluminal abscess

Traveler's Diarrhea
- **Bacterial causes:** *E coli* (most commonly ETEC), *Shigella, C jejuni, Salmonella, Aeromonas, Plesiomonas shigelloides,* noncholera *Vibrio*
- **Nonbacterial causes:** *Rotavirus* (Mexico), *Norovirus* (Mexico), *Giardia* (North America, Russia), *Cryptosporidium, Cyclospora,* and (rarely) *Entamoeba*

---

[*] American Medical Association. MMWR Recomm Rep. 2004 Apr 16;53(RR-4):1-33.

- **High-risk areas:** Developing countries of Latin America, Asia, Africa, and the Middle East
- **Intermediate-risk areas:** Southern Europe and some Caribbean islands
- **Low-risk areas:** United States, Canada, northern Europe, Australia, New Zealand

Noninfectious Considerations

- **Secretory diarrhea:** Carcinoid syndrome, Zollinger-Ellison syndrome, medullary carcinoma of the thyroid, villous adenoma of the rectum, vasoactive intestinal peptide-secreting pancreatic adenoma
- **Inflammatory diarrhea:** Inflammatory bowel disease, ischemic colitis, radiation enteritis, eosinophilic gastroenteritis

Management and Empiric Therapy of Diarrhea

Community-Acquired Diarrhea

- Rehydration for initial management
- Stool culture (with fever, bloody stools, or abdominal pain) for *Salmonella*, *Shigella*, *Campylobacter*, and *E coli* O157:H7; consider testing for community-acquired *C difficile*
- Empiric therapy (pending cultures) with a fluoroquinolone or (for suspected fluoroquinolone-resistant *Campylobacter*) a macrolide
- Avoid antimicrobial therapy if *E coli* O157:H7 is suspected (eg, bloody diarrhea with hemolytic uremic syndrome)

Traveler's Diarrhea

- Rehydration is goal of initial management
- No fever or blood in stool
  - Mild diarrhea of 1-2 loose stools per day: No treatment or treatment with only bismuth or loperamide
  - Moderate to severe diarrhea of >2 loose stools per day: Hydration plus bismuth or loperamide; add a fluoroquinolone for high-stool output (to shorten duration of diarrhea); rifaximin is also an option
- Fever, blood in stool, abdominal pain: A fluoroquinolone for 3 days; stool culture if possible

Persistent (>7 Days) Diarrhea

- Stool examination for *Giardia*, *Cryptosporidium*, *Cyclospora*, *Isospora*, and other parasites
- Consider noninfectious causes for culture-negative prolonged inflammatory diarrhea (eg, inflammatory bowel disease)

Clostridium Difficile Infection–Associated Diarrhea

Table 67 Treatment Guidelines for *Clostridium difficile* Infection

Disease Classification	Treatment Regimen[a]
Initial episode	
Mild to moderate: Leukocytes <15×10⁹/L or unchanged creatinine	metronidazole 500 mg oral tid for 10-14 days
Severe uncomplicated: Leukocytes ≥15×10⁹/L or creatinine increased by 50%	vancomycin 125 mg oral qid for 10-14 days
Severe complicated, no ileus: Plus hypotension, shock, megacolon, or perforation; severe colitis on CT scan	vancomycin 500 mg oral qid plus metronidazole 500-750 mg IV q8h Consider colectomy for severe disease as appropriate
Severe complicated, with ileus: Plus hypotension, shock, megacolon, or perforation; severe colitis on CT scan	vancomycin 500 mg oral or by NGT qid plus metronidazole 500-750 mg IV q8h and vancomycin (intracolonic) rectal enema 500 mg in 100 mL saline qid Retention enema: An 18-inch Foley catheter with a 30-mL balloon is inserted into the rectum; the balloon is inflated and vancomycin is instilled; the catheter is clamped for 60 minutes, then deflated and removed Consider colectomy for severe disease as appropriate
First recurrence	Re-treat with initial regimen that was effective; if severe, use the appropriate treatment regimen outlined above
Second recurrence	Treat infection then vancomycin taper or pulse regimen[b]: For mild to moderate or severe uncomplicated, treat with vancomycin 125 mg oral qid for 10-14 days, followed by a vancomycin taper with 125 mg bid for 7 days vancomycin 125 mg oral qid for 10-14 days, then 125 mg bid for 7 days, then 125 mg daily for 7 days, then 125 mg every 2-3 days for 2-8 weeks For severe-complicated, treat as for initial episode or first recurrence, followed by a vancomycin taper as above

Table 67 Treatment Guidelines for *Clostridium difficile* Infection[a] (*Cont'd.*)

Disease Classification	Treatment Regimen
Multiple relapses	Longer tapering of vancomycin dosage: vancomycin 500 mg qid for 10-14 days followed by rifaximin 400 mg tid for 14 days
	IV immunoglobulin 400 mg/kg once
	Fecal replacement therapy
	Other options

[a] Fidaxomicin is a new FDA-approved drug that may result in fewer recurrences for non-NAP1 strains. Due to its high cost, its role is not yet clearly defined.

[b] Tedesco FJ, et al. Am J Gastroenterol. 1985 Nov;80(11):867-8.

Adapted from Ask Mayo Expert. *Clostridium difficile* infection [Mayo Clinic Intranet]. Mayo Foundation; c2010. [cited 2011 Jul 29] [2 screens]. Used with permission of Mayo Foundation for Medical Education and Research.

Suggested Reading

Cohen SH, et al. Infect Control Hosp Epidemiol. 2010 May;31(5):431-55.
Gerding DN, et al. Clin Infect Dis. 2008 Jan 15;46(Suppl 1):S32-42.

Intra-Abdominal Infections

Peritonitis and Polymicrobial Intra-Abdominal Infections

Elements of Diagnosis

Primary Peritonitis (Spontaneous Bacterial Peritonitis)

- Peritoneal infection without an obvious source
- Adult patients with cirrhosis and ascites (higher risk: gastrointestinal [GI] bleeding, previous spontaneous bacterial peritonitis [SBP], or low protein concentration in ascitic fluid) or, occasionally, congestive heart failure, malignancy, or connective tissue disease
- Pediatric patients with postnecrotic cirrhosis, nephrotic syndrome, or urinary tract infections
- Ascitic fluid with >250/mm^3 polymorphonuclear neutrophils; fever; diffuse abdominal pain; clinical presentation may be more insidious with progressive ascites

Secondary Peritonitis

- Peritoneal infection, commonly by communication with GI or genitourinary (GU) tract (eg, due to perforation, trauma, pelvic inflammatory disease [PID]); suppurative or obstructive biliary tract infection; abdominal abscess
- Fever, marked abdominal pain, tenderness to palpation (focal or diffuse, often with rebound tenderness and muscle rigidity), peripheral and peritoneal fluid leukocytosis
- Prompt abdominal and pelvic computed tomography (CT) scan (optimal for identification of source and definition of treatment); possible surgical options

Peritonitis in Patients With Peritoneal Dialysis[a]

- Peritoneal infection usually is caused by contamination of the catheter by common skin organisms; other causes include catheter exit-site infections, subcutaneous-tunnel infections, transient bacteremia, contamination of the dialysate delivery system, and transmural migration through an intact intestinal wall or vaginal leak
- Fever, abdominal pain, tenderness to palpation (focal or diffuse), nausea or vomiting, diarrhea, cloudy effluent with leukocyte count >100 cells/mm^3, peripheral leukocytosis, effluent Gram stain (9-50%), positive culture (90-95%)

Peritoneal, Retroperitoneal, or Pelvic Abscess

- Numerous potential sources such as primary or secondary peritonitis (especially due to enteric perforation), appendicitis, diverticulitis, inflammatory bowel disease, PID, postabdominal or pelvic surgery (eg, repair of enteric or biliary anastomotic leak; splenectomy)

[a] Li PK, et al. Perit Dial Int. 2010 Jul-Aug;30(4):393-423.

- Commonly due to polymicrobial infections (especially from enteric or GU source); monomicrobial infections (eg, hematogenous seeding of devitalized tissue; retroperitoneal extension of vertebral osteomyelitis)
- Clinical presentation typically is based on location and source of infection
- Abdominal CT (ideal) or ultrasound can define location and potential source, and can aid percutaneous drainage

Appendicitis

- Most common in older children and young adults in their teens and 20s
- Early symptoms are nonspecific and may include periumbilical or epigastric pain. Later, when the parietal peritoneum becomes inflamed, more focused right lower quadrant pain develops.
- Any stage of infection may be accompanied by mild fever, anorexia, and nausea or vomiting. Guarding or rebound tenderness may occur on examination.
- Pain in the right flank, right back, or right upper quadrant may occur when the inflamed appendix is retrocecal or when appendicitis occurs during pregnancy (2nd and 3rd trimesters)
- Diagnosis is by clinical examination, observation, diagnostic laparoscopy (8-25% negative appendectomy rate), or imaging with CT of the abdomen, with ultrasonography (in young women, children, or pregnant women), or with magnetic resonance imaging
- Treatment of acute appendicitis is surgical appendectomy
- More prolonged, broadened antimicrobial therapy is indicated in acute appendicitis with perforation, abscess formation, and chronic and recurrent appendicitis; surgery or drainage may be needed

Diverticulitis

- Increased dietary fiber and exercise inversely correlate with incidence of diverticulosis; diverticulitis indicates inflammation from microscopic or macroscopic perforation of a diverticulum into pericolic fat
- Left lower quadrant pain is common, whereas right-sided diverticulitis occurs in only 1-2% (more common in Asians); bleeding may occur
- CT of the abdomen is the diagnostic procedure of choice. Findings consistent with diverticulitis include pericolic fat stranding (98%), diverticula (84%), bowel wall thickening (70%), and phlegmon or abscess formation. Ultrasound can exclude gynecologic abnormalities in women of childbearing age. Colonoscopy can rule out cancer, inflammatory bowel disease, irritable bowel disease, or other conditions that mimic diverticulitis.
- Uncomplicated diverticulitis can usually be managed with antibiotics alone, although as many as one-third of patients will have another episode. Lack of response with antimicrobial therapy within 48-72 hours should prompt additional investigations.
- Complicated diverticulitis includes perforation, uncontrolled sepsis, lack of response to antibacterial therapy, obstruction, abscess, or fistula (to bladder or vagina); typical management is with both surgery and antimicrobial therapy
- Surgery is generally advised after a first attack of complicated diverticulitis or after 2 or more episodes of uncomplicated diverticulitis

Table 68 Treatment of Peritonitis and Polymicrobial Intra-Abdominal Infections

Syndrome and Common Pathogens	First-Line Treatment	Alternate Treatment
Primary peritonitis		
Escherichia coli, Klebsiella, Streptococcus pneumoniae, other streptococci, and *Enterococcus*	ceftriaxone, cefotaxime, cefepime, or levofloxacin[a] for 10-14 days (shorter duration is often successful); SBP recurrence is common	A carbapenem, piperacillin/tazobactam, ticarcillin/clavulanate, moxifloxacin (use moxifloxacin with caution in patients with ESLD)
Secondary peritonitis		
Enteric flora, commonly polymicrobial (eg, Enterobacteriaceae,[b] other aerobic gram-negative bacilli, *Bacteroides,* other anaerobic bacteria; occasionally aerobic gram-positive bacteria and *Candida*	piperacillin/tazobactam; ticarcillin/clavulanate; a carbapenem; a fluoroquinolone plus metronidazole; a 2nd-, 3rd-, or 4th-gen cephalosporin plus metronidazole; or ampicillin/sulbactam plus a fluoroquinolone[a]; tigecycline	
	Surgical debridement or drainage may be required	
	Duration of treatment is variable and based on source and surgical intervention, if any	
	For immunocompromised or unstable patients, or for patients with recent antibacterial therapy, consider adding fluconazole (for *Candida*) until microbiology is defined	
Peritoneal dialysis peritonitis		
Gram-positive bacteria (60-80%): *Staphylococcus epidermidis, S aureus, Streptococcus,* diphtheroids	Intraperitoneal antibiotic therapy is superior to IV therapy and is dosed either intermittently (once daily per exchange) or continuously (all exchanges) (see Table 69 "Antibiotic Dosage for Peritonitis During Peritoneal Dialysis in Anuric Patients" treatment duration is 10-21 days; clinical improvement can be expected within 48-96 hours	See Table 69 "Antibiotic Dosage for Peritonitis During Peritoneal Dialysis in Anuric Patients"
Gram-negative bacteria (15-30%): *E coli, Klebsiella, Enterobacter, Proteus, Pseudomonas*		

Table 68 Treatment of Peritonitis and Polymicrobial Intra-Abdominal Infections (Cont'd.)

Syndrome and Common Pathogens	First-Line Treatment	Alternate Treatment
Less common pathogens: *Candida, Acinetobacter*, anaerobes, atypical mycobacteria (*M chelonae* or *M fortuitum*), *M tuberculosis, Aspergillus fumigatus, Nocardia asteroides, Fusarium*	Indications for catheter removal: Relapsing or refractory peritonitis, intraperitoneal abscess, refractory exit-site or tunnel infection; fungal peritonitis Consider catheter removal if patient is not responding to therapy for multiple enteric organisms or if patient has mycobacterial peritonitis	
Abdominal abscess		
Depends on location and suspected source (usually polymicrobial if source is the intestinal tract)	Percutaneous catheter drainage or surgical debridement to evacuate devitalized or avascular infected material, define microbiology, and determine duration of antimicrobial therapy Initial therapy same as for secondary peritonitis Targeted antimicrobial therapy based on culture data and suspected source	
Appendicitis		
Acute, uncomplicated (with luminal obstruction)	Immediate surgery and perioperative antimicrobial prophylaxis: cefazolin plus metronidazole; cefoxitin; or cefotetan	Other standard surgical wound prophylaxis regimens
Appendicitis		
With perforation or abscess formation (same as for secondary peritonitis above)	Same as for secondary peritonitis above	
Diverticulitis	Consider surgery for repeated episodes, perforation, or fistula; otherwise, treat same as for secondary peritonitis above	

[a] Resistance to quinolones is increasing; they should not be used empirically unless hospital survey indicates >90% susceptibility for *E coli*. (Solomkin JS, et al. Clin Infect Dis. 2010 Jan 15;50[2]:133-164. Erratum in: Clin Infect Dis. 2010 Jun 15;50[12]:1695.)

[b] Enterobacteriaceae group includes *E coli, Klebsiella, Enterobacter, Citrobacter, Serratia, Yersinia, Salmonella*, and *Shigella*.

Table 69 Antibiotic Dosage for Peritonitis During Peritoneal Dialysis in Anuric Patients[a]

Medication	Dose by Type of Peritoneal Dialysis	
	Intermittent (per Exchange, Once Daily)	Continuous (All Exchanges)
Aminoglycosides		
gentamicin	0.6 mg/kg	LD: 8 mg/L
		MD: 4 mg/L
tobramycin	0.6 mg/kg	LD: 8 mg/L
		MD: 4 mg/L
Cephalosporins		
cefazolin	15 mg/kg	LD: 500 mg/L
		MD: 125 mg/L
cefepime	1 g	LD: 500 mg/L
		MD: 125 mg/L
ceftazidime	1.0-1.5 g	LD: 500 mg/L
		MD: 125 mg/L
cefotaxime	1 g	LD: 500 mg/L
		MD: 125 mg/L
Penicillins		
ampicillin	ND	MD: 125 mg/L
oxacillin	ND	MD: 125 mg/L
penicillin G	ND	LD: 50,000 mg/L
		MD: 25,000 mg/L
piperacillin	ND	LD: 500 mg/L
		MD: 250 mg/L
Antifungals		
amphotericin B deoxycholate	NA	1.5 mg/L
fluconazole	200 mg/L IP q24-48h	
Others		
ciprofloxacin	ND	LD: 50 mg/L
		MD: 25 mg/L
vancomycin	15-30 mg/kg every 5-7 days	LD: 1,000 mg/L
		MD: 25 mg/L

Table 69 Antibiotic Dosage for Peritonitis During Peritoneal Dialysis in Anuric Patients[a] (Cont'd.)

Medication	Dose by Type of Peritoneal Dialysis	
	Intermittent (per Exchange, Once Daily)	Continuous (All Exchanges)
aztreonam	ND	LD: 1,000 mg/L
		MD: 250 mg/L
TMP-SMX	ND	LD: 320/1,600 mg/L oral
		MD: 80/400 mg/L oral daily
ampicillin/sulbactam	2 g q12h	LD: 1,000 mg/L
		MD: 100 mg/L
imipenem	1 g q12h	LD: 250 mg/L
		MD: 50 mg/L

[a] Anuric is defined as <100 mL/day urine output; for patients with >100 mL/day urine output, increase dose by 25%.

Adapted from Li PK, et al. Perit Dial Int. 2010 Jul-Aug;30(4):393-423. Used with permission.

Hepatobiliary Infections

Elements of Diagnosis

Cholecystitis and Cholangitis

- **Cholecystitis:** Inflammation of the gallbladder: 20-50% complicated by infection. Gallstone disease is the most common cause of cholecystitis in the United States. Complications include gangrenous cholecystitis, emphysematous cholecystitis, gallbladder empyema, pyogenic liver abscess, and bacteremia. Murphy sign (ie, inhibition of inspiration by pain during palpation over gallbladder) is often present and may be produced by ultrasound transducer probing the gallbladder.
- **Cholangitis:** Inflammation or infection of the common bile duct, commonly associated with obstruction or strictures of the biliary tract. Symptoms include fever and continuous right upper quadrant abdominal pain.
  - **Acute or ascending cholangitis:** Charcot triad (right upper quadrant or epigastric abdominal pain, fever or chills, and jaundice [50-70%]); with hypotension and confusion (Reynold pentad) (<14%)
- Abdominal ultrasound frequently establishes diagnosis. Abnormal findings include thickened (>4 mm) gallbladder wall, pericholecystic fluid, and intramural gas or ductal dilatation suggestive of cholecystitis. Common bile duct dilatation or visible obstruction may suggest

cholangitis. A HIDA (hepatobiliary iminodiacetic acid) scan can be helpful if ultrasound is nondiagnostic: Failure of the gallbladder to accumulate the marker is highly suggestive of acute cholecystitis caused by obstruction of the cystic duct. Abdominal CT may also identify gallstones within the cystic duct, gallbladder distention and mural thickening, and enhancement of the liver adjacent to the gallbladder ("rim sign") or ductal obstruction.

Viral Hepatitis

- **Hepatitis A virus (HAV):** Fecal-oral spread (by contaminated food or water); usually self-limiting; acute viral hepatitis in 40-60% of infections (more common in adults); fulminant disease in 8% of patients; no chronic infection. Prevention: HAV vaccine. Postexposure prophylaxis: HAV immunoglobulins are recommended for patients <12 months or >40 years of age and for those with immunosuppressive conditions, chronic liver disease, or HAV vaccine allergy; and HAV vaccine is recommended for immunocompetent patients 12 months to 40 years old.
- **Hepatitis B virus (HBV):** Transmission is typically by intravenous (IV) route or contaminated needlestick, through birth from an infected mother, or by sexual contact; acute hepatitis develops in 30-40% of infections; chronic disease in 10-25%; increased risk of cirrhosis and hepatocellular carcinoma occurs with chronic HBV disease. Prevention: HBV vaccine series. Postexposure prophylaxis: HBV immunoglobulins and HBV vaccine series, depending on HBV infection status of source and recipient's HBV vaccination status (see section on "Occupational Postexposure Prophylaxis and Management," page 317).
- **Hepatitis C virus (HCV):** Transmission is typically by IV or contaminated needlestick; sexual transmission less common but possible; chronic HCV disease in 85%, with cirrhosis developing in 20% of those patients within 20 years; hepatocellular carcinoma risk is increased with HCV-mediated cirrhosis. No HCV vaccine or immunoglobulins currently available.
- **Hepatitis D virus (HDV):** HDV consists of a defective RNA virus that uses hepatitis B surface antigen as its structural shell (requires HBV coinfection or superinfection in patients with chronic HBV infection). More aggressive liver disease occurs when HDV superinfects patients with chronic HBV infection, with development of chronic hepatitis in ≥75% and cirrhosis in 70-80%.
- **Hepatitis E virus:** HEV is not a chronic disease. It occurs by fecal-oral transmission (usually by contaminated water). Pregnant women have 15-25% mortality, especially in 3rd trimester.

Hepatosplenic Candidiasis

- Manifestation of chronic disseminated candidiasis; more common in patients with hematologic malignancies after prolonged chemotherapy-associated neutropenia
- Common presentation includes persistent fever despite antibacterial agents, especially with recovering neutrophils; occasional right upper quadrant abdominal pain, anorexia, and nausea or vomiting

- Diagnosis is by abdominal CT or magnetic resonance imaging (most sensitive), which shows characteristic multiple small nodular hypolucent lesions throughout the liver and spleen during neutrophil recovery; lesions are commonly absent with neutropenia

Hepatic Abscess (Chronic Disseminated Candidiasis)

- Sources include intestinal infections with portal circulation (40-50%; eg, pylephlebitis from diverticulitis, pancreatitis, omphalitis, irritable bowel disease, postoperative infection), biliary duct system infections (cholangitis caused by intraductal stones, tumor, occluded stent), bacteremia (5-10% [infective endocarditis, line sepsis]), contiguous infections (5-10%), trauma (0-5%), or idiopathic (20-40%).
- Bacterial or pyogenic hepatic abscesses generally occur with acute fever and right upper quadrant abdominal pain. Amebic abscesses are similar to pyogenic abscesses, resulting in fever, dull right upper quadrant pain, and GI symptoms (15-35%: nausea or vomiting, abdominal cramping, or diarrhea).
- Diagnosis is by abdominal CT or ultrasound (preferred with suspected biliary disease) for diagnostic aspiration (Gram stain, aerobic or anaerobic culture) and to define treatment options. Blood cultures are 50% positive.
- Amebic abscesses: *E histolytica* serology; aspirate not usually required (unless no response to treatment or to exclude secondary bacterial infection, or risk of rupture).

Splenic Abscess

- Sources include hematogenous seeding (eg, infective endocarditis and other endovascular infections, often in the presence of emboli or hemoglobinopathy), trauma, or contiguous extension from adjacent infected tissue.
- Clinical presentation can be quite variable; fever, abdominal pain, and splenomegaly may all be present. Persistent fever or bacteremia is suspicious for infective endocarditis.
- Abdominal CT or ultrasound for diagnosis and to define treatment options

Table 70 Treatment of Hepatobiliary Infections

Common Pathogens	First-Line Treatment	Alternate Treatment
Cholecystitis and cholangitis		
Enterobacteriaceae[a] and other aerobic gram-negative bacilli; enterococci and other gram-positive bacteria; occasionally *Bacteroides* and other anaerobes	Piperacillin/tazobactam; ticarcillin/clavulanate; a carbapenem; a fluoroquinolone[b] plus metronidazole; a 2nd-, 3rd-, or 4th-gen cephalosporin plus metronidazole; or ampicillin/sulbactam plus a fluoroquinolone	Monotherapy with a 2nd-, 3rd-, or 4th-gen cephalosporin; a fluoroquinolone[b]; or tigecycline
Less common (biliary tract): *Clonorchis sinensis, Opisthorchis felineus, O viverrini, Fasciola hepatica*	Acute cholecystitis: Gangrene or perforation suspected: Immediate cholecystectomy with intraoperative cholangiogram	
	Unstable patients: Delay definitive surgery (cholecystotomy preferred)	
	Acute cholangitis: Drainage of biliary tract endoscopically (ERCP has 90% success), surgically, or transcutaneously	
	Treatment of parasites affecting biliary tree	
Viral hepatitis		
HAV	Supportive care	
HBV	Pegylated IFN, entecavir, lamivudine, emtricitabine, adefovir, tenofovir, telbivudine	IFN
HCV	Pegylated IFN plus ribavirin and plus either boceprevir or telaprevir	IFN plus ribavirin or pegylated IFN monotherapy

Table 70 Treatment of Hepatobiliary Infections (*Cont'd.*)

Common Pathogens	First-Line Treatment	Alternate Treatment
Hepatosplenic candidiasis	Stable disease: oral fluconazole	
Candida albicans most common	Acutely ill: amphotericin B lipid complex induction, followed by oral fluconazole; or an echinocandin followed by oral fluconazole	amphotericin B deoxycholate effective but more toxic than amphotericin B lipid complex
Hepatic abscess (often polymicrobial)		
Common: *E coli*, *Klebsiella*, *Streptococcus anginosus* group, *Enterococcus*, other viridans streptococci, *Bacteroides*	Pyogenic liver abscesses require drainage: Surgical or percutaneous; antimicrobial therapy covering suspected pathogens while awaiting microbiology results (see section above on "Cholecystitis and Cholangitis")	
Uncommon: Other Enterobacteriaceae, *Pseudomonas*, *S aureus*, β-hemolytic streptococci, other anaerobes	Pyogenic liver abscesses require drainage: Surgical or percutaneous; antimicrobial therapy covering suspected pathogens while awaiting microbiology results (see section above on "Cholecystitis and Cholangitis")	
Entamoeba histolytica	Amebic liver abscess (*E histolytica*): Typically does not require drainage; metronidazole or tinidazole and an agent (eg, paromomycin) to eliminate enteric carrier state	
Splenic abscess		
S aureus, *S anginosus* group, other streptococci, *E coli*, *Salmonella*, anaerobes	Empiric antibiotic selection depends on suspected source and should cover common pathogens; consider splenectomy for complex multifocal, *Candida*, or multiloculated bacterial abscess and percutaneous drainage for localized abscess, although antifungal therapy may be sufficient for *Candida* abscesses	
Other: Fungi (*Candida*, *Aspergillus*) in immunocompromised patients; *Mycobacterium tuberculosis*		

[a] Enterobacteriaceae group includes *E coli*, *Klebsiella*, *Enterobacter*, *Citrobacter*, *Serratia*, *Yersinia*, *Salmonella*, and *Shigella*.

[b] Resistance to quinolones is increasing; they should not be used empirically unless hospital survey indicates >90% susceptibility for *E coli*. (Solomkin JS, et al. Clin Infect Dis. 2010 Jan 15;50[2]:133-64. Erratum in: Clin Infect Dis. 2010 Jun 15;50[12]:1695.)

Management of the Febrile Neutropenic Patient

Elements of Diagnosis

- **Fever:** Single oral temperature of ≥38.3°C (101°F) or a temperature of ≥38.0°C (100.4°F) for ≥1 hour
- **Neutropenia:** A neutrophil count of <500 cells/mm³ or one that is expected to fall below 500/mm³ over the next 48 hours

Common Pathogens

- Bacteria
  - Enterobacteriaceae (eg, *Escherichia coli*, *Klebsiella*, *Enterobacter*)
  - Nonfermenting gram-negative bacilli (eg, *Pseudomonas aeruginosa*, *Acinetobacter*, *Stenotrophomonas maltophilia*)
  - Gram-positive cocci (eg, *Staphylococcus aureus*, coagulase-negative staphylococci[a], streptococci, enterococci)
  - Gram-positive bacilli (eg, *Bacillus*, *Corynebacterium*)[a]
- Fungi
  - *Aspergillus*
  - Agents causing mucormycosis (eg, *Rhizopus*, *Mucor*)
  - Less common organisms (eg, *Fusarium*, *Scedosporium*)

Diagnostic Evaluation

- Review exposure history, recent anti-infective therapy, and medications
- Conduct physical examination with particular attention to the pharynx, skin, intravenous (IV) access sites, lungs, sinuses, mouth, esophagus, and perianal area
- Run laboratory tests, including complete blood cell count, liver function tests, and creatinine
- Obtain blood and urine cultures
- Order other cultures on the basis of clinical circumstances
- Obtain a chest radiograph
- Conduct site-specific imaging studies, as indicated
- Consider *Aspergillus* galactomannan and/or (1,3)-β-D-glucan testing in high-risk patients

Risk Assessment

High-Risk Patients

- Anticipate prolonged (>7 days) and profound neutropenia (ANC ≤100 cells/mm³ following cytotoxic chemotherapy (commonly encountered with hematologic malignancy treatment regimens)
- Significant comorbid conditions include hypotension, new pulmonary infiltrate or hypoxemia, new-onset abdominal pain or neurologic changes, intravascular catheter infection, or symptomatic mucositis

---

[a] Recovery of these organisms in blood culture usually suggests an IV catheter infection.

- Evidence of hepatic insufficiency (aminotransferases >5× normal values) or renal insufficiency (Cl$_{Cr}$ <30 mL/min)

Low-Risk Patients
- Neutropenia is expected to resolve in ≤7 days (common with solid tumor chemotherapy regimens)
- Absence of any high-risk comorbidities
- Normal hepatic and renal function

Initial Empiric Therapy

High-Risk Patients
- **Initial therapy:** Direct at aerobic and facultative gram-negative bacilli
  - Monotherapy is recommended with an antipseudomonal β-lactam agent (eg, cefepime, a carbapenem,[b] piperacillin/tazobactam); ceftazidime is less reliable for monotherapy[c]
  - Modification of the initial empiric regimen (eg, addition of an aminoglycoside or a fluoroquinolone) should be considered for severely ill patients or those likely to be infected with antibiotic-resistant organisms
  - Prior fluoroquinolone prophylaxis precludes the use of fluoroquinolones for initial empiric therapy
- **Add vancomycin,[d] if there is:**
  - Clinically suspected catheter-associated infection
  - Known colonization with MRSA or with penicillin- or cephalosporin-resistant pneumococci
  - Blood culture positive for gram-positive organisms
  - Hypotension or other signs of severe sepsis
  - Soft tissue infection
  - Health care–associated pneumonia documented radiographically
  - Recent or current fluoroquinolone prophylaxis
- **Include coverage for anaerobic bacteria (eg, metronidazole, meropenem, imipenem, piperacillin/tazobactam) if there is:**
  - Evidence of perianal infection
  - Presence of necrotizing gingivitis
  - Recovery of anaerobic bacteria in culture
  - Potential intra-abdominal infection (eg, neutropenic colitis)

Low-Risk Patients
- Consider cautious outpatient management with oral or IV antibiotics after a period of observation of ≥4 hours

---

[b] Appropriate carbapenems include meropenem, doripenem, or imipenem/cilastatin; ertapenem does not have reliable activity against *Pseudomonas* or other nonfermenting gram-negative bacilli.
[c] Prolonged use of ceftazidime may induce or select for β-lactamase production, leading to antibiotic resistance in certain gram-negative organisms such as *Enterobacter*, *E coli*, or *Klebsiella*. In addition, ceftazidime provides suboptimal activity against gram-positive organisms when compared with cefepime or the carbapenems.
[d] In patients known to be colonized with vancomycin-resistant enterococci, linezolid or daptomycin should be used in place of vancomycin, pending culture and sensitivity data.

- Recommended oral regimen is ciprofloxacin plus amoxicillin/clavulanate every 8 hours[e]
- IV antibiotic regimens are the same as those used for high-risk patients

Pathogen-Directed Therapy

- Base antibiotic selection on in vitro susceptibility data
- Consider combination therapy (eg, a β-lactam plus an aminoglycoside) for severe infection due to *P aeruginosa* or other resistant gram-negative organisms pending susceptibilities
- Use linezolid or daptomycin in place of vancomycin for patients colonized with vancomycin-resistant organisms until susceptibility data become available
- Discontinue vancomycin after 48-72 hours if cultures are negative for gram-positive organisms

Persistent Fever Despite Empiric Antibiotic Therapy

- If patient is stable, continue with same antibacterial program
- If a new infection is identified, adjust antibiotic therapy accordingly
- If patient is unstable or clinically worsening, broaden antibacterial regimen to cover possible resistant gram-negative, gram-positive, anaerobic, or fungal infection
- Identification of a documented infection and susceptibilities should guide changes to the initial empiric antibiotic regimen
- Consider addition of an antifungal agent (eg, voriconazole, an amphotericin B product,[f] an echinocandin) in high-risk patients who remain febrile for 4 days after initiation of empiric antibacterial therapy (for patients who have been receiving antifungal prophylaxis with an azole, use either an amphotericin B product[g] or caspofungin)
- Repeat diagnostic clinical examination (including computed tomography scan of the chest and/or abdomen to assess for a possible occult fungal infection or an intra-abdominal process such as neutropenic enterocolitis)

Duration of Antibiotic Therapy

- **Stop empiric anti-infective therapy when neutrophil count is ≥500 cells/mm^3 and rising daily if there is/are:**
  - No evidence of focal infection
  - Negative findings on cultures

---

[e] Use with caution in patients who have recently received quinolone treatment or prophylaxis.
[f] Amphotericin B products include liposomal amphotericin B, amphotericin B lipid complex, and amphotericin B deoxycholate.
[g] An amphotericin product is preferable for patients who have been receiving voriconazole prophylaxis or if the clinical situation suggests possible mucormycosis.

- For documented infections, the duration of therapy is dictated by the particular organism and the site of the infection (generally 10-14 days); appropriate antibiotics should continue at least until ANC >500 cells/mm³
- Stable patients with unexplained but resolved fever who remain afebrile for 4-5 days may have empiric antibiotics switched to a fluoroquinolone prophylaxis for the duration of the neutropenia

Other Considerations

- In patients with a history of a type 1 allergic reaction to penicillin, consider use of aztreonam or ciprofloxacin[e] for coverage of gram-negative organisms in combination with vancomycin or clindamycin
- For patients with a history of vancomycin allergy, consider use of linezolid or daptomycin
- Guide choice of empiric anti-infectives by local or institutional antibiotic resistance profiles
- Remove catheters from patients with intravascular catheter infections due to S aureus, gram-negative bacilli, fungi, or mycobacteria; catheter removal is also recommended for tunnel infection, septic thrombosis or emboli, hemodynamic instability, or bacteremia persisting for >48 hours
- Consider granulocyte transfusions only in unusual circumstances (eg, disseminated *Fusarium* infection)
- Fluoroquinolone prophylaxis should be considered for high-risk patients with expected durations of prolonged and profound neutropenia
- Primary antifungal prophylaxis
  - Should be given against *Candida* to allogeneic HSTC patients and those undergoing myeloablative chemotherapy
  - Can be considered against *Aspergillus* for selected patients >13 years of age who are undergoing intensive chemotherapy for AML/MDS in whom the risk of invasive aspergillosis is substantial
- Secondary antifungal prophylaxis with a mold-active agent is recommended in patients with prior invasive aspergillosis, anticipated prolonged neutropenic periods of at least 2 weeks, or a prolonged period of neutropenia immediately prior to HSCT

Suggested Reading

Freifeld AG, et al. Clin Infect Dis. 2011;52(4):e56-e93.

Sexually Transmitted Diseases[a]

Elements of Diagnosis

Urethritis

- Abrupt-onset, purulent urethral discharge and dysuria are more common with *Neisseria gonorrhoeae* than with *Chlamydia trachomatis* and other nongonococcal urethritis (NGU) pathogens
- Mucopurulent or purulent urethral discharge and dysuria, which can occur with any pathogen, often impede clinical distinction
- Gram stain of urethral discharge shows >5 leukocytes per high-power field (HPF)
- Positive leukocyte esterase test on first-void urine
- Presence of gram-negative diplococci on stain or culture does not exclude coinfection with other pathogens
- Coinfection with *N gonorrhoeae* and *C trachomatis* or *Ureaplasma urealyticum* occurs in 15-20% of heterosexual men with urethritis
- Nucleic acid amplification tests for *N gonorrhoeae* and *C trachomatis* can be performed on urine specimens, obviating the need for urethral swab specimens

Cervicitis

- Mucopurulent or purulent endocervical discharge
- Gram stain of cervical discharge shows >10 leukocytes per HPF
- Most common in adolescent females
- Patients commonly present without symptoms
- Coinfection common with *N gonorrhoeae* and *C trachomatis* or *U urealyticum*
- Abdominal pain and adnexal tenderness may signify pelvic inflammatory disease

Vaginitis

- Clinical clues include vaginal discharge, vulvar pruritus, dyspareunia
- Microscopic examination with coverslip can reveal motile trichomonads and clue cells
- KOH (potassium hydroxide) preparation enables identification of *Candida* as yeast or pseudohyphae
- Positive (strong fishy odor) whiff test with KOH is characteristic of trichomoniasis and bacterial vaginosis (BV)
- Vaginal fluid pH is >4.5 with either trichomoniasis or BV

Genital Ulcerative Diseases

- **Syphilis:** Average incubation period of 21 days; painless ulcer (chancre); nontender, nonfluctuant adenopathy in primary syphilis

[a] Workowski KA, Berman S; Centers for Disease Control and Prevention (CDC). MMWR Recomm Rep. 2010 Dec 17;59(RR-12):1-110. Erratum in: MMWR Recomm Rep. 2011 Jan 14;60(1):18. Dosage error in article text.

- **Chancroid:** Incubation period of 2-7 days; painful ulcers; fluctuant adenopathy
- **Genital herpes:** Incubation period of 2-7 days; multiple vesicles; painful ulcers; can recur
- **Lymphogranuloma venereum:** Variable incubation period; characteristic groove sign (lymphadenopathy above and below inguinal ligament); fluctuant buboes that can rupture
- **Donovanosis (granuloma inguinale):** Variable incubation period; painless ulcers; scar formation

Common Pathogens and Clinical Characteristics

Urethritis: Urethral Discharge and Dysuria (Common)

- ***N gonorrhoeae* urethritis:** discharge purulent
- **NGU:** Symptoms less abrupt; more mucoid discharge; more common than gonorrhea in the US and other developed countries
  - ***C trachomatis:*** Most common NGU pathogen (15-40% of cases)
  - ***Mycoplasma genitalium:*** 15-25% NGU cases in US
  - **Less common (1-5%)**
    - Herpes simplex virus
    - *U urealyticum*
    - *Trichomonas vaginalis*

Cervicitis: Possible Cervical Discharge or Asymptomatic

- Same pathogens as urethritis
- Human papillomavirus (HPV)

Vaginitis: Vaginal Discharge, Vaginal Irritation

- **BV:** 30-45% of cases; replacement of normal vaginal hydrogen peroxide–producing lactobacilli with anaerobic bacteria (eg, *Bacteroides, Mobiluncus, Peptostreptococcus, Gardnerella vaginalis,* and *Mycoplasma hominis*)
  - **Vaginal discharge:** Moderate amount; gray or white; homogeneous and adherent; pH >4.5
  - **Addition of KOH (whiff test):** Positive
  - **Microscopy examination (KOH wet mount):** Clue cells present; few leukocytes
- ***Candida:*** 20-25% of cases; controversial vaginal sexually transmitted disease (STD) pathogen
  - **Vaginal discharge:** Scant or moderate; white, clumped, adherent; pH 4.0-4.5
  - **Whiff test:** Negative (no fishy odor)
  - **Microscopy examination (KOH wet mount):** Pseudohyphae often present; few leukocytes
- ***T vaginalis:*** 15-20% of cases
  - **Vaginal discharge:** Profuse; green-yellow; homogeneous; frothy; pH 5.0-6.0
  - **Whiff test:** Positive (fishy odor present)
  - **Microscopy examination (KOH wet mount):** Motile trichomonads; many leukocytes

Genital Ulcerative Disease: Cutaneous Ulcerations, Commonly With Adenopathy

- *Treponema pallidum:* Syphilis
  - **Lesions:** Usually painless and solitary; occasionally multiple; sharply demarcated border; indurated with red or smooth base
  - **Lymphadenopathy:** Unilateral or bilateral; nontender; firm
- *Haemophilus ducreyi:* Chancroid
  - **Lesions:** Multiple, painful, nonindurated or mildly indurated; erythematous border with rough yellow-gray base
  - **Lymphadenopathy:** Usually unilateral; tender; may suppurate
- Herpes simplex virus
  - **Lesions:** Multiple painful lesions; may coalesce; nonindurated, smooth, erythematous lesions
  - **Lymphadenopathy:** Usually bilateral; firm and tender
- **L1, L2, L3 serovars of *C trachomatis:*** Lymphogranuloma venereum
  - **Lesions:** Usually single; variable pain; nonindurated
  - **Lymphadenopathy:** Unilateral or bilateral; firm, tender; frequently suppurative; groove sign is common
- *Calymmatobacterium granulomatis:* Donovanosis; granuloma inguinale
  - **Lesions:** Solitary or multiple rolled or elevated rough lesions; usually nontender
  - **Lymphadenopathy:** Pseudoadenopathy; inguinal swelling

Table 71 Pathogen-Directed Therapy

Clinical Situation	First-Line Treatment	Alternate Treatment
Urethritis and cervicitis[a]		
N gonorrhoeae[b]	**EITHER**	**One of the following:**
	ceftriaxone 250 mg IM once	ceftizoxime 500 mg IM once; **OR**
	OR	cefotaxime 500 mg IM once; **OR**
	cefixime[c] 400 mg oral once	
	Note: fluoroquinolones are no longer recommended for treatment of gonococcal infections in US because of widespread resistance	cefoxitin 2 mg IM once with probenecid 1g oral; **OR**
		cefpodoxime[c] 400 mg oral once; **OR**
		cefuroxime axetil[c] 1 g oral once; **OR**

Table 71 Pathogen-Directed Therapy (*Cont'd.*)

Clinical Situation	First-Line Treatment	Alternate Treatment
		spectinomycin[c] 2 g IM once; **OR**
		azithromycin 2 g oral once[d]
C trachomatis and other NGU pathogens	**EITHER** azithromycin 1 g oral once **OR** doxycycline 100 mg oral bid for 7 days	One of the following: erythromycin base 500 mg oral qid for 7 days; **OR** erythromycin ethylsuccinate 800 mg oral qid for 7 days; **OR** ofloxacin 300 mg oral bid for 7 days; **OR** levofloxacin 500 mg oral q24h for 7 days
Recurrent or persistent urethritis or cervicitis (ensure that both *N gonorrhoeae* and NGU pathogens were treated appropriately)		
M genitalium[e] and *U urealyticum*	azithromycin or erythromycin regimen (dosing as above for *C trachomatis* and other NGU pathogens)	
T vaginalis	metronidazole 2 g oral once **OR** tinidazole 2 g oral once	
Vaginitis		
BV	One of the following: metronidazole 500 mg oral bid for 7 days; **OR** metronidazole gel 0.75% 5 g intravaginal daily for 5 days; **OR** clindamycin cream 2% 5 g intravaginal for 7 days	One of the following: tinidazole 2 g oral daily for 3 days; **OR** tinidazole 1 g oral daily for 5 days; **OR** clindamycin 300 mg oral bid for 7 days; **OR** clindamycin ovules 100 mg intravaginal daily for 3 days; **OR** boric acid (intravaginal) 600 mg once daily for 2 wk

(Continues)

Table 71 Pathogen-Directed Therapy (*Cont'd.*)

Clinical Situation	First-Line Treatment	Alternate Treatment
Candida	Intravaginal agents: butoconazole, clotrimazole, miconazole, nystatin, tioconazole, terconazole Oral systemic agents: fluconazole 150 mg once; itraconazole 200 mg once	
T vaginalis	**One of the following:** metronidazole 2 g oral once; **OR** tinidazole 2 g oral once	metronidazole 500 mg oral bid for 7 days
Genital ulcerative disease		
Primary syphilis	benzathine penicillin G 2.4 million units IM once	**One of the following:** doxycycline 100 mg oral bid for 14 days; **OR** tetracycline 500 mg oral qid for 14 days; **OR** ceftriaxone 1 g IV or IM daily for 10-14 days; **OR** azithromycin 2 g oral once (failures and increasing resistance reported)
Chancroid (*H ducreyi*)	**One of the following:** azithromycin 1 g oral once; **OR** ceftriaxone 250 mg IM once; **OR** ciprofloxacin 500 mg oral bid for 3 days; **OR** erythromycin base 500 mg oral qid for 7 days	
HSV		
First episode	**One of the following:** acyclovir 400 mg oral tid or 200 mg 5 times daily for 7-10 days; **OR** valacyclovir 1 g oral bid for 7-10 days; **OR** famciclovir 250 mg oral tid for 7-10 days	

Table 71 Pathogen-Directed Therapy (*Cont'd.*)

Clinical Situation	First-Line Treatment	Alternate Treatment
Recurrent disease	**One of the following:**	
	acyclovir 400 mg tid or 800 mg bid for 5 days or 800 mg tid for 2 days; **OR**	
	valacyclovir 500 mg bid for 3 days or 1 g oral daily for 5 days; **OR**	
	famciclovir 125 mg orally bid for 5 days or 500 mg once followed by 250 mg oral bid for 2 days or 1 g oral bid for 1 day only	
Suppressive therapy	**One of the following:**	
	acyclovir 400 mg oral bid; **OR**	
	valacyclovir 500 mg to 1 g oral daily; **OR**	
	famciclovir 250 mg oral bid	
LGV	doxycycline 100 mg oral bid for 21 days	**EITHER**
		erythromycin base 500 mg oral qid for 21 days
		OR
		azithromycin 1 g oral once weekly for 3 wk
Donovanosis	doxycycline 100 mg oral bid for ≥3 wk (until complete resolution)	**One of the following:**
		ciprofloxacin 750 mg oral bid for ≥3 wk (until complete resolution); **OR**
		erythromycin base 500 mg oral qid for ≥3 wk (until complete resolution); **OR**
		azithromycin 1 g oral once weekly for >3 wk; **OR**
		TMP-SMX 1 DS tab bid for ≥3 wk

[a] Unless excluded by laboratory testing, treat for BOTH *N gonorrhoeae* and *C trachomatis* and other NGU pathogens.

[b] Nondisseminated.

[c] Should not be used to treat pharyngeal gonococcal infection.

[d] Reserved for very select patients intolerant to other options; active against most *N gonorrhoeae* and NGU pathogens (no additional NGU treatment warranted); GI tolerance a concern with 2-g dose; lower doses and other macrolides not recommended.

[e] *M genitalium* has better response rate to azithromycin than to doxycycline.

Other Conditions

Human Papillomavirus

- Types 6 and 11: Condyloma acuminatum (anogenital warts); most common viral STD in the US
- Types 16, 18, 31, 33, and 35: Cervical infection; oncogenic association with cervical cancer
- Most HPV infections are clinically asymptomatic; gynecologic examination with Papanicolaou test recommended
- HPV vaccine is now available for adolescents and young adults

Molluscum Contagiosum: Benign Disease Caused by Poxviridae Virus

- Classically 2- to 10-mm dome-shaped papules, often with central umbilication
- Treatment is local curettage or cryotherapy

Pelvic Inflammatory Disease: Endometriosis, Salpingitis, Tubo-Ovarian Abscess, Pelvic Peritonitis

- Clinical diagnosis with findings of cervical motion tenderness; uterine and/or adnexal tenderness
- When associated with cervicitis, *N gonorrhoeae* and *C trachomatis* are primary pathogens
- Anaerobic bacteria and *Streptococcus* may contribute
- Treatment: IV regimen
  - First-line treatment
    - cefotetan 2 g IV every 12 hours or cefoxitin 2 g IV every 6 hours plus doxycycline 100 mg IV or oral every 12 hours
    - clindamycin 900 mg IV every 8 hours plus gentamicin 2 mg/kg IV load then gentamicin 1.5 mg/kg IV every 8 hours (or single daily dose of gentamicin 3-5 mg/kg can be substituted)
  - Alternate treatment
    - ampicillin/sulbactam 3 g IV every 8 hours plus doxycycline 100 mg IV every 12 hours
- Treatment: Non-IV regimen
  - ceftriaxone 250 mg IM once, or cefoxitin 2 g IM with probenecid 1 g oral once; combined with doxycycline 100 mg oral twice daily for 14 days with or without metronidazole 500 mg oral twice daily for 14 days
  - Another select 3rd-gen cephalosporin (eg, ceftizoxime or cefotaxime) plus doxycycline 100 mg oral twice daily for 14 days with or without metronidazole 500 mg oral twice daily for 14 days
  - An alternative oral option includes levofloxacin 500-750 mg (if infection with *N gonorrhoeae* is excluded) with metronidazole 500 mg 3 times daily for 14 days

Pediculosis Pubis

- First-line treatment
  - permethrin 1% cream or pyrethrins with piperonyl butoxide; apply to affected area for 10 minutes and then wash off
- Alternate treatment
  - ivermectin 250 mcg/kg oral; repeat in 2 weeks
  - malathion 0.5% lotion; apply to affected area for 8-12 hours and then wash off

Scabies

- First-line treatment
  - permethrin 5% cream; apply for 8-14 hours to all areas of body from neck down and then wash off
  - ivermectin 200 mcg/kg oral; repeat in 2 weeks
- Alternate treatment
  - lindane 1% (1 oz of lotion or 30 g of cream); apply thinly to all areas of body from neck down and then wash off after 8 hours

Note

- Avoid fluoroquinolones and doxycycline during pregnancy
- Avoid metronidazole during 1st trimester of pregnancy; metronidazole may cause a disulfiram-like reaction when taken with alcohol

Tuberculosis

Mycobacterium tuberculosis Complex

General Information

- Group of mycobacteria causing tuberculosis (TB) in mammals
- Composed of *Mycobacterium tuberculosis*, *M bovis*, *M africanum*, *M microti*, *M canetti*, and *M mungi*; producing similar clinical TB in mammals
  - *M tuberculosis* causes TB in humans, whereas other species predominantly cause disease in animals
- *M bovis*
  - *M bovis* occasionally can produce disease in humans who consume unpasteurized milk
  - Progressive infection in immunosuppressed patients can occur with attenuated bacille Calmette-Guérin (BCG) *M bovis* through either BCG vaccination or BCG bladder irrigations
  - Resistant to pyrazinamide

New *M tuberculosis* Diagnostic Tests

- **Serum interferon-γ release assay (IGRA):** *M tuberculosis* antigen-specific interferon (IFN)-γ release assays: QuantiFERON-TB Gold In-Tube (QFT-GIT; Cellestis Ltd, Melbourne, Australia) and T-SPOT.TB (Oxford Immunotec Ltd, Oxford, United Kingdom)
  - Detect IFN-γ release from specific, previously sensitized, memory T cells by in vitro stimulation by *M tuberculosis*–specific proteins (eg, ESAT-6 and CFP10)
  - Identify patients infected with *M tuberculosis* (either active disease or inactive or latent disease)
  - Differentiate *M tuberculosis* infection from previous BCG vaccination and most nontuberculous mycobacteria infections
  - False-positive results possible with *M marinum*, *M kansasii*, and *M szulgai* infections
  - IGRAs may be used in the same clinical setting as the tuberculin (TB) skin test (also called TST, PPD [purified protein derivative], or the Mantoux test); as with the TST, if active TB is suspected, additional diagnostic testing (eg, chest radiographs, sputum collection for appropriate stains and cultures, human immunodeficiency virus [HIV] testing) should be performed while awaiting the IGRA results.
- **Nucleic acid amplification (NAA) assays:** Cobas TaqMan MTB Test (*M tuberculosis* polymerase chain reaction [PCR] test; Roche Molecular Diagnostics, Pleasanton, California) and the Amplified MTD (*Mycobacterium tuberculosis* Direct) Test (Gen-Probe Inc, San Diego, California)
  - Both NAA assays can be used for direct detection of *M tuberculosis* in smear-positive respiratory specimens; the MTD (Roche Molecular Diagnostics) is approved by the US Food and Drug Administration (FDA) for smear-negative respiratory specimens of suspect patients

- Both NAA assays are intended to complement acid-fast bacillus (AFB) smear and mycobacterial culture and to offer a more sensitive and rapid early detection method for active TB
- At Mayo Clinic, an *M tuberculosis* complex PCR is available but it is not yet an FDA-approved test for respiratory, body fluid, tissue, urine, or stool specimens

Treatment of Latent TB Infection in Adults (No Clinical or Radiologic Evidence of Active Disease)

Preferred Treatment
- isoniazid 5 mg/kg daily (300 mg max) oral for 9 months (270 doses minimum)

Alternate Treatment
- rifampin 10 mg/kg daily (600 mg max) oral for 4 months (60 doses minimum)
- isoniazid 5 mg/kg daily (300 mg max) oral for 6 months (180 doses minimum; for patients not able to complete 9 months of therapy)
- isoniazid 900 mg twice weekly (by directly observed therapy [DOT]) for 9 months (76 doses minimum)
- isoniazid 900 mg twice weekly (by DOT) for 6 months (52 doses minimum; for patients not able to complete 9 months of therapy)

Treatment of Pulmonary TB (Active Disease)

- General rules for drug-susceptible *M tuberculosis* isolates
  - All 6-month regimens should contain isoniazid, rifampin, and (initially, for 2 months) pyrazinamide
  - All 9-month regimens should contain isoniazid and rifampin
  - DOT strongly recommended for all patients

Standard Therapy for Drug-Susceptible Pulmonary TB

Option 1
Initiation
- isoniazid, rifampin, pyrazinamide, and ethambutol[a] daily for 8 weeks (56 doses)

---

[a] Discontinue ethambutol if susceptibility data are available and isolate is sensitive to isoniazid, rifampin, and pyrazinamide (all 3 in combination). If pyrazinamide is not used, continue ethambutol for first 2 months for susceptible *M tuberculosis* isolate.

- isoniazid, rifampin, pyrazinamide, and ethambutol[a] 5 days per week[b] for 8 weeks (40 doses)

Continuation Options
- isoniazid and rifampin daily for 18 weeks (126 doses), **OR** 5 days per week[b] for 18 weeks (90 doses)
- isoniazid and rifampin twice weekly for 18 weeks (36 doses)[c]
- isoniazid[c] and rifapentine[d] once weekly for 18 weeks (18 doses)

Option 2

Initiation
- isoniazid, rifampin, pyrazinamide, and ethambutol[a] daily for 2 weeks (14 doses), then isoniazid, rifampin, pyrazinamide, and ethambutol[a] twice weekly for 6 weeks (12 doses)[c]
- isoniazid, rifampin, pyrazinamide, and ethambutol[a] 5 days per week[b] for 2 weeks (10 doses), then twice weekly for 6 weeks (12 doses)

Continuation Options
- isoniazid and rifampin twice weekly for 18 weeks (36 doses)[c]
- isoniazid[c] and rifapentine[d] once weekly for 18 weeks (18 doses)

Option 3

Initiation
- isoniazid, rifampin, pyrazinamide, and ethambutol[a] 3 times weekly for 8 weeks (24 doses)[c]

Continuation Options
- isoniazid and rifampin 3 times weekly for 18 weeks (54 doses)[c]

Option 4 (for Pregnant Patients or Those Intolerant of pyrazinamide[e,f])

Initiation
- isoniazid, rifampin, and ethambutol[a] daily for 8 weeks (56 doses)
- isoniazid, rifampin, and ethambutol[a] 5 days per week for 8 weeks (40 doses)

Continuation Options
- isoniazid and rifampin daily for 31 weeks (217 doses)
- isoniazid and rifampin 5 days per week[b] for 31 weeks (155 doses)
- isoniazid and rifampin twice weekly for 31 weeks (62 doses)[c]

---

[b] Five-day-a-week administration should be given by DOT.
[c] Increase doses of isoniazid, pyrazinamide, and ethambutol when these drugs are given 1-3 times per week instead of daily. The rifampin dose is the same whether given daily or intermittently.
[d] The continuation phase of treatment may consist of isoniazid plus rifapentine once weekly for 4 months (by DOT) for HIV-negative patients with noncavitary pulmonary TB and negative sputum smears at completion of the initial 2-month treatment.
[e] For pregnant patients: Use of pyrazinamide is not recommended in the US by the Centers for Disease Control and Prevention (CDC) unless the patient is HIV positive or drug resistance is suspected or confirmed, and streptomycin should be avoided. Streptomycin can be harmful to the fetus; the effects of pyrazinamide on the fetus have not been studied well enough for the CDC to recommend its use during pregnancy.
[f] Pregnant women taking isoniazid should also receive vitamin B_6.

Treatment Duration (Pulmonary Disease With Susceptible *M tuberculosis* Isolate)

- 2-Month induction phase
- 4-Month continuation phase for most patients (6-month total treatment)
- 7-Month continuation phase recommended for 3 groups of patients (9-month total treatment)
  - Patients with cavitary disease on initial chest radiographs who have a positive sputum culture after 2 months of initial phase treatment
  - Patients whose initial phase of treatment did not contain pyrazinamide
  - Patients transitioned to once-weekly treatment with isoniazid and rifapentine in the continuation phase of therapy and who have a positive sputum culture after 2 months of initial phase treatment

Special Circumstances

- **HIV coinfection:** Consult an HIV expert
  - rifampin-based regimens generally not recommended with most protease inhibitors or nonnucleotide reverse transcriptase inhibitors[g]
  - rifabutin causes less hepatic cytochrome P450 enzyme induction than rifampin and may be used in place of rifampin (with dosing adjustments[h]) to reduce adverse drug-to-drug interactions
  - The use of once-weekly isoniazid plus rifapentine during the continuation phase is contraindicated for HIV-positive patients because of an unacceptably high rate of treatment failure or relapse (often with rifamycin-resistant organisms)
  - Twice-weekly treatment, either as part of the initial phase or the continuation phase, is not recommended for HIV-positive patients with CD4 <100/mcL
- **Drug-resistant TB:** Consult a TB expert, because composition of an effective treatment regimen depends on the type and number of drugs that the *M tuberculosis* isolate is resistant to. Adverse side effects are more common with 2nd-line TB drugs, which require close monitoring.
- **Culture-negative TB (2 treatment options)**
  - isoniazid, rifampin, pyrazinamide, and ethambutol daily for 6 months (preferred)
    - Use of all 4 drugs for duration of therapy is justified because of possible drug resistance
    - If source patient (index case) is known to have a drug-susceptible isolate, then pyrazinamide and ethambutol may be stopped after 2 months

---

[g] Exceptions to this rule include ritonavir and efavirenz.

[h] Information on rifamycins and antiretroviral dosing can be found at http://www.cdc.gov/tb/publications/guidelines/TB_HIV_Drugs/default.htm (Managing Drug Interactions in the Treatment of HIV-Related Tuberculosis) [cited 2011 Jan 27].

- isoniazid, rifampin, pyrazinamide, and ethambutol for first 2 months, followed by isoniazid and rifampin for 2 more months (4-month total treatment)
- **Indications for use of vitamin B$_6$ (pyridoxine) with isoniazid:**
  - Alcoholism
  - Diabetes mellitus
  - Malnutrition
  - HIV infection
  - Preexisting peripheral neuropathy
  - Pregnancy (including 2 months postpartum)
  - Seizure disorder
  - Uremia

Table 72 Treatment of Extrapulmonary TB

Duration of TB Treatment by Location of Drug-Susceptible Disease	Use of Corticosteroids
6 Months	
Disseminated disease in adults	No
Genitourinary disease	No
Lymph nodes	No
Pericardial disease	Yes[a]
Peritoneal disease	No
Pleural disease	No
6-9 Months	
Bones and joints (nonvertebral)	No
9 Months	
Disseminated disease in children	No
9-12 Months	
CNS disease/meningitis	Yes[b,c]
Vertebral disease	No

[a] Usual prednisone dosing for pericarditis (adults): 60 mg/day for 4 weeks, followed by 30 mg/day for 4 weeks, then 15 mg/day for 2 weeks, and then 5 mg/day for 1 week.

[b] Adjunctive dexamethasone is recommended for all patients with CNS TB, particularly those with a decreased level of consciousness or TB meningitis.

[c] Usual dexamethasone dose for CNS TB in adults is 12 mg/day for 3 weeks, which is then tapered over the following 3 weeks.

Data from Blumberg HM, et al. Am J Respir Crit Care Med. 2003 Feb 15;167(4):603-62.

Nontuberculosis Mycobacterial Infections

Mycobacteria Classification, Identification, and Diagnosis

Runyon Classification of Nontuberculosis Mycobacteria (NTM)

- **Group I (photochromogens):** Produces pigment in light: *Mycobacterium kansasii, M marinum, M simiae*
- **Group II (scotochromogens):** Produces pigment in dark: *M scrofulaceum, M szulgai, M xenopi, M gordonae*
- **Group III (nonphotochromogens):** No pigment: *M avium-intracellulare* complex (MAC), *M haemophilum, M ulcerans, M malmoense, M terrae* complex
- **Group IV (rapidly growing mycobacteria):** *M fortuitum, M chelonae, M abscessus*

Laboratory or Diagnostic Testing

- Microbial stains
  - **Acid-fast bacilli (AFB) stain (Ziehl-Neelsen or Kinyoun carbolfuchsin):** Red-staining mycobacteria on blue-green background
    - Beaded ("barber pole") appearance with *M kansasii*
    - *Nocardia* and *Rhodococcus* will also stain weakly AFB positive
  - **Auramine-rhodamine stain (fluorescence microscopy):** More sensitive than AFB stain; less specific
- Culture: Both broth and solid media
- Rapid mycobacteria identification tests
  - **HPLC (high-performance liquid chromatography):** Identifies differing species by specific mycolic acid fingerprint patterns
  - **DNA probe:** Available for identifying *M tuberculosis, M gordonae, M kansasii,* and MAC
  - **BACTEC NAP Test (BD [Becton, Dickinson and Company], Franklin Lakes, New Jersey):** Inhibits growth of *M tuberculosis* but not NTM strains
- The serum interferon-γ release assay (IGRA), which is used to detect infection with *M tuberculosis,* is usually negative for NTM infections except those caused by *M kansasii, M marinum,* or *M szulgai*

Specialized Diagnostic Criteria for NTM Pulmonary Disease

- **Note:** All criteria are required, because many NTM can be isolated as environmental contaminants or airway commensals or as minimal disease
  - Appropriate clinical pulmonary symptoms

- Radiographic findings include nodular or cavitary opacities on chest radiographs or computed tomography (CT) scans with multifocal bronchiectasis and multiple small nodules or nodular infiltrates
- NTM culture growth from 2 or more sputum samples or 1 bronchial wash or lavage; **OR** from tissue biopsy showing granulomatous inflammation or AFB present on staining with NTM growth in culture; **OR** from tissue biopsy showing granulomatous inflammation or AFB present on staining with NTM growth in culture of 1 or more sputum or bronchial samples; **AND** exclusion of other diagnoses (with any of the preceding findings)

Major Syndromes of Select NTM Mycobacteria

Pulmonary Disease

- **Most common:** MAC, M kansasii, M abscessus
- **Less common:** M fortuitum, M szulgai, M xenopi (in areas of Canada, United Kingdom, and Europe), M malmoense (in Scandinavia and other areas of northern Europe), M celatum, M asiaticum, and M shimodii

Skin, Soft-Tissue, and Bone or Joint Disease

- **Cutaneous disease:** M marinum, rapidly growing mycobacteria (ie, M fortuitum, M chelonae, M abscessus), M ulcerans
- **Tenosynovitis of hand:** M marinum, MAC, rapidly growing mycobacteria, M kansasii, M terrae, M szulgai, M malmoense, M xenopi
- **Postsurgical wound infections:** Commonly caused by rapidly growing mycobacteria

Lymphadenitis

- **Note:** Localized head and neck NTM lymphadenitis is predominantly a disease of children aged 1-5 years that is caused primarily by MAC, M scrofulaceum, and, in northern Europe, M malmoense
- **Note:** M tuberculosis accounts for 90% of mycobacterial lymphadenitis in adults and for many cases in children living in regions where tuberculosis (TB) is endemic

Disseminated Disease (Typically in Immunosuppressed Patients)

- **Corticosteroid use, transplant recipients, hematologic malignancies**
  - **Fever of unknown origin:** MAC
  - **Multiple skin or subcutaneous abscesses:** M kansasii, M chelonae, M abscessus, M haemophilum, M scrofulaceum
- **Human immunodeficiency virus (HIV):** Typically CD4 counts <50/mcL
  - **Bacteremia:** MAC (most common bacterial bloodstream pathogen in AIDS patients)
  - M kansasii (associated with pulmonary disease), M haemophilum (associated with skin, soft tissue, bone, and joint infections)

Select Nontuberculosis Mycobacteria

M avium-intracellulare **Complex (MAC)**

General Information: Pulmonary Disease

- **Risk factors or associations with pulmonary MAC disease**
  - α_1-Antitrypsin deficiency
  - Ciliary dyskinesia
  - Cystic fibrosis
  - Gastroesophageal reflux disease
  - Prior pulmonary histoplasmosis
  - Slender body habitus with pectus excavatum
- **Course:** High variability in pulmonary disease and rates of disease progression; patients with minimal pulmonary disease may not require treatment
- **Diagnosis:** Pulmonary MAC diagnosed by combination of active symptoms, radiologic findings on chest radiograph (or CT scan), and positive MAC cultures
- **Posttreatment–recurring MAC disease:** Not uncommon, especially with chronic lung disorders (eg, bronchiectasis)

Clinical Disease

- Immunocompetent patients
  - Pulmonary disease
    - **Fibrocavitary type:** May appear similar to TB with predominance of upper lobe cavitary disease; about 50% of cases
      - Typically men; heavy smoking, alcoholism; aged <60 years
      - Higher MAC organism burden; AFB stain commonly positive
      - Monomicrobial MAC infection more common
    - **Nodular bronchiectasis type:** Presence of bronchiectasis with nodular disease; 40% of cases
      - Typically women; nonsmoking, no alcoholism; mean age, 70 years
      - Lower MAC organism burden; AFB smear commonly negative
      - Polymicrobial infections common (ie, coexisting MAC, *P aeruginosa*, rapidly growing NTM, *Aspergillus*, *Nocardia*, and other MAC substrains)
  - Hypersensitivity-like pulmonary disease
    - **Common association with hot tubs:** Especially common with indoor hot tubs ("hot tub lung")
    - **Patients:** Often relatively young and healthy; chest CT scan may show diffuse infiltrate with ground-glass opacities
  - Head or neck lymphadenitis (ie, cervical); predominantly a pediatric infection in children aged 1-5 years
  - Cutaneous disease with external hypersensitivity reactions; rarely disseminated
- HIV, AIDS, or immunosuppressed patients
  - **Disseminated disease:** Fever, night sweats, weight loss; hepatosplenomegaly common; positive blood cultures in more than 90% of patients; CD4 counts usually less than 50/mcL
  - **Enteric disease:** Enteritis, colitis, malabsorption
  - **Pulmonary disease:** Less common

Treatment of Pulmonary MAC Disease

- Combination therapy for at least 12 months of negative sputum cultures while undergoing treatment
  - **First-line treatment:** Preferably use a 3-drug therapy of clarithromycin (or azithromycin) plus ethambutol and either rifampin or rifabutin
    - Daily therapy (for cavitary or severe disease) or thrice-weekly therapy
    - Consider addition of thrice-weekly amikacin or streptomycin for first 2-3 months for severe and extensive (especially cavitary) disease
    - Susceptibility testing recommended initially only for clarithromycin; no other susceptibility testing correlated with clinical outcome
    - Follow monthly mycobacteria sputum cultures
    - A 2-drug treatment with clarithromycin (or azithromycin) plus ethambutol may be acceptable in select mild cases but generally is not recommended because of potential risk for macrolide resistance
  - **Alternate treatment:** Consider moxifloxacin, levofloxacin, amikacin, ethionamide, possibly linezolid
  - **Pulmonary hygiene optimization:** With chronic lung disease or bronchiectasis: Flutter valve, postural drainage, β-agonist inhaler; mucolytic agents (possibly)

Treatment of Hypersensitivity MAC Lung Disease

- Remove source of exposure (eg, avoid contaminated hot tub)
- Moderate to severe cases: Consider corticosteroid taper (4-8 weeks) or combination drug therapy for shorter periods (3-6 months) or both

Treatment of Children With NTM Cervical Lymphadenitis (MAC, M scrofulaceum)

- Excisional surgery without chemotherapy
- Combination drug therapy if surgical excision is incomplete

Treatment of Disseminated MAC Disease (Advanced HIV or AIDS)

- Combination therapy with daily clarithromycin (or azithromycin) plus ethambutol and preferably also including either rifabutin or rifampin
- Duration of therapy in HIV-positive patients: Lifelong or consider discontinuing after at least 12 months in asymptomatic patients with sustained increase in CD4 counts >100/mcL for more than 6 months after starting or modifying highly active antiretroviral therapy
- Avoid adverse drug interactions (eg, rifabutin or rifampin and select antiretroviral drugs) in HIV patients (for more information, see the Centers for Disease Control and Prevention Web site[a])

---

[a] Managing Drug Interactions in the Treatment of HIV-Related Tuberculosis [online]. National Center for HIV/AIDS, Viral Hepatitis, STD, and TB Prevention, Division of Tuberculosis Elimination. Atlanta (GA) December 2007: Centers for Disease Control and Prevention. [cited 2011 Feb 28]. Available from: http://www.cdc.gov/tb/publications/guidelines/TB_HIV_Drugs/PDF/tbhiv.pdf.

M kansasii

General Information

- **Appearance:** Long, banded or beaded on AFB stain
- **Geographic predominance:** Midwestern and southwestern US; isolated from soil, natural water supplies, tap water

Clinical Disease

- **Pulmonary disease:** Thin-walled cavities are common on chest radiographs, although noncavitary and nodular bronchiectasis disease can occur
- **Lymphadenitis:** Especially cervical lymph node involvement
- **Granulomatous skin lesions, erythema nodosum**
- **Bone, joint, and soft tissue infections**

Treatment

- **First-line treatment:** Use rifampin plus both ethambutol and isoniazid for at least 12 months of negative sputum cultures in pulmonary disease; rifampin is the cornerstone of treatment and is the only drug associated with in vitro resistance and clinical failure
- **Alternate treatment (ie, if rifampin resistant or intolerant):** clarithromycin, moxifloxacin, amikacin, streptomycin, sulfamethoxazole

M marinum

General Information

- Known as "swimming pool granuloma" or "fish tank granuloma"; associated with exposure to salt water, freshwater, fish tanks, and swimming pools
- Infection acquired by skin inoculation; preferential growth in cooler 27-32°C areas of body (ie, extremities)

Clinical Disease

- **Cutaneous disease:** Granulomatous skin lesions; nodules commonly in line of lymphatic drainage ("ascending" appearance similar to that of cutaneous sporotrichosis)
  - Typically appears on extremities (eg, elbows, knees, dorsum of feet and hands)
  - May be solitary, grouped, or widespread

Treatment: Variable Approaches (Typically Less Virulent Mycobacteria)

- **Skin and soft tissue infection:** Use 2 active drugs for 3-4 months (typically 1-2 months after symptoms resolve); single-drug therapy may be an alternate approach for minimal disease in select cases (not generally recommended)
- **Tenosynovitis and joint disease:** May require debridement with combination drug therapy for 4-6 months
- **First-line drug treatment:** Use clarithromycin (or azithromycin) plus ethambutol; rifampin can be added for bone and other more serious forms of disease
- **Alternate drug treatment:** Consider trimethoprim-sulfamethoxazole (TMP-SMX); minocycline or doxycycline; moxifloxacin or ciprofloxacin

M leprae: Leprosy, Hansen Disease

General Information

- *M leprae* grows best at cooler (33°C) temperatures and has a predilection for cooler areas of the body
- Found mainly in the tropics and subtropics; man is its only host, and infection is spread by direct contact (eg, close household contact; nasal discharge from infected patient is most common mode of transmission)
- Organism is **NOT** cultured from laboratory media; diagnosis is made clinically with supporting tissue histology and microbial stains

Clinical Syndromes

- **Lepromatous leprosy:** Symmetric nodules (widely distributed), thickened dermis; cooler areas of body mostly affected; nasal collapse (ie, saddle-nose deformity); ear lobes; skin biopsy shows many bacilli
- **Tuberculoid leprosy:** Few hypopigmented anesthetic macules with distinct borders; distal hypoesthesia with selective loss of pain and temperature most common; peripheral nerves may become enlarged and palpable; prominent neurologic involvement; skin biopsy shows only a few bacilli
- **Other Clinical Findings of Leprosy**
  - Peripheral neuritis: Ulnar nerve tropism leads to clawing of 4th and 5th fingers with decreased motor skill ("claw hand") and decreased sensory and fine touch; may be associated with skin lesions
  - Nasal collapse
  - Renal amyloidosis
  - Uveitis, glaucoma
  - Gynecomastia (due to decreased testosterone)
- **Reversal reactions:** Clinical disease produced by change in host's immune response to *M leprae*
  - **Type 1 reactions:** Induced by cell-mediated immunity
    - **Upgrading reactions:** Typically seen in patients with borderline lepromatous disease who undergo a shift toward more tuberculoid (paucibacillary) forms; may develop after induction of therapy
    - **Downgrading reactions:** Occur with transformation from tuberculoid to more lepromatous (multibacillary) form; often develop in absence of therapy
    - **Note:** Both reactions may appear similar clinically and may contain erythema and edema of existing skin lesions with painful neuropathy and ulceration; treat severe reactions with a corticosteroid taper
  - **Type 2 reactions:** Immune complex–mediated; including erythema nodosum leprosum
    - Immune complex–mediated vasculitis; often ulceration with damage to nerves
    - Treatment options include nonsteroidal anti-inflammatory drugs (NSAIDs), corticosteroids, clofazimine, thalidomide

Treatment

- **Paucibacillary disease:** dapsone plus rifampin for 6-12 months
- **Multibacillary disease:** dapsone plus both rifampin and clofazimine for 12-24 months

The Rapidly Growing Mycobacteria: *M fortuitum, M chelonae, M abscessus*

General Information
- Typical growth in liquid media within 3-7 days
- Water, soil, and nosocomial pathogens; flourish in warm humid environments (eg, hot tubs, water piping)
- Typically appear AFB-stain positive, but can be weakly staining or even AFB-stain negative
- Can infect healthy, immunocompetent patients
- Geographic predominance in southeastern US, along Gulf Coast (from Florida to Texas), Hawaii

Clinical Disease
- Pulmonary disease
  - Occurs typically in patients with underlying chronic lung disease; bronchiectasis
  - *M abscessus* is most common and most difficult-to-treat mycobacterial disease
  - Chest radiograph typically shows multilobar, patchy reticulonodular infiltrate with upper lobe predominance; cavitation less common (15% of cases)
- Skin and soft tissue infection
  - Usually related to trauma or surgery; develops into wound infection; abscesses common
  - Cutaneous infections and hypersensitivity reactions (eg, due to contaminated hot tubs or pedicure equipment)
- Bone and joint infections
  - Secondary to trauma or previous orthopedic surgery
- Less common: Keratitis, lymphadenitis

Treatment
- Selection and duration of combination therapy depend on pathogen, host, syndrome, and susceptibility to available drugs
- *M fortuitum* is typically susceptible to more antibiotic options than other rapidly growing mycobacteria
- *M chelonae* is less susceptible to cefoxitin and usually more susceptible to tobramycin than to amikacin
- *M abscessus* (especially pulmonary disease) is commonly multidrug resistant and difficult to treat successfully; it is more susceptible to amikacin and cefoxitin but relatively resistant to tobramycin
- Drugs active against rapidly growing mycobacteria vary depending on organism and susceptibilities but may include clarithromycin, azithromycin, amikacin (or tobramycin), cefoxitin, imipenem, moxifloxacin, linezolid, minocycline, and tigecycline
- Other drugs that may possess some activity (especially against *M fortuitum*) include doxycycline and sulfonamide
- Surgery is generally indicated for abscesses, extensive infections, and removal of associated foreign material, and for localized *M abscessus* pulmonary infections
- Duration of therapy varies, depending on severity and species; 4-6 months for skin and soft tissue infections, 6 months (with surgical debridement) for bone and joint infections, and 12 months (or longer)

of negative sputum cultures for pulmonary infections (*M abscessus* pneumonitis may require surgery)

Other Less Common Rapidly Growing Mycobacteria

- *M smegmatis* group (*M smegmatis*, *M wolinskyi*, *M goodii*)
  - Clinical disease (uncommon); associated with lymphadenitis, osteomyelitis, postsurgical wound infections, intravenous catheter infections
  - Treatment considerations include amikacin, TMP-SMX, doxycycline, moxifloxacin, imipenem, ethambutol, and possibly cefoxitin; in vitro group resistance to clarithromycin and other macrolides
- *M immunogenum*
  - Typically from contaminated water source
  - Commonly drug resistant; treatment considerations include clarithromycin and amikacin

M scrofulaceum

Clinical Disease

- Cervical lymphadenitis in young children
- Chronic cutaneous disease
- Pulmonary disease (less common)

Treatment

- Can be multidrug resistant; considerations include clarithromycin, azithromycin, fluoroquinolones
- Surgical excision for localized lymphadenitis and cutaneous disease

M haemophilum

General Information

- Wide geographical distribution (Europe, United Kingdom, Israel, Africa, Fiji, Australia, Canada, and US)
- More common and pronounced disease in immunocompromised patients (eg, transplant recipients, patients taking chronic corticosteroids, HIV-positive or AIDS patients)
- Fastidious in vitro growth; special in vitro growth requirements for hemin- or iron-containing compounds; growth at cooler (32°C) temperatures
- Commonly AFB-stain positive from tissue, but cultures may be negative

Clinical Disease

- Cutaneous lesions (most common), typically over the extremities; can be chronic
- Lymphadenitis can occur in healthy children
- Septic arthritis
- Disseminated disease may occur in immunosuppressed patients

Treatment

- Consider clarithromycin, rifampin, rifabutin, ciprofloxacin, amikacin; variable activity with doxycycline, kanamycin, TMP-SMX
- Isolated lymphadenitis in children and immunocompetent patients may be treated with surgical excision alone

M terrae Complex: M terrae, M triviale, M nonchromogenicum, M hiberniae

Clinical Disease

- **Localized tenosynovitis:** Typically affects upper extremities, including hands, wrists, fingers; often occurs in association with trauma
- **Less common:** Pulmonary disease (can produce cavitary disease); genitourinary and gastrointestinal infections

Treatment

- Consider clarithromycin, azithromycin, ethambutol, rifampin, fluoroquinolones, linezolid
- Surgery may be required

M xenopi

General Information

- Obligate thermophile; enhanced growth at 42°C (commonly isolated from hot water taps and showerheads)

Clinical Disease

- Chronic pulmonary disease (common in Canada, the United Kingdom, and other parts of Europe)
- Patients typically have underlying chronic lung disease; upper lobe cavitary disease (common); cavities may be large

Treatment

- Poor correlation between in vitro susceptibility testing and clinical response
- Consider clarithromycin, moxifloxacin, rifampin, and ethambutol; role of isoniazid is unclear and may not be beneficial

M ulcerans

General Information

- Tropical rain forests of Africa, Australia, southwestern Asia, and South and Central America; Papua New Guinea; Malaysia
- Optimal growth at cooler (28-33°C) temperatures; predilection for extremities; prolonged incubation period (>3 months); slow growth

Clinical Disease

- African Buruli ulcer or Australian Bairnsdale ulcer; cutaneous, necrotic, painless; progressive, granulomatous; may involve large areas of skin; can become disfiguring
- Associated with minor penetrating trauma and concurrent or subsequent contact with contaminated soil or water

Treatment

- Difficult in more advanced stages
- Consider clarithromycin, often with rifampin, ethambutol, some aminoglycosides; possibly TMP-SMX, tetracycline
- Wound debridement with skin grafting may be required

M szulgai

General Information
- M szulgai infections are rare and generally not considered contaminants; infections usually occur in immunosuppressed patients (eg, HIV-positive patients or transplant recipients); AFB stain may show some banding (similar to that for M kansasii)

Clinical Disease
- Pulmonary disease has a presentation similar to that of TB
- Extrapulmonary disease includes osteomyelitis, joint infection, and skin and soft tissue infections

Treatment
- Consider isoniazid, rifampin, and pyrazinamide
- Alternates include moxifloxacin, clarithromycin, azithromycin

M malmoense

General Information
- Northern Europe (2nd most common NTM isolate from sputum and cervical lymph nodes of children), Finland, Zaire, Japan; rare in US but sometimes found in Florida, Texas, Georgia

Clinical Disease
- Pulmonary disease
- Lymphadenitis
- Other (less common) conditions include tenosynovitis, cutaneous disease, disseminated disease

Treatment
- Poor correlation between in vitro susceptibility testing and clinical response
- Consider combination of isoniazid, rifampin, and ethambutol; possibly add clarithromycin or a fluoroquinolone or both

Other Mycobacteria

M celatum
- Can cross-react with acridinium ester–labeled DNA probe used to identify M tuberculosis (AccuProbe; Gen-Probe, Inc, San Diego, California)
- Respiratory disease (eg, immunosuppressed patients), uncommon isolate
- Typically susceptible to clarithromycin, azithromycin, fluoroquinolones, rifabutin

M genavense
- Disseminated disease in immunosuppressed patients (eg, HIV-positive or AIDS); closely resembles disseminated MAC
  - Involvement of blood, marrow, liver, spleen, enteric tissue
  - Splenomegaly common
- Difficult to grow in culture; requires supplemented media
- Usually susceptible to clarithromycin, azithromycin, fluoroquinolones, amikacin, rifampin, rifabutin

M gordonae

- Commonly isolated from tap water ("tap water bacillus")
- Ubiquitous in nature and most commonly regarded as nonpathogenic or as a specimen contaminant
- Less common pulmonary and disseminated disease reported in immunocompromised and AIDS patients

M mucogenicum

- Central venous catheter infections with secondary bloodstream infections; less common peritoneal dialysis catheter infections
- Common contaminant in isolates from respiratory secretions
- Usually susceptible to amikacin, clarithromycin, cefoxitin, fluoroquinolones, minocycline, doxycycline, TMP-SMX, and imipenem

M simiae

- Geographic locales include Israel, Cuba, and southwestern US (Texas, Arizona, New Mexico)
- Clinical disease not common; infection usually develops in immunosuppressed patients or in those with chronic lung disease, commonly as pulmonary disease or (less commonly) as intra-abdominal infection
- Susceptibility drug data may not correlate with clinical outcome
- Consider clarithromycin, moxifloxacin, TMP-SMX

Suggested Reading

De Groote MA, Huitt G. Clin Infect Dis. 2006 Jun 15;42(12):1756–63. Epub 2006 May 11.
Griffith DE, et al. Am J Respir Crit Care Med. 2007 Feb 15;175(4):367–416. Erratum in: Am J Respir Crit Care Med. 2007 Apr 1;175(7):744-5.

Fungal Infections

Select Taxonomy

Yeasts
- *Candida*
- *Cryptococcus neoformans* and *C gattii*
- Other: *Saccharomyces, Trichosporon,* etc

Dimorphic Fungi

Two different growth forms: Outside the body (25°C), they grow as a mold, producing hyphae and having asexual reproduction of spores; inside the body (37°C), they grow in a yeast form
- *Histoplasma capsulatum*
- *Blastomyces dermatitidis*
- *Coccidioides immitis* and *C posadasii*
- *Paracoccidioides brasiliensis*
- *Sporothrix schenckii*
- *Penicillium marneffei*

Filamentous Fungi
- *Aspergillus*
- Agents of mucormycosis and entomophthoromycosis

Select Fungi

Candida

Risk Factors for Localized, Mucocutaneous Candidiasis, and Invasive or Disseminated Disease
- Folliculitis
- Prolonged intensive care unit stay with *Candida* colonization of multiple nonsterile sites
- Prolonged use of systemic antibacterial agents
- Central venous catheters
- Parenteral nutrition
- Bowel perforation and surgery involving the intestinal wall
- Immunosuppressive conditions, including diabetes mellitus and corticosteroid use
- Burn wounds
- Estrogen therapy, oral contraceptive use, pregnancy (vaginal candidiasis)

Clinical Diseases
- **Oral thrush:** More typical in immunosuppressed patients (eg, human immunodeficiency virus [HIV], corticosteroids)
  - **Pseudomembranous:** White, creamy plaques on inflamed base (eg, palate, tongue, buccal mucosa)

- **Hyperplastic:** Candidal leukoplakia; white lesions that do not wipe off but respond to therapy
- **Erythematous (atrophic):** Spotty or confluent red patches (often underdiagnosed)
- **Angular cheilitis (perlèche):** Erythema and fissures at corner of mouth
- **Esophagitis:** More common in immunosuppressed patients although occasionally occurs in immunocompetent patients; odynophagia and/or dysphagia common; usually presents with oral thrush although can be separate
- **Vaginitis (vaginal candidiasis):** Associated with pregnancy, use of high-estrogen oral contraceptives, uncontrolled diabetes mellitus, tight-fitting clothing, antibiotics, and dietary factors
  - Affects 75% of childbearing women
  - 40% of affected women have a 2nd episode; 5% have recurrent disease (>4 episodes per year)
- **Cutaneous syndromes**
  - **Intertriginous infection:** In warm moist areas of the body, more common among patients with diabetes or obesity
  - **Folliculitis**
  - **Balanitis:** Infection of the glans penis; *Candida* infection may also involve scrotum
  - **Paronychial infection:** Swelling, tenderness, erythema around nail
  - **Disseminated:** Macronodular lesions; lesions resembling ecthyma gangrenosum
- **Urinary candidiasis:** Colony count from urine culture is not directly predictive of urinary tract infection; clinical judgment required
- **Disseminated disease (acute or subacute)**
  - **Candidemia:** Fourth most common cause of nosocomial bloodstream infections in US; only 25% of patients with extensive organ disease have positive blood cultures
  - **Ocular candidiasis:** Incidence secondary to candidemia is variable and may in part depend on source and timing of antifungal therapy
  - **Meningitis:** Especially in patients with intravenous (IV) drug abuse; postneurosurgery and central nervous system (CNS) shunt infections
  - **Osteomyelitis:** Usually from hematogenous dissemination
  - **Peritonitis:** From peritoneal dialysis, bowel surgery, or perforated bowel
  - **Endocarditis:** Most common form of fungal infective endocarditis; large vegetations typical
- **Hepatosplenic candidiasis:** Chronic disseminated candidiasis
  - Typically seen in patients with hematologic malignancies; postchemotherapy with prolonged neutropenia
  - May present as persistent fever with neutropenia, without focal signs or symptoms, unresponsive to antibacterial therapy; ultrasound and computed tomography (CT) results may be normal initially during the period of neutropenia
  - With recovery from neutropenia, fever continues with elevation of liver enzymes (especially alkaline phosphatase); abdominal ultrasound, CT, or magnetic resonance imaging commonly shows

multiple small, round, hypoechoic or low-attenuated lesions scattered throughout the liver and spleen; lesions can later calcify

- Predominantly a clinical and radiographic diagnosis; liver biopsy is commonly false-negative; blood cultures are usually negative

Treatment: Depends on Syndrome and Type of Candida

- **Oral thrush:** Oral nystatin, clotrimazole troches, oral fluconazole
- **Esophagitis:** Oral fluconazole, other azoles,[a] or an echinocandin[b]; for refractory disease, use an amphotericin B product
- **Vaginitis:** Topical or oral azole[a] therapy
- **Candidemia**
  - **Nonneutropenic host:** fluconazole[c] or an echinocandin[b]; an amphotericin B product for refractory disease; for uncomplicated candidemia, treat for 2 weeks after last positive blood culture and improved symptoms
  - **Neutropenic host:** An echinocandin, an amphotericin B product, fluconazole[c] (not recommended for initial therapy in patients with recent azole exposure), voriconazole
- **Chronic disseminated candidiasis:** fluconazole[c] or an amphotericin B product; alternate treatments include other azoles[a] and echinocandins[b]; treatment duration is typically months for clinical response and radiographic maturation (multiple scattered, low-attenuation foci can persist despite successful therapy because of focal scarring and chronic inactive granulomatous changes)
- **Additional treatment information:** See guidelines for treatment of candidiasis (Pappas PG, et al. Clin Infect Dis. 2009 Mar 1;48[5]:503–35)

Cryptococcus

General Information and Endemic Areas

- Encapsulated, round yeast 4-6 micrometers; neurotropic fungal infection
- Common sources include pigeon and select bird droppings (*C neoformans*); contaminated soil; eucalyptus trees (*C gattii*)
- *C neoformans* is distributed worldwide; commonly found in soil contaminated by pigeon and other bird droppings; accounts for vast majority of cryptococcus infections
- *C gattii* (formerly known as *C neoformans var gattii*) is found on Vancouver Island and in surrounding areas within Canada and the northwest US; high propensity to cause infection in immunocompetent patients; high likelihood of producing CNS and/or pulmonary cryptococcomas; some strains have an elevated MIC (minimal inhibitory concentration) to azoles

---

[a] The azole class of antifungal agents includes fluconazole, itraconazole, voriconazole, posaconazole.
[b] The echinocandin class of antifungal agents includes caspofungin, anidulafungin, micafungin.
[c] Use fluconazole for susceptible *Candida* (eg, *C albicans, C tropicalis, C parapsilosis*).

Clinical Disease: Typically in Immunosuppressed Patients
- **Pulmonary cryptococcosis:** Lungs are the portal of entry and the most common site of infection; can readily disseminate to other organs (especially CNS)
- **CNS disease:** Includes meningitis, meningoencephalitis, cerebral cryptococcomas; clinical symptoms may be acute (eg, headache, fever, nuchal rigidity), subacute, or chronic (eg, altered mental status, headache)
  - **Hydrocephalus or high opening cerebrospinal fluid (CSF) pressure:** >20 cm is common; serial lumbar punctures or ventriculoperitoneal shunts often help reduce spinal and ventricular fluid pressure
  - **Negative prognostic factors:** Abnormal or reduced mental status; CSF cryptococcal antigen titer >1:1,024; CSF leukocytes <20 cells/mcL
- **Cutaneous:** Wide variation in presentation (eg, papules, plaques, cellulitis, tumors); cutaneous cryptococcal lesions signal dissemination; *Cryptococcus* skin papules can resemble molluscum contagiosum
- **Other:** Bone and joint disease; renal disease

Diagnosis
- **Cryptococcal antigen (serum and CSF):** About 95% sensitive for disseminated or meningeal cryptococcal disease; false-positive results can occur with *Trichosporon beigelii* and with *Stomatococcus* and *Capnocytophaga* infections
- **India ink:** Visualization of polysaccharide capsule; 75% sensitivity in CSF cryptococcal disease
- **Cultures:** Blood, CSF, urine
- **Note:** Any patient with a positive serum cryptococcal antigen or a positive blood or urine culture should have a lumbar puncture to rule out CNS cryptococcal disease

Treatment: Selection and Duration of Antifungal Therapy Depend on Location of Disease and Immune Status of Host
See Tables 73-76 below.

Table 73 Cryptococcal Meningoencephalitis in HIV-Infected Patients

Regimen	Duration
Induction therapy[a]	
liposomal amphotericin B 3-4 mg/kg per day or amphotericin B lipid complex 5 mg/kg per day or amphotericin B deoxycholate 0.7-1.0 mg/kg per day; **PLUS** flucytosine 25 mg/kg qid	2 wk
amphotericin B deoxycholate 0.7-1.0 mg/kg per day or liposomal amphotericin B 3-4 mg/kg per day or amphotericin B lipid complex 5 mg/kg per day	4-6 wk

(Continues)

Table 73 Cryptococcal Meningoencephalitis in HIV-Infected Patients (Cont'd.)

Regimen	Duration
Alternates for induction therapy[b]	
amphotericin B product (see above) plus fluconazole 800 mg per day	2 wk
fluconazole plus flucytosine	8 wk
fluconazole ≥800 mg per day (some experts favor 1,200 mg per day if used alone)	10-12 wk
itraconazole[c] 200 mg bid	10-12 wk
Consolidation therapy	
fluconazole 400 mg per day	≥8 wk
Maintenance (suppressive) therapy	
fluconazole 200 mg per day	≥1 y
Alternates for maintenance therapy	
itraconazole[c] 400 mg per day	≥1 y
amphotericin B deoxycholate[c] 1 mg/kg per wk (less effective than azoles)	≥1 y

Notes
- Monitor CSF opening pressure, as repeat lumbar punctures may be needed
- Can stop maintenance therapy (during effective HAART) in HIV patients with CD4 >100 cells/mcL and undetectable (or very low) HIV viral load for ≥3 mo after completing a minimum 12-month course of antifungal therapy
- Restart antifungal maintenance therapy if CD4 count drops <100 cells/mcL

[a] Begin HAART 2-10 weeks after the start of initial antifungal treatment.

[b] In unique clinical situations when primary recommendations are not available, alternate regimens may be considered but are not encouraged.

[c] Inferior to primary recommendation; follow serum levels.

Adapted from Perfect JR, et al. Clin Inf Dis. 2010 Feb 1:50(3):291–322. Used with permission.

Table 74 Cryptococcal Meningoencephalitis in Organ Transplant Recipients

Regimen	Duration
Induction therapy[a]	
liposomal amphotericin B 3-4 mg/kg per day or amphotericin B lipid complex 5 mg/kg per day; **PLUS** flucytosine 25 mg/kg qid	2 wk

Table 74 Cryptococcal Meningoencephalitis in Organ Transplant Recipients (*Cont'd.*)

Regimen	Duration
Alternates for induction therapy	
liposomal amphotericin B 6 mg/kg per day or amphotericin B lipid complex 5 mg/kg per day or amphotericin B deoxycholate[b] 0.7 mg/kg per day	4-6 wk
Consolidation therapy	
fluconazole 400-800 mg per day	8 wk
Maintenance (suppressive) therapy	
fluconazole 200-400 mg per day	6 mo to 1 y
Note	
• Monitor CSF opening pressure, as repeat lumbar punctures may be needed	

[a] Immunosuppressive management may require sequential or stepwise reductions.

[b] Many transplant recipients have been successfully treated with amphotericin B deoxycholate; however, there is considerable risk of added renal dysfunction with calcineurin inhibitor use and the effective dose is imprecise.

Adapted from Perfect JR, et al. Clin Inf Dis. 2010 Feb 1:50(3):291–322. Used with permission.

Table 75 Cryptococcal Meningoencephalitis in HIV-Negative, Nontransplant Patients (Data Limited)

Regimen	Duration
Induction therapy	
liposomal amphotericin B 3-4 mg/kg per day, or amphotericin B lipid complex 5 mg/kg per day, or amphotericin B deoxycholate 0.7-1.0 mg/kg per day; **PLUS** flucytosine 25 mg/kg qid	≥4 wk[a,b]
amphotericin B deoxycholate[c] 0.7-1.0 mg/kg per day	≥6 wk[a,b]
amphotericin B product plus flucytosine 25 mg/kg qid	2 wk[b,d]
Consolidation therapy	
fluconazole[e] 400-800 mg/day	8 wk
Maintenance therapy	
fluconazole 200 mg/day	6-12 mo

[a] Four weeks of induction therapy is appropriate for patients with meningitis who have no neurologic complications and no significant underlying diseases or immunosuppression, and for whom the CSF culture after 2 weeks of treatment does not yield viable yeasts.

[b] For prevention of early relapse after induction therapy, fluconazole consolidation and maintenance therapy are recommended.

[c] For flucytosine-intolerant patients.

[d] For patients who have a low risk of therapeutic failure as determined by diagnosis of early cryptococcal infection, no severe immunosuppression, and an excellent clinical response to initial 2-week antifungal combination therapy.

[e] A higher dosage of fluconazole (800 mg per day) is recommended for patients with normal renal function who undergo the 2-week induction regimen.

Adapted from Perfect JR, et al. Clin Inf Dis. 2010 Feb 1:50(3):291–322. Used with permission.

Table 76 Nonmeningeal Cryptococcosis

Regimen	Duration
Pulmonary disease in immunosuppressed and immunocompetent patients	
Mild-to-moderate pulmonary cryptococcosis: fluconazole 400 mg per day	6-12 mo
Severe pulmonary cryptococcosis: Same as for CNS disease	12 mo
Patients with nonmeningeal, nonpulmonary cryptococcosis	
Cryptococcemia: Same as for CNS disease	12 mo
Nonpulmonary, non-CNS disease, single-site disease without fungemia in immunocompetent host: fluconazole 400 mg per day	6-12 mo

Note

Follow-up monitoring of serum cryptococcal antigens during therapy is not consistently helpful in predicting outcome.

- In immunosuppressed patients with pulmonary cryptococcosis, CNS involvement should be ruled out by spinal fluid evaluation.
- In immunocompetent patients with pulmonary cryptococcosis, a spinal fluid evaluation should be considered to rule out asymptomatic CNS involvement. However, in such patients with asymptomatic pulmonary nodule or infiltrate, no symptoms of CNS infection, and a negative or very low serum cryptococcal antigen, the spinal fluid evaluation is not required.
- itraconazole, voriconazole, or posaconazole can be used for pulmonary cryptococcosis in patients intolerant to fluconazole.

Adapted from Perfect JR, et al. Clin Inf Dis. 2010 Feb 1:50(3):291–322. Used with permission.

Histoplasma capsulatum

General Information

- Intracellular yeast 1-2×3 micrometers; calcium deposits are common in tissue (eg, lungs, liver, spleen)
- *H capsulatum* prevalence is associated with soil contaminated with bird and bat droppings, chicken and other bird roosts, and caves

Endemic Areas

- Found worldwide, but more common in the Mississippi and Ohio river valleys, in the south-central United States, and in parts of Central and South America, Africa, and southeast Asia

Clinical Disease

- **Acute pulmonary histoplasmosis:** Often self-limiting patchy pneumonitis; hilar and mediastinal adenopathy is common; lung infiltrate can be diffuse with heavier exposure or immunosuppression; erythema nodosum may be present
- **Histoplasmoma:** Small calcified lung nodules (inactive), often with hilar calcification; may persist after resolution of primary infection
- **Chronic pulmonary histoplasmosis:** Usually upper lobes, often cavities; can mimic tuberculosis radiologically; cavitary findings are often called "marching cavity" because the cavities gradually enlarge in >50% of cases

- **Mediastinal lymphadenitis and mediastinal granuloma:**
  Granulomatous inflammation and enlargement of mediastinal lymph
  nodes, which can occasionally produce secondary airway compression
  or superior vena cava syndrome
- **Fibrosing mediastinitis:** Exaggerated inflammatory response leads
  to extensive fibrotic tissue deposition in mediastinum; can result
  in hypoxemia, dysphagia, and superior vena cava syndrome; limited
  treatment options include surgery
- **Disseminated histoplasmosis (ie, extrapulmonary spread,
  progressive):** Can involve multiple sites
  - **Adrenal gland disease:** May lead to adrenal insufficiency
  - **Hepatosplenomegaly:** Lesions may later calcify
  - **Cutaneous lesions:** Erythematous maculopapular lesions
  - **Ocular disease:** 2 general forms
    - Choroiditis in association with progressive, disseminated
      histoplasmosis
    - Presumed ocular histoplasmosis (POHS): Postinfectious
      inflammatory syndrome with choroidal retinal scars
  - **Bone marrow disease:** Leukopenia, anemia, thrombocytopenia
  - **Infective endocarditis, pericarditis**
  - **CNS disease:** Can present as basilar meningitis or cerebral mass
    lesions
  - **Oropharyngeal ulcers:** Usually occur with disseminated disease

Diagnosis
- **Culture**
- **Serology:** Serologic testing is insensitive and commonly negative with
  active disease; low serology titers are less specific for disease but may
  be helpful if >1:32 or positive for H or M bands
- **Tissue staining**
- ***Histoplasma* antigen:** From urine, blood, CSF

Table 77 Treatment of Histoplasmosis

Type of Histoplasmosis	Severe Disease	Mild to Moderate Disease
Pulmonary		
Acute	liposomal amphotericin B 3 mg/kg per day or amphotericin B lipid complex 5 mg/kg per day or amphotericin B deoxycholate 0.7-1.0 mg/kg per day for 1-2 wk, followed by itraconazole[a] 200 mg bid for 12 wk corticosteroid supplementation (optional)[b]	For symptoms of ≤4 wk: None For symptoms of >4 wk: itraconazole[a] 200 mg 1-2 times per day for 6-12 wk
Chronic cavitary	itraconazole[a] 200 mg 1-2 times per day for 12-24 mo	Same as for severe disease

(Continues)

Table 77 Treatment of Histoplasmosis (*Cont'd.*)

Type of Histoplasmosis	Severe Disease	Mild to Moderate Disease
Disseminated	liposomal amphotericin B 3 mg/kg per day, amphotericin B lipid complex 5 mg/kg per day, or amphotericin B deoxycholate 0.7-1.0 mg/kg per day for 1-2 wk; followed by itraconazole[a] 200 mg bid for at least 12 mo[c,d]	itraconazole[a] 200 mg bid for at least 12 mo[c]
Meningitis	liposomal amphotericin B 5 mg/kg per day for 4-6 wk, followed by itraconazole[a] 200 mg 2-3 times per day for at least 12 mo	Same as for severe disease
Mediastinal lymphadenitis	itraconazole[a,e] 200 mg 1-2 times per day for 6-12 wk in patients with symptoms that warrant treatment with corticosteroids or with symptoms lasting >4 wk	Mild symptoms of <4 wk: None
Mediastinal granuloma	Symptomatic patients: itraconazole[a] 200 mg 1-2 times per day for 6-12 wk	None in asymptomatic patients
Fibrosing mediastinitis	Antifungal treatment not usually indicated; stenting of obstructed vessels may be useful Select cases[f]: itraconazole[a] 200 mg 1-2 times per day for 3 mo	Same as for severe disease
Pericarditis	corticosteroids and itraconazole[a,e] 200 mg 1-2 times per day for 6-12 wk Hemodynamic compromise: Pericardial drainage	NSAIDs for 2-12 wk
Rheumatologic	corticosteroids plus itraconazole[a,e] 200 mg 1-2 times per day for 6-12 wk	NSAIDs for 2-12 wk

[a] Give itraconazole as a loading dose (200 mg tid) for 3 days followed by 200 mg bid thereafter (or once daily with mild disease). Monitoring serum itraconazole levels is recommended after 2 weeks to ensure adequate enteric drug absorption. Alternate azoles with either less activity or less published clinical data include fluconazole, voriconazole, and posaconazole.

[b] Effectiveness of corticosteroids is controversial.

[c] Therapy should be continued until *Histoplasma* antigen concentration is <2 units/mL in urine or serum. Antigen levels should be followed for 12 months after therapy has ended to monitor for early relapse of infection.

[d] Lifelong suppressive therapy may be required in AIDS patients without adequate immune reconstitution (eg, response to HAART) and in other significantly immunosuppressed patients if immunosuppression cannot be reversed.

[e] If corticosteroids are used to treat pericarditis, concurrent use of itraconazole is recommended to reduce the risk of progressive infection.

[f] Therapy is controversial and probably ineffective except in cases of mediastinal lymphadenitis or mediastinal granuloma misdiagnosed as fibrosing mediastinitis.

Adapted from Wheat LJ, et al. Clin Infect Dis. 2007 Oct 1;45(7):807–25. Epub 2007 Aug 27. Used with permission.

Blastomyces dermatitidis

General Information

- Thick-walled, broad-based budding yeasts 5-15 micrometers; common association with riverbanks, soil, decaying matter, wood

Endemic Areas

- South-central, southeastern, and midwestern US; St Lawrence river basin

Clinical Disease

- **Pulmonary disease:** Acute or chronic pneumonia; chronic infection (common) can last 2-6 months with weight loss, night sweats, and occasional cavitation
- **Skin disease:** Most common extrapulmonary finding; can present as verrucous or ulcerative lesions; subcutaneous nodules or "cold abscesses," black pepper–like lesions, or eschar formation
- **Osteomyelitis:** Occurs in up to 25% of extrapulmonary cases; noncaseating granulomas with suppuration and necrosis
- **Genitourinary infection:** Prostatitis, epididymo-orchitis
- **CNS infection:** Rare; more common in immunosuppressed patients

Diagnosis

- **Culture**
- **Tissue staining:** Characteristic broad-based budding yeasts
- **Serology:** Serologic testing is insensitive and can be negative with active disease
- ***Blastomyces* antigen:** Urine, blood

Table 78 Treatment of Blastomycosis

Type of Blastomycosis	Severe Disease	Mild to Moderate Disease
Pulmonary	liposomal amphotericin B or amphotericin B lipid complex 3-5 mg/kg per day or amphotericin B deoxycholate[c] 0.7-1.0 mg/kg per day for 1-2 wk, followed by itraconazole[a] 200 mg bid for 6-12 mo	itraconazole[a] 200 mg 1-2 times per day for 6-12 mo[b]
Disseminated	liposomal amphotericin B or amphotericin B lipid complex 3-5 mg/kg per day or amphotericin B deoxycholate[c] 0.7-1.0 mg/kg per day for 1-2 wk followed by itraconazole[a] 200 mg bid for 12 mo	itraconazole[a] 200 mg 1-2 times per day for 6-12 mo Osteoarticular disease: Treat for 12 mo

(Continues)

Table 78 Treatment of Histoplasmosis (*Cont'd.*)

Type of Blastomycosis	Severe Disease	Mild to Moderate Disease
CNS infection	liposomal amphotericin B or amphotericin B lipid complex 5 mg/kg per day for 4-6 wk (preferred) followed by an oral azole[d] for at least 1 y	Same as for severe disease
Immunosuppressed patients[e]	liposomal amphotericin B or amphotericin B lipid complex 3-5 mg/kg per day or amphotericin B deoxycholate 0.7-1.0 mg/kg per day for 1-2 wk followed by itraconazole[a] 200 mg bid for 12 mo[f]	Same as for severe disease

[a] Give itraconazole as a loading dose (200 mg tid) for 3 days followed by 200 mg bid thereafter (or once daily for mild disease). Monitoring serum itraconazole levels is recommended after 2 weeks to ensure adequate enteric drug absorption.

[b] Spontaneous cure without treatment can occur in some immunocompetent patients with mild disease; however, consideration should be given to treating all infected patients to prevent extrapulmonary dissemination.

[c] The entire course of therapy with amphotericin B deoxycholate can be given to a total of 2 g; however, most clinicians prefer to use step-down itraconazole therapy after the patient's condition improves. Liposomal amphotericin B and amphotericin B lipid complex have fewer adverse effects.

[d] Step-down therapy can be done with fluconazole 800 mg per day, itraconazole 200 mg 2-3 times per day, or voriconazole 200-400 mg bid. Longer treatment may be required for immunosuppressed patients.

[e] Includes transplant recipients or patients with HIV infection, hematologic malignancies, or other forms of immunosuppression.

[f] Life-long suppressive treatment may be required in patients with AIDS without adequate immune reconstitution (eg, response to HAART) and in other immunosuppressed patients if immunosuppression cannot be reversed.

Data from Chapman SW, et al. Clin Infect Dis. 2008 Jun 15;46(12):1801–12.

Coccidioides immitis and *C posadasii*
General Information
- Large, round spherules 20-80 micrometers containing many small endospores
- *Coccidioides* flourish just below the surface of desert soil, and outbreaks have been associated with dust storms and construction projects
- Persons of African or Filipino ancestry and immunosuppressed patients are at increased risk for disseminated disease

Endemic Areas
- Desert southwestern US, Mexico, Central America, and Argentina

Clinical Disease
- **Acute coccidioidomycosis or primary disease:** Often self-limiting
  - **Pulmonary disease:** See below
  - **Immune-mediated syndromes**
    - Migratory polyarthralgia (nondeforming), "desert rheumatism"
    - Erythema nodosum (more frequent in women), erythema multiforme ("the bumps")
  - **Valley fever:** Symptoms same as above plus fever, myalgia, malaise, peripheral blood eosinophilia
- **Pulmonary disease:** Cough, pleurisy, fever, and weight loss 1-3 weeks after exposure; hilar adenopathy, pleural effusion, or cavitation
  - **Residual pulmonary nodules:** Affects about 4% of patients after primary pneumonia
  - **Coccidioidal pulmonary cavities:** Typically thin-walled cavities (affects 2-8% of adults)
  - **Ruptured cavities:** Bronchopleural fistula can form; dyspnea and chest pain are common; can occur in young, healthy patients; not associated with immunosuppression
  - **Chronic fibrocavitary pneumonia:** Can occur in patients whose primary pneumonia fails to resolve
  - **Diffuse, reticulonodular pneumonia:** Affects immunosuppressed patients
- **Extrapulmonary disease**
  - **Cutaneous disease:** Most common site of dissemination; granulomas; subcutaneous abscesses; plaques with wart-like appearance
  - **Osteomyelitis and joint infections:** Typically in weight-bearing joints
  - **Meningitis and CNS disease:** Basilar disease; hydrocephalus is common; CSF eosinophilia is common
  - **Other (less common) sites:** Endocrine glands, eyes, liver, kidneys, genitalia, prostate, peritoneal cavity

Diagnosis
- **Culture**
- **Tissue staining:** Identify characteristic spherules containing endospores
- **Serology:** Can be false-negative early in disease
  - **Complement fixation:** Height of complement fixation titer can correlate with disease extent and response to therapy; serial or longitudinal complement fixation testing should be done consistently in the same laboratory
  - **Immunodiffusion**
  - **Enzyme immunoassay**
- **Note:** Peripheral blood eosinophilia may be present

Treatment
- Antifungal treatment options include the following:
  - fluconazole 400 mg/day (higher dosing can be used initially for CNS disease)
  - itraconazole 200 mg tid for 3 days followed by 200 mg bid thereafter. Monitoring serum itraconazole levels is recommended after 2 weeks to ensure adequate enteric drug absorption

- liposomal amphotericin B or amphotericin B lipid complex 3-5 mg/kg per day; or amphotericin B deoxycholate 0.7-1.0 mg/kg per day
- voriconazole and posaconazole are alternate azoles with anti-*Coccidioides* activity but with less published clinical experience
- Relapse is common, especially for meningitis
- **Pulmonary disease**
  - **Acute, uncomplicated pulmonary disease:** May be observed without treatment; however, treatment is recommended with either fluconazole or itraconazole for 3-6 months for the following:
    - Immunosuppressive conditions
    - Significant and/or persisting pulmonary or extrapulmonary symptoms; loss of >10% body weight; chest radiograph with infiltrates in over half of lung or in both lungs
    - Consider treatment in patient with serum complement fixation titer >1:16
  - **Diffuse or progressive pulmonary disease:** Administer amphotericin B product initially, followed by fluconazole or itraconazole for at least 1 year
  - **Pulmonary nodule (asymptomatic):** Monitor without treatment; follow radiologically for 2 years to ensure no progression
  - **Pulmonary cavity**
    - **Asymptomatic:** Most authorities would not treat (but patients should be followed clinically and radiologically)
    - **Symptomatic:** Antifungal therapy warranted (variable duration); check for bacterial superinfection; surgical resection considered in select cases
    - **Ruptured coccidioidal cavity in pleural space:** Well-recognized complication; surgical resection and antifungal therapy recommended (variable duration)
  - **Chronic fibrocavitary pneumonia:** Antifungal therapy for at least 1 year and surgery for refractory lesions or hemoptysis
- **Osteoarticular disease:** Antifungal therapy with surgical debridement; variable treatment duration (eg, 6-12 months), depending on disease location, extent, and response to therapy (eg, monitor erythrocyte sedimentation rate, C-reactive protein, and anti-*Coccidioides* complement fixation serologic titers)
- **Meningitis and other CNS infections**
  - Therapy with fluconazole (400-1,000 mg daily) is preferable (consider beginning with fluconazole 800-1,000 mg daily); alternate treatments include IV or intrathecal amphotericin B product, voriconazole, and itraconazole
  - For patients who respond to azole therapy, consider continuation of azole treatment indefinitely to prevent relapse
  - Patients who do not respond initially to systemic treatment may be candidates for intrathecal amphotericin B therapy 0.1-1.5 mg per dose ranging from daily to weekly therapy
  - Monitor for associated CNS vasculitis

Paracoccidioides brasiliensis

General Information
- Reproduces by multiple, budding "pilot wheel" (South American blastomycosis)
- Most cases are found in men (15:1)

Endemic Areas
- Latin America from Mexico to Argentina; especially Brazil, Colombia, Argentina, and Venezuela

Clinical Disease
- **Lungs:** Usual portal of entry; patchy or confluent infiltrate; bullae can form; 2 types
  - **Juvenile form:** More chronic course; more severe prognosis; minimal respiratory symptoms
  - **Adult form:** More clinically significant respiratory symptoms; better outcome
- **Mucosal ulcerations:** Mouth, lips, gums, tongue, palate (granulomatous appearance), nose
- **Skin:** Warty, ulcerative lesions; crusting; granulomatous
- **Lymphadenopathy:** Cervical, axillary, mesenteric, mediastinal

Treatment
- Either itraconazole or ketoconazole for at least 6 months (≥12 months for more severe disease)
- sulfonamides (eg, sulfadiazine, trimethoprim-sulfamethoxazole)
- amphotericin B product (in combination therapy)
- Additional active drugs but with less clinical experience include posaconazole and voriconazole

Sporothrix schenckii

General Information
- Oval- or cigar-shaped budding yeast at 37°C
- Common in soil, plants, or plant products such as straw, wood, sphagnum moss, and thorny plants
- Infection commonly due to mild skin trauma (eg, contact with plants or rose thorns while gardening) with potential lymphatic or hematogenous spread); less commonly by inhalation

Clinical Disease
- **Cutaneous infection:** By local skin trauma
  - **Plaque sporotrichosis:** Nontender plaque
  - **Lymphocutaneous sporotrichosis:** Multiple nodular lesions following lymphatic path
  - Tissue biopsy with stain and culture important to exclude *Mycobacterium marinum* and *Nocardia*, which can have a similar clinical appearance
- **Extracutaneous disease**
  - **Osteoarticular disease:** *S schenckii* infection has a distinct predilection for joints (chronic arthritis)
  - **CNS disease:** Typically produces chronic meningitis
  - **Pulmonary disease:** Subacute or chronic; cavitation usually in upper lobes

Treatment

- **Lymphocutaneous and cutaneous disease:** First-line treatment is itraconazole for 3-6 months; alternate treatments include high-dose terbinafine-saturated solution of potassium iodide, fluconazole (less effective), and local hyperthermia
- **Pulmonary sporotrichosis:** Chronic cavitary fibronodular disease
  - Treat with amphotericin B product or itraconazole
  - Surgical resection may be required, especially with cavitary disease
- **Osteoarticular disease:** First-line treatment is itraconazole (for at least 1 year); alternate treatments include amphotericin B product or fluconazole
- **Meningeal disease:** Treat with amphotericin B product
- **Severe or disseminated disease:** IV amphotericin B product; change to itraconazole as patient's condition stabilizes and improves

Aspergillus

General Information

- Filamentous, narrow, nonpigmented, septated hyphae with branching at 45° angles
- Angioinvasive pattern
- **Laboratory testing:** Blood and CSF cultures rarely yield *Aspergillus*; galactomannan antigen (serum, bronchial lavage, or wash); serum (1,3)-β-D-glucan; tissue examination
- **Definitive diagnosis:** Requires both histopathologic evidence (eg, invasive hyphae) and positive *Aspergillus* culture
- Tissue morphology of branching, septated hyphae is not specific for *Aspergillus* and is also characteristic of *Fusarium*, *Pseudallescheria boydii*, and agents of phaeohyphomycosis; Zygomycetes may also have similar appearance but with minimal or no septa

Clinical Disease and Treatment

- **Active antifungal agents:**
  - liposomal amphotericin B 3-5 mg/kg per day,[a] amphotericin B lipid complex 5 mg/kg per day, or amphotericin B deoxycholate 0.7-1.0 mg/kg per day
  - voriconazole IV 6 mg/kg every 12 hours for 1 day followed by 4 mg/kg bid or 200 to 300 mg oral bid
  - itraconazole 200 mg oral tid for 3 days followed by 200 mg bid thereafter. Monitoring serum itraconazole levels is recommended after 1-2 weeks to ensure adequate enteric drug absorption; dose adjustments may be required.
  - posaconazole[b] 200 mg oral qid or 400 mg oral bid. Monitoring serum posaconazole levels is strongly recommended after 1-2 weeks to ensure adequate enteric drug absorption.
  - caspofungin 70 mg IV once, then 50 mg IV daily
  - anidulafungin[b] 200 mg IV once, then 100 mg IV daily
  - micafungin[b] 100-150 mg IV daily

---

[a] Many providers favor 5 mg/kg per day dosing of liposomal amphotericin B for treatment of invasive aspergillosis in patients with normal renal function

[b] Not approved for treatment of invasive aspergillosis

- **Invasive aspergillosis**
- **Invasive pulmonary aspergillosis:** Angioinvasive disease typically in immunosuppressed patients (eg, neutropenia); hemoptysis and pulmonary hemorrhage are common
  - **Chest radiograph (variable):** Nodular or wedge-shaped pleural densities; cavities may occur later
  - **Chest CT (variable):** Nodular lesions; halo sign may be present early (area of low attenuation surrounding nodular lung lesion); later a crescent sign might appear (air crescent near periphery of lung nodule caused by contracted lung tissue); both halo and crescent signs are nonspecific and are also seen in mucormycosis and other filamentous fungal diseases
  - **Treatment:** voriconazole preferred; alternates include amphotericin B product, posaconazole, itraconazole, echinocandins
    - Optimal duration for invasive pulmonary aspergillosis varies (minimum of 6-12 weeks; commonly longer); continue during period(s) of immunosuppression and until pulmonary lesions resolve
    - After successful treatment of aspergillosis, resume antifungal therapy in patients receiving additional (induction or consolidation) chemotherapy, undergoing transplantation, or beginning other significant forms of immunosuppression
    - Surgical resection of isolated lesion (eg, large or cavitary) considered in select patients who require additional chemotherapy or transplantation
    - Role of combination therapy remains unclear (under investigation); in select cases, it is considered salvage therapy
    - *Aspergillus terreus* is less susceptible to amphotericin B therapy and more responsive to voriconazole, posaconazole, itraconazole, or echinocandins
- **Chronic necrotizing pulmonary aspergillosis (CNPA):** Slowly progressive, chronic inflammatory destruction with local fungal tissue invasion in patients with underlying structural lung disease and low-grade immunosuppression (eg, due to diabetes mellitus, low-dose corticosteroids, connective tissue diseases); diagnosis is often delayed
  - **Chest imagining (variable):** Cavitary disease with mycetoma occurs in about 50% of patients
  - **Treatment:** Typically prolonged oral azole or amphotericin B product therapy; adjunct surgical resection in select cases (eg, hemoptysis, large cavities)
- **Acute invasive sinus aspergillosis:** Rapidly progressive disease in neutropenic patients with spread to contiguous structures, including eyes and brain
  - **Diagnosis:** Urgent endoscopic inspection in neutropenic patient with biopsy and culture of suspicious mucosal lesions to document tissue invasion and identify invasive fungus species
  - **Treatment:** Combined medical and surgical debridement approach; voriconazole preferred if *Aspergillus* confirmed (eg, not mucormycosis); amphotericin B product for initial or empiric treatment if fungal species is not yet confirmed. Alternates include

posaconazole, itraconazole, or an echinocandin, depending on fungus type and extent of disease.

- **Chronic invasive sinusitis:** May occur in immunocompetent or mildly immunocompromised patients; slower progression of months to years
  - **Diagnosis:** Endoscopic inspection with biopsy and culture
  - **Treatment:** Surgical debridement and drainage; antifungal therapy for significant invasive disease
- **CNS aspergillosis:** Abscess, meningitis, epidural abscess, subarachnoid hemorrhage
  - Disease development by hematogenous dissemination or direct extension of sinus infection
  - **Treatment:** Preferably voriconazole (if mucormycosis is excluded); alternates include amphotericin B product, itraconazole, posaconazole; surgery may be required for diagnosis and determination of adjunct medical therapy; debride as much of lesion as possible
- **Endocarditis (large vegetations)**
  - Vegetations (large, high embolization risk) are more common on prosthetic valves but also are reported on healthy native valves; blood cultures are rarely positive despite high-grade endovascular infection
  - **Treatment:** Early surgical resection or valve replacement with antifungal therapy; voriconazole or amphotericin B product recommended; lifelong antifungal therapy should be considered
- **Bone and joint aspergillosis**
  - Vertebrae and disks are most common hematogenous locations of infection; localized disease through trauma
  - **Treatment:** Combination surgical debridement and medical therapy: voriconazole preferred; alternates include amphotericin B product, posaconazole, itraconazole, echinocandins
- **Ocular aspergillosis:** Rapidly progressive disease (ophthalmologic emergency)
  - **Endophthalmitis:** Diagnosis by vitreal aspiration
    - **Treatment:** Intravitreal amphotericin B with pars plana vitrectomy (when appropriate) with IV amphotericin B product; intravitreal and/or systemic voriconazole
  - **Keratitis:** Locally invasive corneal infection
    - **Treatment:** Topical amphotericin B eye drops; other adjunct therapies include intracameral injection of amphotericin B (into anterior chamber); oral, systemic, or intracameral voriconazole; itraconazole
- **Saprophytic aspergillosis**
  - **Pulmonary aspergilloma:** Noninvasive or minimally invasive fungal mass that exists in lung cavity (eg, in old tuberculosis cavities); patients usually have chronic pulmonary disease; overlap exists between fungal colonization and tissue invasion
  - **Chronic cavitary pulmonary aspergillosis:** Slowly progressive (years); typically consists of multiple cavities that may coalesce; may contain an aspergilloma; typically no visible or significant hyphae invasion of tissue; hemoptysis can occur

- **Treatment:** Systemic antifungal therapy with voriconazole or itraconazole
- ***Aspergillus* otomycosis:** Both colonization with tissue irritation (common) and localized invasion (usually with immunosuppression or anatomical defect present) can occur
  - **No tissue invasion:** Local cleaning measures, cerumen removal, topical therapy
  - **Tissue invasion:** Systemic antifungal therapy with surgical evaluation
- ***Aspergillus* airway colonization:** Common in patients with chronic structural lung disease, chronic obstructive pulmonary disease, bronchiectasis; does not require treatment

- Allergic *Aspergillus* disease
  - **Allergic bronchopulmonary aspergillosis:** A type of hypersensitivity pneumonitis
    - **Diagnosis:** Constellation of asthma, peripheral blood eosinophilia, precipitating antibodies to *Aspergillus*, scratch test reactivity to *Aspergillus* antigen, elevated serum IgE (immunoglobulin E), history of pulmonary infiltrates (transient or fixed) and central bronchiectasis; supporting findings include repeat *Aspergillus* culture growth from sputum, history of brown plugs or flecks in sputum, elevated IgE concentration against *Aspergillus* antigen, and Arthrus reaction (late skin reaction) to *Aspergillus* antigen
    - **Chest radiographs:** May show transient areas of consolidation, more commonly in upper lobes; "fleeting shadows" are common
    - **Treatment:** Primary treatment is with corticosteroids; oral antifungal therapy may be a useful adjunct as a steroid-sparing agent
  - **Allergic *Aspergillus* sinusitis:** Typically affects immunocompetent patients, common history of asthma or polyps, chronic disease (months to years) common; note that allergic fungal sinusitis not specific to *Aspergillus* can be produced by environmental exposures to dematiaceous and other fungi
    - **Diagnosis:** Endoscopic findings of allergic mucin (identified grossly or histopathologically) with fungal elements but without fungal tissue invasion
    - **Treatment:** Endoscopic drainage if obstruction is present; itraconazole can be used as an adjunct; possible role for nasal or systemic corticosteroids in select patients; antibacterial agents if secondary bacterial infection present

Additional information available in Walsh TJ, et al. Clin Infect Dis. 2008 Feb 1;46(3):327–60

Agents of Mucormycosis

General Characteristics

- **Appearance:** Broad nonseptate (or few septate) hyphae with right-angle branches; Gomori methenamine silver stain is less reliable for identification of mucormycosis; possibly add periodic acid–Schiff reaction stain if hematoxylin-eosin tissue stain is suggestive of fungal infection

- **Angioinvasive organism:** Leads to tissue infarction and necrosis (eg, in sinuses or lungs); typically in immunosuppressed patients (eg, with prolonged neutropenia); disease progression can be rapid
- **Course:** Grows best in low-pH, high-glucose environment (eg, diabetic ketoacidosis) and is associated with deferoxamine treatment
- **Species common with human infection:** *Rhizopus, Cunninghamella, Mucor, Syncephalastrum, Rhizomucor, Apophysomyces, Absidia,* and *Saksenaea*

Clinical Disease (Usually in Immunocompromised Patients)
- **Rhinocerebral infection:** Most common clinical presentation of mucormycosis
  - Initial acute sinusitis with necrosis of nasal septum and turbinates; rapid spread to contiguous structures (eg, palate, orbits, brain)
  - Secondary CNS infection common with 80-90% mortality
- **Pulmonary:** Angioinvasive disease of pulmonary vessels with secondary necrosis and hemorrhage; can appear in similar fashion to aspergillosis including radiographic halo and air crescent signs
- **Other organ system involvement:** Cutaneous (eg, skin trauma or inoculation, tissue necrosis, black eschar); gastrointestinal mucormycosis (less common) with involvement of stomach (58%) and colon (32%); renal mucormycosis; isolated involvement of CNS
- **Treatment:** Can be difficult without immunologic recovery
  - liposomal amphotericin B or amphotericin B lipid complex 5-7.5 mg/kg per day, or amphotericin B deoxycholate 1 mg/kg per day
  - posaconazole 200 mg oral qid or 400 mg oral bid. Monitoring of serum posaconazole levels is strongly recommended after 1-2 weeks to ensure adequate enteric drug absorption.
  - Prompt surgical debridement is required for rhinocerebral disease; ideal for other sites, if possible

Antiretroviral Therapy for HIV Infection

Elements of Diagnosis and Clinical Issues Related to Starting Therapy

- Obtain confirmatory human immunodeficiency virus (HIV) testing by rapid test or enzyme-linked immunosorbent assay (ELISA); optimally repeat HIV viral load (VL) and CD4 T-cell (CD4) count 2 times before initiation of therapy; a substantial change in CD4 count is generally >30%
- Perform VL immediately before treatment initiation (or change in therapy) and again 2-8 weeks later; for the latter, the optimal decrease would be at least 1 log
- Conduct resistance testing for acute HIV infection, for chronic HIV infection before initiation of therapy, and (if HIV VL >1,000 copies/mL) for virologic failure or suboptimal response
- Obtain baseline testing of HIV VL, CD4 count, complete blood cell count (CBC), chemistries (eg, renal and liver function, lipids, glucose), urinalysis, sexually transmitted disease testing, serologies (for cytomegalovirus [CMV], toxoplasmosis, and hepatitis), tuberculin test, chest radiograph, urinalysis, Papanicolaou test, and (as appropriate) specific opportunistic infection testing
- Obtain patient history of vaccinations, HIV risk factors, probable exposures, allergies, substance abuse, psychiatric history, opportunistic infections, cardiac risk factors, pregnancy or lactation status, current medications (including alternative or herbal medications), history of previous antiretrovirals, results of previous resistance testing, medication adherence issues, and social issues that may affect adherence
- Perform extensive counseling about implications of the diagnosis, transmission risk factors, and prognosis. Patients initiating antiretroviral treatment should be willing and able to commit to lifelong treatment. They should understand the risks and benefits of therapy, and the importance of adherence. Patients may choose to postpone therapy, or the provider may decide to defer therapy on the basis of clinical and psychosocial factors.
- Review potential drug interactions before initiating therapy or adding any new medication
- Drug-specific testing: Obtain HLA-B*5701 testing if considering abacavir therapy. Obtain tropism testing if considering maraviroc therapy. Obtain a pregnancy test in women of childbearing age if considering efavirenz.
- Focus on treatment goals of reducing HIV-related morbidity or mortality, improving quality of life, restoring or preserving immune function, and maximally and durably suppressing HIV VL

Table 79 Indications for Antiretroviral Therapy

Clinical Category	CD4 Count	Plasma Viral RNA, Copies/mL	Recommendation
Symptomatic (eg, AIDS-defining illness, severe symptoms)	Any value	Any value	Treat
Asymptomatic	CD4 <500/mcL	Any value	Treat
Asymptomatic	CD4 >500/mcL	Any value	Treatment is reasonable but negotiable; discuss pros and cons of early treatment vs waiting
Pregnant patients (regardless of symptoms)	Any value	Any value	Treat pregnant patients to prevent mother-to-child transmission; preferred agents are lopinavir/ritonavir and zidovudine/lamivudine
			Refer to USDHHS guidelines for detailed information
Coinfected with HBV	Any value	Any value	Treat (if therapy for HBV is indicated)
			tenofovir plus either emtricitabine or lamivudine should be part of treatment program
HIV-related nephropathy	Any value	Any value	Treat

Adapted from Panel on Antiretroviral Guidelines for Adults and Adolescents [Internet]. Department of Health and Human Services. Jan 10, 2011 [cited 2011 Mar 14]. Available from: http://aidsinfo.nih.gov/ContentFiles/AdultandAdolescentGL.pdf.

Table 80 Preferred Antiretroviral Agents for Treatment-Naive HIV Patients Who Are Not Pregnant[a,b]
(Individualize the antiretroviral regimen on the basis of patient- and drug-specific factors.)

Preferred regimens

- **NNRTI-based regimen**
  - efavirenz/tenofovir/emtricitabine (coformulated)
- **Integrase-inhibitor–based regimen**
  - raltegravir plus tenofovir/emtricitabine (coformulated)
- **PI-based regimens** *(in alphabetical order)*
  - Boosted atazanavir plus tenofovir/emtricitabine (coformulated)
  - Boosted darunavir plus tenofovir/emtricitabine (coformulated)
- **Preferred regimen for pregnant women**
  - lopinavir/ritonavir (coformulated) plus zidovudine/lamivudine (coformulated)

Alternate regimens

- **NNRTI-based regimens** *(in alphabetical order)*
  - efavirenz plus **EITHER** abacavir[c]/lamivudine (coformulated) **OR** zidovudine/lamivudine (coformulated)
  - nevirapine plus zidovudine/lamivudine (coformulated)
- **PI-based regimens** *(in alphabetical order)*
  - Boosted atazanavir plus **EITHER** abacavir[c]/lamivudine (coformulated) **OR** zidovudine/lamivudine (coformulated)
  - Boosted fosamprenavir plus 1 of the following: abacavir[c]/lamivudine (coformulated); **OR** zidovudine/lamivudine (coformulated); **OR** tenofovir/emtricitabine (coformulated)
  - lopinavir/ritonavir (coformulated) plus 1 of the following: abacavir[c]/lamivudine (coformulated); **OR** zidovudine/lamivudine (coformulated); **OR** tenofovir/emtricitabine (coformulated)

Acceptable but less satisfactory regimens[d]

- **NNRTI-based regimen**
  - efavirenz plus didanosine and **EITHER** lamivudine **OR** emtricitabine
- **PI-based regimens**
  - atazanavir plus ritonavir and **EITHER** abacavir[c]/lamivudine (coformulated) **OR** zidovudine/lamivudine (coformulated)
- **Integrase-inhibitor regimen**
  - raltegravir plus **EITHER** abacavir[c]/lamivudine (coformulated) **OR** zidovudine/lamivudine (coformulated)
- **CCR5 antagonist–based regimens**
  - maraviroc plus zidovudine/lamivudine (coformulated)
  - maraviroc plus **EITHER** tenofovir/emtricitabine (coformulated) **OR** abacavir[c]/lamivudine (coformulated)

---

[a] Adapted from Panel on Antiretroviral Guidelines for Adults and Adolescents [Internet]. Department of Health and Human Services. Jan 10, 2011 [cited 2011 Mar 14]. Available from: http://aidsinfo.nih.gov/ContentFiles/AdultandAdolescentGL.pdf.

[b] Specific combinations of drugs are preferred in the USDHHS guidelines.

[c] Use abacavir only if HLA-B*5701 test is negative.

[d] These regimens are less satisfactory than preferred regimens or more definitive data are needed to support their use.

Table 81 Nucleoside or Nucleotide Reverse Transcriptase Inhibitors (NRTIs): Select Characteristics

Medication	Usual Adult Dose (Without Organ Dysfunction)	Dosing Instructions
abacavir (Ziagen)	300 mg bid or 600 mg daily	Take without regard to food
	No dose adjustment needed for renal dysfunction	
	Adjust dosage with liver disease; contraindicated with severe liver disease	
abacavir 600 mg plus lamivudine 300 mg (coformulated [Epzicom])	1 tab once daily	Take without regard to food
	Cl_{Cr} <50 mL/min: Give separately with renal-adjusted dosing as per individual agents	
abacavir 300 mg plus lamivudine 150 mg and zidovudine 300 mg (coformulated [Trizivir])	If >40 kg: 1 tab bid	Take without regard to food
	Cl_{Cr} <50 mL/min: Give separately with renal-adjusted dosing as per individual agents	

Adverse Effects	Metabolism or Excretion Route and Pharmacokinetic Drug Interaction Potential[a,b]
All patients initiating abacavir should be confirmed as HLA-B*5701 negative because of increased risk of hypersensitivity reaction (fever, malaise, GI effects, rash, respiratory symptoms, and elevated transaminases and creatine kinase, respiratory symptoms) with the HLA-B*5701 allele that can be severe or fatal (usually within days to 6 wk after initiation of abacavir)	Hepatic metabolism by alcohol dehydrogenase or glucuronyl transferase, with renal excretion of metabolites
	May inhibit or be affected by other drugs that inhibit alcohol dehydrogenase or UDP-glucuronyl transferase
Rechallenge after hypersensitivity reaction is contraindicated because of possibly severe or fatal consequences	Alcohol increases abacavir levels
GI intolerance, fever, malaise, headache, increased transaminases	
Possible increased risk of myocardial infarction	
Possible shorter time to virologic failure in patients with VL >100,000 compared to that with other NRTIs	
NRTI class side effects: Fat redistribution; lactic acidosis and hepatomegaly with steatosis (infrequent)	
Pregnancy category C	
See individual agents	See individual agents
See individual agents	See individual agents

(Continues)

Table 81 Nucleoside or Nucleotide Reverse Transcriptase Inhibitors (NRTIs): Select Characteristics (*Cont'd.*)

Medication	Usual Adult Dose (Without Organ Dysfunction)	Dosing Instructions
didanosine (Videx EC)	If ≥60 kg: EC capsules: 400 mg once daily	Take on empty stomach
	With tenofovir: 250 mg once daily	
	If <60 kg: EC capsules: 250 mg once daily	
	With tenofovir: 200 mg once daily	
	Cl_{cr} <60 mL/min: Reduce dose	
efavirenz 600 mg plus emtricitabine 200 mg and tenofovir 300 mg (coformulated [Atripla])	1 tab once daily	Do not take with high-fat meal
	Cl_{cr} <50 mL/min: Give separately in renal-adjusted dosing as per individual agents	Take at bedtime at least to start with
emtricitabine (Emtriva)	200 mg once daily	Take without regard to food
	Cl_{cr} <50 mL/min: Reduce dose	
emtricitabine 200 mg plus tenofovir 300 mg (coformulated [Truvada])	1 tab once daily	Take without regard to food
lamivudine (Epivir)	If ≥50 kg: 150 mg bid or 300 mg once daily	Take without regard to food
	If <50 kg: 2 mg/kg bid	
	Cl_{cr} <50 mL/min: Reduce dose	

Adverse Effects	Metabolism or Excretion Route and Pharmacokinetic Drug Interaction Potential[a,b]
Pancreatitis, peripheral neuropathy, GI intolerance; also associated with portal hypertension and esophageal varices	50% renally cleared
	tenofovir can significantly increase didanosine levels; reduce didanosine dose
Fatal lactic acidosis has been reported in pregnant patients receiving stavudine plus didanosine; avoid combination, especially in pregnancy	ribavirin can increase didanosine exposure and risk of toxicity; use combination with caution
NRTI class side effects: Fat redistribution; lactic acidosis and hepatomegaly with steatosis	methadone can decrease didanosine levels; consider dose increase
Pregnancy category B	hydroxyurea can increase potential for toxicity; avoid concomitant use
	Use cautiously with drugs that cause neuropathy
	Avoid combination of stavudine and didanosine because of increased risk of lactic acidosis
See individual agents	See individual agents
Generally well tolerated; headache, diarrhea, nausea, rash; generally mild skin discoloration (hyperpigmentation on palms or soles)	Renal excretion
Active against HBV; may see flare on discontinuation	
NRTI class side effects: Fat redistribution; lactic acidosis and hepatomegaly with steatosis (infrequent)	
Pregnancy category B	
See individual agents	See individual agents
Generally well tolerated; headache, nausea, diarrhea, abdominal pain, rash, pancreatitis in pediatric patients (rare in adults)	Renal excretion; adjust dosage for renal insufficiency or failure
Active against HBV; may see flare on discontinuation	

(Continues)

Table 81 Nucleoside or Nucleotide Reverse Transcriptase Inhibitors (NRTIs): Select Characteristics (*Cont'd.*)

Medication	Usual Adult Dose (Without Organ Dysfunction)	Dosing Instructions
lamivudine (Epivir) (continued)		
lamivudine 150 mg plus zidovudine 300 mg (coformulated [Combivir]) **Preferred NRTI backbone in pregnant women**	1 tab bid Cl$_{Cr}$ <50 mL/min: Give separately in renal-adjusted dosing as per individual agents	Take without regard to food
stavudine (Zerit)	If ≥60 kg: 40 mg bid If <60 kg: 30 mg bid Cl$_{Cr}$ <50 mL/min: Reduce dose	Take without regard to food
tenofovir (Viread)	300 mg once daily Cl$_{Cr}$ <50 mL/min: Reduce dose	Take without regard to food

Adverse Effects	Metabolism or Excretion Route and Pharmacokinetic Drug Interaction Potential[a,b]
NRTI class side effects: Fat redistribution; lactic acidosis and hepatomegaly with steatosis (infrequent)	
Pregnancy category C	
See individual agents	See individual agents
Peripheral neuropathy, GI intolerance, headache, insomnia, pancreatitis, hyperlipidemia, ascending neuromuscular weakness	50% renally cleared
	Increased risk of pancreatitis, neuropathy, hepatotoxicity, and lactic acidosis when combined with didanosine
Fatal lactic acidosis reported in pregnant patients receiving stavudine plus didanosine; avoid combination in pregnancy	
NRTI class side effects: Fat redistribution or lipoatrophy; lactic acidosis and hepatomegaly with steatosis (higher frequency with stavudine)	
Pregnancy category C	
Mild GI complaints, asthenia, headache; renal dysfunction including Fanconi syndrome; osteomalacia	Renally cleared
	Can substantially increase didanosine levels; reduce didanosine dose
Active against HBV; flare may occur on discontinuation	Can decrease atazanavir levels; use atazanavir in combination with ritonavir
NRTI class side effects: Fat redistribution; lactic acidosis and hepatomegaly with steatosis (infrequent)	Concomitant therapy with ritonavir, lopinavir, atazanavir, or didanosine can increase tenofovir levels and toxicity; monitor closely
Pregnancy category B	cidofovir, ganciclovir, and valganciclovir can compete for tubular secretion; monitor closely

(*Continues*)

Table 81 Nucleoside or Nucleotide Reverse Transcriptase Inhibitors (NRTIs): Select Characteristics (Cont'd.)

Medication	Usual Adult Dose (Without Organ Dysfunction)	Dosing Instructions
zidovudine (Retrovir)	300 mg bid Cl$_{cr}$ <15 mL/min: Reduce dose	Take without regard to food

[a] Drug interactions listed here are not all-inclusive and do not include drugs with overlapping toxicities.

[b] See individual drug package insert and other resources for specific drug interactions.

Adapted from Panel on Antiretroviral Guidelines for Adults and Adolescents [Internet]. Department of Health and Human Services. Jan 10, 2011 [cited 2011 Mar 14]. Available from: http://aidsinfo.nih.gov/ContentFiles/AdultandAdolescentGL.pdf.

Table 82 Non-Nucleoside Reverse Transcriptase Inhibitors (NNRTIs): Select Characteristics

Medication	Usual Adult Dose (Without Organ Dysfunction)	Dosing Instructions
delavirdine (Rescriptor)	400 mg tid	Take without regard to food
efavirenz (Sustiva)	600 mg once daily (preferably at bedtime to start)	Take with or without food; avoid high-fat meals, which can increase bioavailability (by up to 50%)

Adverse Effects	Metabolism or Excretion Route and Pharmacokinetic Drug Interaction Potential[a,b]
Macrocytic anemia or neutropenia; malaise, GI intolerance, insomnia, asthenia; myalgia, myopathy	Hepatic metabolism with renal clearance of metabolites
NRTI class side effects: Fat redistribution; lactic acidosis and hepatomegaly with steatosis	ribavirin can inhibit phosphorylation and activation of zidovudine
Pregnancy category C	

Adverse Effects	Metabolism or Excretion Route and Pharmacokinetic Drug Interaction Potential[a,b]
Skin rash (common); can usually treat through but may be serious in some cases	Hepatic metabolism
Mild headache, fatigue, GI complaints, increased transaminases	Substrate for CYP3A4[c,d] and CYP2D6
Pregnancy category C	Can inhibit CYP3A4,[e] CYP2D6, CYP2C9, and CYP2C19
	Avoid H_2-receptor antagonists or PPIs
Rash (can usually treat through if mild)	Hepatic metabolism
CNS symptoms (eg, dizziness, light-headedness, nightmares, feelings of disengagement, impaired concentration, agitation); can be minimized by taking at bedtime and often subside after 2-4 wk	Substrate for CYP3A4[c,d]
	Can induce or inhibit CYP3A4[e]
	Can decrease methadone levels or effects; titrate dose
Case reports of psychosis, delusional thoughts, suicidal ideation, and depression (more frequent in patients with history of mental illness)	Accelerates the metabolism of protease inhibitors and many other drugs
Increased transaminases, especially in patients with hepatitis	
Mild increase in cholesterol and triglycerides in some patients	
False-positive urine screening test for marijuana	

(Continues)

Table 82 Non-Nucleoside Reverse Transcriptase Inhibitors (NNRTIs): Select Characteristics (*Cont'd.*)

Medication	Usual Adult Dose (Without Organ Dysfunction)	Dosing Instructions
efavirenz (Sustiva) (continued)		
efavirenz 600 mg plus emtricitabine 200 mg and tenofovir 300 mg (coformulated [Atripla])	1 tab once daily Cl_{Cr} <50 mL/min: Give separately in dosing as per individual agents	Take on an empty stomach (or not with high-fat meal); take at bedtime to start with
etravirine	200 mg bid	Take after a meal, not on an empty stomach
nevirapine (Viramune)	200 mg once daily for 14 days then either 200 mg immediate release bid or 400 mg XR once daily Contraindicated with significant liver disease	Start with 2-wk lead-in of reduced dose to reduce incidence of rash Autoinduction occurs and stabilizes at 2-4 wk Take without regard to food
rilpivirine (Edurant)	25 mg daily	Take with food

ᵃ Drug interactions listed here are not all-inclusive and do not include drugs with overlapping toxicities.

ᵇ See individual drug package insert and other resources for specific drug interactions.

Adverse Effects	Metabolism or Excretion Route and Pharmacokinetic Drug Interaction Potential[a,b]
Pregnancy category D (avoid in pregnant patients or patients likely to become pregnant)	
See individual agents	See individual agents
Rash (usually resolves without discontinuing etravirine but can occasionally be serious)	Substrate for CYP3A4, CYP2C9, and CYP2C19
Nausea and diarrhea	Induces CYP3A4 and inhibits CYP2C9 and CYP2C19
Elevated transaminases particularly in patients with HBV or HCV	Many interactions with other antiretrovirals; interactions with many anticonvulsants and other medications
Lipid and glucose elevation can occur	
Pregnancy category B	
Rash (can usually treat through if mild); rare serious cutaneous reactions (eg, Stevens-Johnson syndrome)	Hepatic metabolism
	Substrate for CYP3A4[c,d]
Severe and fatal cases of hepatitis reported, particularly in first 18 wk; risk of hepatotoxicity may increase with elevated transaminases, history of HBV or HCV, CD4 >250/mcL in women, and CD4 >400/mcL in men; if hepatitis occurs, discontinue nevirapine permanently; during first 8 wk, monitor patients intensively for serious cutaneous reactions and signs of hepatotoxicity	Induces CYP3A4[e]
	Decreases methadone levels
	Decreases oral contraceptive levels; use alternate method of birth control
Pregnancy category C	
Higher virologic failure with VL>100,000	Hepatic metabolism
Headache, insomnia, and rash	Substrate for CYP 3A4[c,d]
Depression	Avoid concomitant use of PPIs and space apart from H$_2$ receptor antagonists
Prolonged QT interval possible	Avoid coadministration with QT-prolonging medications

(*Continues*)

Table 82 Non-Nucleoside Reverse Transcriptase Inhibitors (NNRTIs): Select Characteristics (*Cont'd.*)

[c] Abbreviated list of CYP3A4 **inducers** that can decrease serum levels of substrates for CYP3A4 (eg, PIs, NNRTIs): rifampin, rifabutin, rifapentine, carbamazepine, phenobarbital, phenytoin, nevirapine, efavirenz, St. John's wort.

[d] Abbreviated list of CYP3A4 **inhibitors** that can potentially increase serum levels of substrates for CYP3A4 (eg, PIs, NNRTIs): PIs, erythromycin, clarithromycin, azole antifungals, amiodarone, cimetidine, grapefruit juice.

[e] Abbreviated list of CYP3A4 **substrates** (serum levels can be increased by CYP3A4 inhibitors such as PIs and decreased by CYP3A4 inducers such as nevirapine or efavirenz): benzodiazepines (avoid midazolam or triazolam; lorazepam can be used with PIs); statins (avoid use of lovastatin or simvastatin with PIs; pravastatin and fluvastatin do not significantly interact with PIs, and atorvastatin and rosuvastatin can be used with caution and monitoring); dihydropyridine calcium channel blockers; ergot alkaloids (avoid with PIs); sildenafil, vardenafil, and tadalafil (dose reduction of erectile dysfunction drugs needed with PIs); some antiarrhythmics (eg, amiodarone, lidocaine, quinidine); warfarin; pimozide (avoid with PIs); rifabutin (may need dose alterations of 1 or both drugs); some antidepressants and anticonvulsants (eg, carbamazepine, phenytoin, phenobarbital); immunosuppressants (eg, cyclosporine, tacrolimus, sirolimus); azole antifungals.

Adapted from Panel on Antiretroviral Guidelines for Adults and Adolescents [Internet]. Department of Health and Human Services. Jan 10, 2011 [cited 2011 Mar 14]. Available from: http://aidsinfo.nih.gov/ContentFiles/AdultandAdolescentGL.pdf.

Table 83 Select Characteristics of PIs

Medication	Usual Adult Dose (Without Organ Dysfunction)	Dosing Instructions
atazanavir (Reyataz)	400 mg once daily; **OR**	Take with food
	300 mg atazanavir plus 100 mg ritonavir, both once daily	
	Use boosted regimen with ritonavir when combined with tenofovir, efavirenz, or nevirapine	
	Use 400 mg atazanavir plus 100 mg ritonavir, daily in patients receiving efavirenz, in pregnant women, and in patients who either are also taking tenofovir or receiving an H_2 receptor antagonist	
	Dosage adjustment needed with liver disease; use of atazanavir is contraindicated with severe liver disease	
darunavir (Prezista)	Treatment-naive or experienced patients but with no darunavir resistance mutations:	Take with food
	800 mg with 100 mg plus ritonavir, both once daily	

Adverse Effects	Metabolism or Excretion Route and Pharmacokinetic Drug Interaction Potential[a,b]
Increased indirect bilirubin (usually asymptomatic), jaundice, GI effects (less frequent with boosted ritonavir), rash, nephrolithiasis	Hepatic metabolism
	Substrate for CYP3A4[c,d]
	Can inhibit CYP3A4,[e] CYP1A2, and CYP2C9
Prolonged PR interval, 1st-degree heart block in some patients	Levels decreased by tenofovir; use atazanavir plus ritonavir; atazanavir can also increase tenofovir levels (monitor for adverse effects)
PI class side effects[f]; atazanavir has less effect on glucose and lipids than that of other PIs	
Pregnancy category B	Space apart from antacids, avoid use with PPIs and H₂ receptor antagonists (or use boosted atazanavir and space apart from H₂ antagonist)
Diarrhea, nausea, and headache; elevated transaminases; rash (contains a sulfonamide moiety, so use with caution in patients with sulfonamide allergy)	Hepatic metabolism
	Substrate for CYP3A4[c,d]
	Inhibitor of CYP3A4[e]
PI class side effects[f]	Many drug interactions
Pregnancy category B	Increases levels of pravastatin and other statins

(Continues)

Table 83 Select Characteristics of PIs (*Cont'd.*)

Medication	Usual Adult Dose (Without Organ Dysfunction)	Dosing Instructions
darunavir (Prezista) (continued)	At least 1 resistance mutation: 600 mg with 100 mg plus ritonavir, both bid Avoid with severe liver disease	
fosamprenavir (Lexiva)	Treatment-naive patients: 1,400 mg bid **OR** 1,400 mg plus ritonavir 200 mg, both once daily; **OR** 700 mg plus ritonavir 100 mg, both bid PI-experienced patients: Use 700 mg plus ritonavir 100 mg, both bid; coadministration with efavirenz: Use boosted regimen with ritonavir Adjust dosage with liver disease	Take without regard to food
indinavir (Crixivan)	800 mg q8h With ritonavir: 800 mg plus ritonavir 100 mg or 200 mg, both bid With efavirenz or nevirapine: 1,000 mg q8h Adjust dosage with liver disease	Take on empty stomach or with light meal, unless given with ritonavir Drink >48 oz water daily to decrease risk of nephrolithiasis
lopinavir 200 mg/ ritonavir 50 mg (coformulated; Kaletra)	400 mg plus ritonavir 100 mg (2 tab) bid; **OR** 800 mg plus ritonavir 200 mg (4 tab once daily); use once-daily regimen only in treatment-naive patients Treatment-experienced patients also on efavirenz or nevirapine: lopinavir 500 mg plus ritonavir 125 mg bid	Take with food

Adverse Effects	Metabolism or Excretion Route and Pharmacokinetic Drug Interaction Potential[a,b]
	Decreases oral contraceptive levels; use alternate method of birth control
vomiting, diarrhea, headache, rash (including rare Stevens-Johnson syndrome); fosamprenavir is a sulfonamide and theoretically has cross-allergenicity with other sulfa drugs	Rapidly converted to amprenavir by cellular phosphatases in the gut
Elevated transaminases	amprenavir is a substrate for CYP3A4[c,d] and can inhibit CYP3A4[e]
PI class side effects[f]	
Pregnancy category C	
Nephrolithiasis (drink >48 oz water daily to decrease risk)	Hepatic metabolism
Increased bilirubin (usually asymptomatic)	Substrate for CYP3A4[c,d]
Headache, nausea, vomiting, diarrhea, rash, increased hepatic transaminases, thrombocytopenia, dry skin and lips, ingrown toenails	Inhibits CYP3A4[e]
PI class side effects[f]	
Pregnancy category C	
GI intolerance, diarrhea, headache, skin rash, asthenia	Hepatic metabolism
Higher incidence of elevated triglycerides and cholesterol than with other PIs	Substrate for CYP3A4[c,d]
Associated with slight increased risk of myocardial infarction	Both lopinavir and ritonavir are potent inhibitors of CYP3A4[e]
PR and QT prolongation have been reported	Decreases methadone levels
Increased transaminases	Decreases oral contraceptive levels; use alternate method of birth control
	Oral solution contains alcohol; avoid with metronidazole or disulfiram

(Continues)

Table 83 Select Characteristics of PIs (*Cont'd.*)

Medication	Usual Adult Dose (Without Organ Dysfunction)	Dosing Instructions
lopinavir 200 mg/ ritonavir 50 mg (coformulated; Kaletra) (continued)	For 3rd trimester of pregnancy: lopinavir 600 mg plus ritonavir 150 mg	
nelfinavir (Viracept)	1,250 mg bid or 750 mg tid Avoid with significant liver disease	Take with food
ritonavir (Norvir)	Use as the sole PI is no longer recommended; when used as a boosting agent with another PI: 100-400 mg in 1-2 divided doses	Whether or not ritonavir is taken with food depends on the other PI it is combined with
saquinavir (Invirase)	saquinavir 1,000 mg with ritonavir 100 mg, both bid Contraindicated with severe hepatic disease	Take with a full meal (or within 2 hours of eating)
tipranavir (Aptivus)	tipranavir 500 mg with ritonavir 200 mg Contraindicated with severe hepatic disease	Take with food

Adverse Effects	Metabolism or Excretion Route and Pharmacokinetic Drug Interaction Potential[a,b]
PI class side effects[f] Pregnancy category C	
Diarrhea (very common), soft stool, nausea, flatulence, rash PI class side effects[f] Pregnancy category B	Hepatic metabolism Substrate for CYP3A4;[c,d] inhibits CYP3A4[e] (induces CYP3A4 occasionally) Decreases oral contraceptive levels; use alternate method of birth control
GI intolerance (dose-related; may resolve with continued therapy); less common when used in low-dose boosting regimen Taste changes, dizziness, headache, somnolence, paresthesia (circumoral and extremities), hepatotoxicity PI class side effects,[f] increased lipids may be more severe with ritonavir vs other PIs Pregnancy category B	Hepatic metabolism Substrate for CYP3A4[c,d] Very potent inhibitor of CYP3A4[e] Inhibits or competes for CYP2C9, CYP2C19, and CYP2D6 Induces CYP1A2 (decreases theophylline levels) Multitude of complex drug-to-drug reactions Decreases methadone levels Decreases oral contraceptive levels; use alternate method of birth control Oral solution contains alcohol
GI intolerance (may subside with continued therapy), diarrhea, headache, asthenia, rash, oral ulcerations, increased transaminases Prolonged QT PI class side effects[f] Pregnancy category B	Hepatic metabolism Substrate for CYP3A4[c,d] Inhibits CYP3A4[e] Levels decreased by dexamethasone
Nausea, vomiting, diarrhea Hypersensitivity (especially in young women): Possible cross-allergy with sulfonamide Hepatotoxicity: Contraindicated with moderate to severe liver disease	Substrate for CYP3A4[c,d] Inhibitor of CYP3A4[e] Many drug-to-drug interactions Decreases oral contraceptive levels; use alternate method of birth control

(Continues)

Table 83 Select Characteristics of PIs (*Cont'd.*)

Medication	Usual Adult Dose (Without Organ Dysfunction)	Dosing Instructions
tipranavir (Aptivus) (continued)		

[a] Drug interactions listed here are not all-inclusive and do not include drugs with overlapping toxicities.

[b] See individual drug package insert and other resources for specific drug interactions.

[c] Abbreviated list of CYP3A4 **inducers** that can decrease serum levels of substrates for CYP3A4 (eg, PIs, NNRTIs): rifampin, rifabutin, rifapentine, carbamazepine, phenobarbital, phenytoin, nevirapine, efavirenz, St. John's wort.

[d] Abbreviated list of CYP3A4 **inhibitors** that can potentially increase serum level of substrates for CYP3A4 (eg, PIs, NNRTIs): PIs, erythromycin, clarithromycin, azole antifungals, amiodarone, cimetidine, grapefruit juice.

[e] Abbreviated list of CYP3A4 **substrates** (serum levels can be increased by CYP3A4 inhibitors such as PIs and decreased by CYP3A4 inducers such as nevirapine or efavirenz): benzodiazepines (avoid midazolam or triazolam; lorazepam can be used with PIs); statins (avoid use of lovastatin or simvastatin with PIs; pravastatin and fluvastatin do not interact with PIs, and atorvastatin and rosuvastatin can be used with caution and monitoring); dihydropyridine calcium channel blockers; ergot alkaloids (avoid with PIs); sildenafil, vardenafil, and tadalafil (dose reduction of erectile dysfunction drugs needed with PIs); some antiarrhythmics (eg, amiodarone, lidocaine, quinidine); warfarin; pimozide (avoid with PIs); rifabutin (may need dose alterations of 1 or both drugs); some antidepressants and anticonvulsants (eg, carbamazepines, phenytoin, phenobarbital); immunosuppressants (eg, cyclosporine, tacrolimus, sirolimus); azole antifungals.

[f] PI class side effects include increased lipids, lipodystrophy, hyperglycemia, hemolytic anemia, and spontaneous bleeding or hematomas with hemophilia.

Adapted from Panel on Antiretroviral Guidelines for Adults and Adolescents [Internet]. Department of Health and Human Services. Jan 10, 2011 [cited 2011 Mar 14]. Available from: http://aidsinfo.nih.gov/ContentFiles/AdultandAdolescentGL.pdf.

Table 84 Fusion Inhibitor: Select Characteristics

Medication	Usual Adult Dose (Without Organ Dysfunction)	Dosing Instructions
enfuvirtide	90 mg SQ bid	Each 108-mg vial should be reconstituted 1:1 with sterile water before injection
		Reconstituted injection should be refrigerated and used within 24 h

[a] Drug interactions listed here are not all-inclusive and do not include drugs with overlapping toxicities.

[b] See individual drug package insert and other resources for specific drug interactions.

Adapted from Panel on Antiretroviral Guidelines for Adults and Adolescents [Internet]. Department of Health and Human Services. Jan 10, 2011 [cited 2011 Mar 14]. Available from: http://aidsinfo.nih.gov/ContentFiles/AdultandAdolescentGL.pdf.

Adverse Effects	Metabolism or Excretion Route and Pharmacokinetic Drug Interaction Potential[a,b]
Fatal and nonfatal intracranial hemorrhages reported	
PI class side effects[f]	
Pregnancy category C	

Adverse Effects	Metabolism or Excretion Route and Pharmacokinetic Drug Interaction Potential[a,b]
Local injection site reactions	Thought to undergo catabolism to constituent amino acids
Possible increased rate of bacterial pneumonia	
Hypersensitivity reaction, nausea and vomiting, diarrhea, peripheral neuropathy	Unlikely to have significant CYP450-related drug interactions
Neutropenia	
Pregnancy category B	

Table 85 Integrase Inhibitor: Select Characteristics

Medication	Usual Adult Dose (Without Organ Dysfunction)	Dosing Instructions
raltegravir (Isentress)	400 mg bid No dosage recommendation available for severe liver disease	Take without regard to food

[a] Drug interactions listed here are not all-inclusive and do not include drugs with overlapping toxicities.
[b] See individual drug package insert and other resources for specific drug interactions.

Table 86 CCR5 Coreceptor Antagonist: Select Characteristics

Medication	Usual Adult Dose (Without Organ Dysfunction)	Dosing Instructions
maraviroc (Selzentry)	300 mg bid For CCR5-tropic virus only: Administer a tropism test before use No dosage recommendations available for severe liver disease	Take without regard to food

[a] Drug interactions listed here are not all-inclusive and do not include drugs with overlapping toxicities.
[b] See individual drug package insert and other resources for specific drug interactions.

Adverse Effects	Metabolism or Excretion Route and Pharmacokinetic Drug Interaction Potential[a,b]
Diarrhea, nausea, and headache most commonly reported in studies	Metabolized by glucuronidation
	Does not affect CYP450 enzymes
Rare myopathy and rhabdomyolysis have been reported (asymptomatic increase in CPK reported)	Levels can be decreased by rifampin and other UGT1A1 inducers; use with caution
Rare hepatic toxicity reported, potentially preceded by symptoms of allergic reaction	
Elevated amylase	

Adverse Effects	Metabolism or Excretion Route and Pharmacokinetic Drug Interaction Potential[a,b]
Cough, fever, upper respiratory infection, rash, musculoskeletal symptoms, abdominal pain, diarrhea, nausea, and dizziness are all commonly reported in studies	Substrate for CYP3A4 and P-glycoprotein
Hepatotoxicity	
Orthostatic hypotension	

Select Opportunistic Infections in Adult Patients With HIV

Pneumocystis jiroveci (Formerly *P carinii*)

- **Risk factors:** Ubiquitous organism; CD4 count <200/mcL; chronic corticosteroid or other immunosuppressive drug therapy
- **Clinical disease**
  - Exertional dyspnea, fever, nonproductive cough, and chest discomfort that gets worse over days to weeks
  - Hypoxemia; chest radiographs vary (most commonly show diffuse bilateral, symmetrical interstitial infiltrate but may be relatively normal early in course and can have atypical presentation)
  - Fulminant pneumonia less common in patients with human immunodeficiency virus (HIV)
  - Concomitant respiratory pathogen not uncommon
  - Immune reconstitution syndrome can be seen (corticosteroids or nonsteroidal anti-inflammatory drugs [NSAIDs] may help)
- **Criteria for starting primary prophylaxis:** CD4 <200/mcL, thrush, or history of AIDS-defining illness
- **Criteria for stopping primary or secondary prophylaxis:** Adequate response to highly active antiretroviral therapy (HAART) with CD4 >200/mcL for ≥3 months

Table 87 Treatment and Prophylaxis of *Pneumocystis jiroveci* (PCP) Infections in HIV Patients

Antimicrobial Therapy	First-Line Treatment	Alternate Treatment
Treatment of active disease (usually 21 days)	**Moderate to severe disease:** TMP-SMX IV 15 mg/kg/24h (TMP component) in divided doses q6-8h for 21 days (can change to oral after clinical improvement)	**Moderate to severe disease:** pentamidine 3-4 mg/kg IV daily; **OR** clindamycin 600-900 mg IV q8h (or clindamycin 300-450 mg oral tid or qid) plus primaquine 15-30 mg oral daily

Table 87 Treatment and Prophylaxis of *Pneumocystis jiroveci* (PCP) Infections in HIV Patients (*Cont'd.*)

Antimicrobial Therapy	First-Line Treatment	Alternate Treatment
Treatment of active disease (usually 21 days) (continued)	If Pao₂ <70 mm Hg or alveolar-arterial oxygen gradient >35 mm Hg, add prednisone (beginning as early as possible and within 3 days of PCP therapy start) 40 mg bid for 5 days, then 40 mg daily for 5 days, then 20 mg daily for 11 days **Mild to moderate disease:** Same daily dose of oral TMP-SMX as above in 3 divided doses; **OR** TMP-SMX DS 2 tab tid	With either option, add prednisone as listed in first-line treatment if criteria are met **Mild to moderate disease:** clindamycin 300-450 mg oral tid or qid plus primaquine 15-30 mg oral daily; **OR** dapsone 100 mg oral daily plus TMP 5 mg/kg oral q8h; **OR** atovaquone 750 mg oral bid
Prophylaxis (primary or secondary)	TMP-SMX 1 DS or SS tab daily	**One of the following:** dapsone 100 mg oral daily or 50 mg oral bid; **OR** dapsone 50 mg oral daily plus pyrimethamine 50 mg oral once weekly and leucovorin 25 mg oral weekly; **OR** dapsone 200 mg oral weekly plus pyrimethamine 75 mg oral weekly plus leucovorin 25 mg oral weekly; **OR** atovaquone 1,500 mg oral daily; **OR** TMP-SMX 1 DS tab 3×/wk; **OR** pentamidine 300 mg Inh monthly

Toxoplasma gondii Encephalitis

- **Risk factors:** CD4 <100/mcL (greatest risk with CD4 <50/mcL), usually represents reactivation (immunoglobulin G [IgG] seropositive); primary disease risk factors are undercooked meat and exposure to cat feces
- **Clinical disease**
  - Most common presentation is focal encephalitis
  - Computed tomogram or magnetic resonance imaging typically shows multiple contrast-enhancing lesions
  - Immune reconstitution syndrome can be seen (corticosteroids or NSAIDs may help)

- **Criteria for starting primary prophylaxis:** Initiate with CD4 <100/mcL and IgG antibody positive for *T gondii*
- **Criteria for stopping prophylaxis:** Adequate response to HAART and
  - **For primary prophylaxis:** CD4 >200/mcL for ≥3 months
  - **For secondary prophylaxis:** Completion of treatment course, resolution of symptoms, and CD4 >200/mcL for ≥6 months

Table 88 Treatment and Prophylaxis of *Toxoplasma gondii* Encephalitis in HIV Patients

Antimicrobial Therapy	First-Line Treatment	Alternate Treatment
Treatment of active disease (at least 6-wk duration)	pyrimethamine 200 mg oral once then 50-75 mg oral daily plus sulfadiazine 1,000-1,500 mg oral q6h and leucovorin 10-20 mg oral daily	**One of the following:** pyrimethamine 200 mg oral once then 50-75 mg oral daily plus leucovorin 10-20 mg oral daily and clindamycin 600 mg IV or oral q6h; **OR** TMP-SMX 5 mg/kg oral bid; **OR** atovaquone 1,500 mg oral bid plus pyrimethamine and leucovorin in the above doses; **OR** atovaquone 1,500 mg oral bid plus sulfadiazine 1,000-1,500 mg oral q6h; **OR** atovaquone 1,500 mg oral bid; **OR** pyrimethamine and leucovorin in the above doses plus azithromycin 900-1,200 mg oral daily
Primary prophylaxis	TMP-SMX 1 DS tab daily	**One of the following:** TMP-SMX 1 SS tab daily; **OR** TMP-SMX 1 SS tab 3×/wk; **OR** dapsone 50 mg oral daily plus pyrimethamine 50 mg oral weekly and leucovorin 25 mg oral weekly; **OR** dapsone 200 mg oral weekly plus pyrimethamine 75 mg oral weekly and leucovorin 25 mg oral weekly; **OR** atovaquone 1,500 mg oral daily with or without both pyrimethamine 25 mg oral daily and leucovorin 10 mg oral daily

Table 88 Treatment and Prophylaxis of *Toxoplasma gondii* Encephalitis in HIV Patients *(Cont'd.)*

Antimicrobial Therapy	First-Line Treatment	Alternate Treatment
Secondary prophylaxis (chronic maintenance therapy)	sulfadiazine 2,000-4,000 mg daily in 2-4 divided doses plus both pyrimethamine 25-50 mg oral daily and leucovorin 10-25 mg oral daily	clindamycin 600 mg oral q8h plus both pyrimethamine 25-50 mg oral daily and leucovorin 10-25 mg oral daily; **OR** atovaquone 750 mg oral q6-12h with or without both pyrimethamine 25 mg oral daily and leucovorin 10 mg oral daily

Mycobacterium avium Complex

- **Risk factors:** Ubiquitous organism; CD4 <50/mcL is greatest risk; can occur at CD4 <100/mcL
- **Clinical disease**
  - Usually disseminated, affecting multiple organs
  - Common symptoms usually include fever, night sweats, weight loss, fatigue, diarrhea
  - Disease can be localized
  - Immune reconstitution syndrome is common
- **Criteria for starting primary prophylaxis:** CD4 <50/mcL
- **Criteria for stopping prophylaxis:** Adequate response to HAART, and
  - **For primary prophylaxis:** CD4 >100/mcL for ≥3 months
  - **For secondary prophylaxis:** Completion of ≥12-month treatment, resolution of symptoms, and CD4 >100/mcL for ≥6 months

Table 89 Treatment and Prophylaxis of *Mycobacterium avium* Complex in HIV Patients

Antimicrobial Therapy	First-Line Treatment	Alternate Treatment
Treatment of active disease (typically ≥12-mo duration): Use at least 2 drugs initially; consider 4-8 wk of corticosteroids if symptoms persist	clarithromycin 500 mg oral bid plus ethambutol 15 mg/kg oral daily with or without rifabutin[a,b] 300 mg oral daily	azithromycin 500-600 mg oral daily (make effort to include either clarithromycin or azithromycin in drug regimen) plus ethambutol 15 mg/kg oral daily **Consider other (3rd or 4th) drug:** rifampin (as active as rifabutin but with more significant antiretroviral drug interactions); **OR**

(Continues)

Table 89 Treatment and Prophylaxis of *Mycobacterium avium* Complex in HIV Patients (*Cont'd.*)

Antimicrobial Therapy	First-Line Treatment	Alternate Treatment
		A newer fluoroquinolone (levofloxacin 500 mg oral daily or moxifloxacin 400 mg oral daily); **OR**
		amikacin 10-15 mg/kg IV daily; **OR**
		streptomycin 1 g IV or IM daily
Primary prophylaxis	azithromycin 1,200 mg oral weekly; **OR**	rifabutin[a,b] 300 mg oral daily
	azithromycin 600 mg oral bid; **OR**	
	clarithromycin 500 mg oral bid	
Secondary prophylaxis (chronic maintenance therapy)	clarithromycin 500 mg oral bid plus ethambutol 15 mg/kg oral daily with or without rifabutin[a,b] 300 mg oral daily	azithromycin 500-600 mg oral daily plus ethambutol 15 mg/kg oral daily

[a] Reduce rifabutin dose to 150 mg 3×/week when used in combination with protease inhibitors.

[b] In combination with efavirenz, rifabutin dose should be increased to 450-600 mg daily or 600 mg 2-3×/week.

Latent Tuberculosis Infection

The tuberculin skin test (TST) is considered positive in HIV-infected patients if TST induration is >5 mm.

A serum interferon-γ release assay (IGRA), including QuantiFERON-TB Gold In-Tube (QFT-GIT, Cellestis Ltd, Melbourne, Australia) and T-SPOT. TB (Oxford Immunotec Ltd, Oxford, United Kingdom), can be used in place of TST. IGRAs are reported as either positive or negative. These tests are more expensive than TST.

Patients are often anergic when their CD4 count is low. With negative TST or indeterminate IGRA results on first test of patients with CD4 <200/mcL, repeat the TST or IGRA after immune reconstitution.

Patients with HIV infection who have ever had a positive TST or IGRA should be treated for latent tuberculosis (TB) infection (LTBI) if not previously treated. Patients with known TB exposure should be treated for LTBI without regard to TST or IGRA results.

Active TB must be ruled out before initiating treatment for LTBI.

Table 90 Treatment of Latent Tuberculosis Infection (LTBI) in HIV Patients

Antimicrobial Therapy	First-Line Treatment	Alternate Treatment
LTBI	isoniazid 300 mg oral daily; **OR**	rifampin 600 mg daily for 4 mo; **OR**
	isoniazid 900 mg twice weekly by DOT plus pyridoxine 50 mg daily for 9 mo	rifabutin (dose adjusted for other drugs) daily for 4 mo
	For persons with known exposure to resistant TB: Consult public health authorities	Note drug-to-drug interactions; dosing adjustment required among rifamycins and most protease inhibitors and NNRTIs

For treatment of active TB, see section on "Tuberculosis" on pages 250-254.

Cryptococcosis

- **Risk factors:** CD4 <50/mcL
- **Clinical disease:** HIV-associated disease is usually subacute meningitis or meningoencephalitis
- Opening pressure is usually high and repeat lumbar puncture is often required to relieve intracranial pressure both with disease and with immune reconstitution syndrome
- **Criteria for starting primary prophylaxis:** Primary prophylaxis is not recommended
- **Criteria for stopping secondary prophylaxis:** Completion of treatment course (12 months) plus CD4 >100/mcL for at least 3 months while on HAART

Table 91 Treatment of Cryptococcosis in HIV Patients[a]

Antimicrobial Therapy	First-Line Treatment	Alternate Treatment
CNS disease	Induction therapy:	Induction therapy:
	liposomal amphotericin B 3-4 mg/kg/day or amphotericin B lipid complex 5 mg/kg/day; either plus flucytosine 100 mg/day in 4 divided doses for ≥2 wk; **OR**	amphotericin B deoxycholate, liposomal amphotericin B, or amphotericin B lipid complex as first-line treatment plus fluconazole 800 mg oral or IV daily with any amphotericin B product

(Continues)

Table 91 Treatment of Cryptococcosis in HIV Patients[a] *(Cont'd.)*

Antimicrobial Therapy	First-Line Treatment	Alternate Treatment
CNS disease (continued)	amphotericin B deoxycholate 0.7-1.0 mg/kg/day plus flucytosine 100 mg/kg oral daily in 4 divided doses for at least 2 wk; **OR**	For patients unable to tolerate amphotericin B: fluconazole 800-1,200 mg IV or oral plus flucytosine 100 mg/kg oral in 4 divided doses daily
	liposomal amphotericin B (3-4 mg/kg/day) or amphotericin B lipid complex 5 mg/kg/day or amphotericin B deoxycholate 0.7-1.0 mg/kg/day for 4-6 wk	If other options are not tolerated or are unavailable:
		Induction therapy: fluconazole 800-2,000 mg daily (if used alone) for 10-12 wk
	Consolidation therapy: (only after ≥2 wk of successful induction therapy):	Consolidation therapy (only after ≥2 wk of successful induction therapy):
	fluconazole 400 mg oral daily for 8 wk	itraconazole solution 800 mg oral daily for 8 wk
Primary prophylaxis	Not routinely recommended	Not routinely recommended
Secondary prophylaxis	fluconazole 200 mg oral lifelong; can consider discontinuation of secondary antifungal prophylaxis or suppression if all criteria are met:	itraconazole 200 mg oral daily
	Completion of ≥12 mo of antifungal therapy	
	Effective antiretroviral therapy (HAART) results in CD4 ≥100/mcL for ≥3 mo	
	HIV viral load is undetectable or sustainably very low	

[a] Additional information, see Perfect JR, et al. Clin Infect Dis. 2010 Feb 1;50(3):291-322.

Cytomegalovirus (CMV) Retinitis

- **Risk factors:** CD4 <50/mcL is greatest risk; can occur at CD4 <100/mcL
- **Clinical disease**
  - Retinitis most common in AIDS patients
  - Colitis, esophagitis, pneumonitis, neurologic disease also possible
  - Immune reconstitution syndrome can be seen (worsening); corticosteroids or NSAIDs may help

- **Criteria for starting primary prophylaxis:** Primary prophylaxis not recommended
- **Criteria for stopping secondary prophylaxis:** Sustained CD4 >100/mcL for ≥3-6 months with no evidence of active disease; should undergo routine eye examinations

Table 92 Treatment and Prophylaxis of Cytomegalovirus Retinitis in HIV Patients

Antimicrobial Therapy	First-Line Treatment	Alternate Treatment
Treatment of active disease	ganciclovir 5 mg/kg IV q12h for 2-3 wk and clinical stabilization,[a] then 5 mg/kg IV daily with ganciclovir ocular implant (change every 6-8 mo); 1 dose of intravitreal ganciclovir can be administered until ocular implant can be placed; **OR** valganciclovir 900 mg oral bid for 2-3 wk and clinical stabilization[a] then once daily, with ganciclovir ocular implant (change every 6-8 mo); 1 dose of intravitreal ganciclovir can be administered until ocular implant is placed. Peripheral lesions: valganciclovir 900 mg oral bid for 14-21 days then 900 mg daily	**One of the following:** ganciclovir 5 mg/kg IV q12h for 2-3 wk then 5 mg/kg IV daily; **OR** ganciclovir 5 mg/kg IV q12h for 2-3 wk then valganciclovir 900 mg oral daily; **OR** foscarnet 60 mg/kg IV q8h or 90 mg/kg q12h for 2-3 wk then 90-120 mg/kg IV daily; **OR** cidofovir 5 mg/kg IV weekly for 2 wk then 5 mg/kg IV every 2 wk with probenecid and saline hydration
Primary prophylaxis	Not routinely recommended	Not routinely recommended
Secondary prophylaxis	valganciclovir 900 mg oral daily; **OR** valganciclovir 900 mg oral daily plus ganciclovir ocular implant until immune recovery, then valganciclovir 900 mg oral daily	**One of the following:** ganciclovir 5 mg/kg IV 5-7×/wk; **OR** foscarnet 90-120 mg/kg IV daily; **OR** cidofovir 5 mg/kg IV every other wk plus oral probenecid 2 g at 3 h before and 1 g at 2 h and at 8 h after cidofovir dose (4 g total)

[a] Clinical stabilization as determined by fundoscopic examination.

Additional Information

- For treatment of non-CNS *Cryptococcus* and other fungal infections, see section on "Fungal Infections" (pages 266-284), which includes Tables 73-78.
- For treatment of *Mycobacterium tuberculosis*, see section on "Tuberculosis" (pages 250-254), which includes Table 72.

Table 93 Recommended Vaccines for Prevention of Opportunistic Infections in Adult HIV Patients

Vaccine	Candidates	Comments
Streptococcus pneumoniae	All patients; consider delaying until CD4 ≥200/mcL	23 Valent *S pneumoniae* vaccine; consider 1 repeat dose in 5 y
Influenza	All patients annually before influenza season	Yearly inactivated influenza vaccine only
HAV	Consider for all patients who are not immune (especially illegal drug users, men who have sex with other men, patients with hemophilia, and patients with liver disease, including HBV or HCV)	HAV vaccine in 2 doses (or combination HAV and HBV vaccine in 3 doses)
HBV	All patients who are not immune	HBV vaccine in 3 doses (or combination HAV and HBV vaccine in 3 doses)

Data from Kaplan JE, et al. MMWR Recomm Rep. 2009 Apr 10;58(RR04):1-198.

Occupational Postexposure Prophylaxis and Management

Important Information for Postexposure Prophylaxis Decisions

Risk of Viral Transmission

Percutaneous Needlestick Exposure From Infected Source

- Human immunodeficiency virus (HIV) transmission risk is about 0.3% (about 1 in 300)
  - About 0.1% after mucous membrane exposure
  - <0.1% after exposure to abraded skin
- Hepatitis B virus (HBV) for nonvaccinated persons when blood from source is:
  - HBsAg (hepatitis B surface antigen) positive **AND** HBeAg (hepatitis B e antigen) positive: HBV transmission risk is about 37-62%
  - HBsAg positive **AND** HBeAg negative: HBV transmission risk is about 23-37%
- Hepatitis C virus (HCV) transmission risk is about 1.8-3% (range, 0-7%)

Body Fluids

- Fluids that pose some degree of risk of HIV, HBV, or HCV transmission: Blood, semen, vaginal secretions, cerebrospinal fluid, synovial fluid, pleural fluid, peritoneal fluid, pericardial fluid, amniotic fluid
- Fluids that do **NOT** pose a risk of HIV, HBV, or HCV transmission: Urine, stool, blood-free saliva, emesis, nasal secretions, tears, sweat

Counseling and Prophylaxis

- Persons exposed to HIV, HBV, or HCV should be offered counseling to promote a full understanding of the risks of viral transmission
- HIV postexposure prophylaxis (PEP) should be started as soon as possible (within hours); any benefit of PEP is significantly decreased when started more than 48 hours after exposure

Information to Document Immediately After Exposure

Clinical Information About Exposure Source

- Known positive HIV, HBV, or HCV source?
- In patients known to be HIV positive: Most recent HIV viral load (VL), current and previous HIV treatment, response to HIV treatment (eg, treatment failure), or suspected drug-resistant virus
- In patients with unknown HIV status: Any clinical findings or previous opportunistic infections indicative of possible HIV infection

Types of Exposure

- Percutaneous (eg, needlestick) vs mucous membrane or abraded skin exposure to blood
- Direct laboratory contact with concentrated virus (eg, in laboratory workers)
- If needlestick injury: Hollow-bore or solid suture needle? Visible blood on needle?
- If mucous membrane or broken skin exposure: Type of infectious fluid (eg, blood) and quantity (eg, a few drops or a splash)

Characteristics of the Exposure

- Date and time of exposure
- Puncture directly into blood vessel?
- Depth of puncture? Was bleeding produced?
- Were any protective barriers (eg, gloves) being worn?

Clinical Information About Exposure Recipient

- HBV vaccination status
- Was wound washed promptly with soap and water?

Table 94 Recommended PEP for HIV-Associated Percutaneous Injuries

	Infection Status of Source	
Type of Exposure	**HIV Positive, Class 1[a]**	**HIV Positive, Class 2[b]**
Less severe[c]	Basic 2-drug PEP	Expanded ≥3-drug PEP
More severe[d]	Expanded ≥3-drug PEP	Expanded ≥3-drug PEP

[a] HIV positive, class 1: Asymptomatic HIV infection or known HIV VL <1,500 copies/mL.

[b] HIV positive, class 2: Symptomatic HIV infection, AIDS, acute seroconversion; known HIV VL ≥1,500 copies/mL.

[c] Examples: Solid needle or superficial injury.

[d] Examples: Large, hollow-bore needle; deep puncture; visible blood on device; needle used in artery or vein of patient.

Adapted from Centers for Disease Control and Prevention. Updated US Public Health Service guidelines for the management of occupational exposures to HIV and recommendations for postexposure prophylaxis. MMWR Recomm Rep. 2005 Sep 30;54(RR-9):1-17.

- Potential for pregnancy, current medications, allergies, and medical conditions

HIV PEP Management

Timing and Duration

- Start HIV PEP as soon as possible after exposure, preferably within hours; beneficial when started within 36 hours of exposure but after 72 hours, benefit is unclear (consult HIV expert)
- Continue HIV PEP for 28 days (4 weeks)

	Infection Status of Source	
HIV Status Unknown	**Source Unknown**	**HIV Negative**
No PEP needed generally; consider 2-drug PEP if source has HIV risk factors	No PEP needed generally; consider 2-drug PEP with likely exposure to HIV-positive person	No PEP needed
No PEP needed generally; consider 2-drug PEP if source has HIV risk factors	No PEP needed generally; consider 2-drug PEP with likely exposure to HIV-positive person	No PEP needed

Table 95 Recommended PEP for HIV-Associated Mucous Membrane Exposures and Nonintact Skin Exposures

Type of Exposure	Infection Status of Source	
	HIV Positive, Class 1[a]	**HIV Positive, Class 2**[b]
Small volume[c]	Consider basic 2-drug PEP	Basic 2-drug PEP
Large volume[d]	Basic 2-drug PEP	Expanded ≥3-drug PEP

[a] HIV positive, class 1: Asymptomatic HIV infection or known HIV VL <1,500 copies/mL.

[b] HIV positive, class 2: Symptomatic HIV infection, AIDS, acute seroconversion; known HIV VL ≥1,500 copies/mL.

[c] Example: A few drops.

[d] Example: A blood splash.

Adapted from Centers for Disease Control and Prevention. Updated US Public Health Service guidelines for the management of occupational exposures to HIV and recommendations for postexposure prophylaxis. MMWR Recomm Rep. 2005 Sep 30;54(RR-9):1-17

HIV PEP Drug Regimens

Basic 2-Drug Regimens
- Truvada (emtricitabine 200 mg/tenofovir 300 mg) 1 tablet once daily
- Combivir (zidovudine 300 mg/lamivudine 150 mg) 1 tablet bid
- tenofovir 300 mg oral once daily plus lamivudine 300 mg oral once daily
- zidovudine 300 mg oral bid plus lamivudine 300 mg oral once daily or lamivudine 150 mg oral bid
- zidovudine 300 mg oral bid plus emtricitabine 200 mg oral once daily
- **Note:** Combination drugs such as Truvada and Combivir decrease pill burden and may improve patient compliance

Expanded (3rd-Drug) Options With 2-Drug Regimen Above
- Kaletra (lopinavir 200 mg/ritonavir 50 mg) 2 tablets oral bid
- atazanavir 300 mg oral once daily plus ritonavir 100 mg oral once daily
- darunavir 800 mg oral once daily plus ritonavir 100 mg oral once daily

Other Drug Combinations
- Other antiretroviral PEP drug combinations can be used (eg, abacavir, fosamprenavir, indinavir, nelfinavir, saquinavir, stavudine, didanosine, nevirapine) if source has drug-resistant HIV or if exposure recipient

Infection Status of Source		
HIV Status Unknown	**Unknown Source**	**HIV Negative**
No PEP needed generally	No PEP needed generally	No PEP needed
No PEP needed generally; consider 2-drug PEP if source has HIV risk factors	No PEP needed generally; consider 2-drug PEP with likely exposure to HIV-positive person	No PEP needed

has drug intolerance; consult HIV expert (see section on additional resources)

HBV PEP Management

Timing and Duration
- When hepatitis B immune globulin (HBIG) is indicated, administer it as soon as possible after exposure (preferably within 24 hours); effectiveness of HBIG beyond 1 week is unclear
- When HBV vaccine is indicated, administer it as soon as possible after exposure (preferably within 24 hours); HBV vaccine can be given simultaneously with HBIG but in a different location (eg, deltoid muscle)

Table 96 Recommended PEP for HBV Exposure

Vaccination Status of Exposed HCP[a]	HBV Antigen or Antibody Status of Source
	HBsAg Positive
Not previously vaccinated	HBIG[b] once and initiate HBV vaccine series
Previously vaccinated	
Known responder[c]	No treatment
Known nonresponder[d]	HBIG once and initiate revaccination or give HBIG twice[e]
HBV antibody response unknown	Test exposed HCP for anti-HBs:
	If adequate, no treatment necessary
	If inadequate, administer HBIG once and give vaccine booster

[a] Persons previously infected with HBV are immune to reinfection and do not require postexposure prophylaxis.

[b] HBIG dose is 0.06 mL/kg IM.

[c] Appropriate protective response to HBV vaccine is defined by quantitative anti-HBs ≥10 milliunits/mL (adequate antibody level).

[d] Inadequate protective response to vaccine is defined by quantitative anti-HBs <10 milliunits/mL (inadequate antibody level).

[e] Two doses of HBIG is preferred for persons who previously completed a second vaccine series but did not develop adequate antibody response.

Adapted from Centers for Disease Control and Prevention. Updated US Public Health Service Guidelines for the Management of Occupational Exposures to HBV, HCV, and HIV and Recommendations for Postexposure Prophylaxis. MMWR Recomm Rep. 2001 Jun 29;50(RR-11):1-54.

HCV Postexposure Management

- There is currently no postexposure immunoglobulin or vaccine for HCV exposure
- Patients with symptomatic acute HCV infection may benefit from antiviral therapy administered after expert consultation

Postexposure HIV, HBV, and HCV Laboratory Monitoring

Source of Exposure

- Test immediately for HIV serology (if HIV positive, check VL and possibly conduct resistance testing if virus is poorly controlled), HBsAg, anti-HBs, and HCV serology

Exposure Recipient

- **HIV serology:** At baseline, 6 weeks, 3 months, and 6 months (consider extending HIV serology testing to 1 year if HCV seroconversion occurs)

HBsAg Negative	**HBV Antigen or Antibody Status of Source**
	HBV Status Unknown (or Not Available for Testing)
Initiate HBV vaccine series	Initiate HBV vaccine series
No treatment	No treatment
No treatment or consider revaccination	If source has known high HBV risk, treat as HbsAg positive
No treatment	Test exposed HCP for anti-HBs:
	If adequate, no treatment necessary
	If inadequate, administer vaccine booster and recheck anti-HBs titer in 1-2 mo

- **If antiretroviral therapy is started for HIV PEP:** Complete blood cell count, liver function tests, and serum creatinine (glucose if protease inhibitor used) at baseline and again after 2 weeks of antiretroviral PEP
- **HBV serology:** At baseline, 4-6 weeks, 3 months, and 6 months (consider alanine aminotransferase [ALT], HBsAg, or HBV DNA if symptoms are consistent with acute infection)
- **HCV serology:** At baseline, 3 months, and 6 months (consider ALT and HCV RNA testing if symptoms are consistent with acute infection)

Suggested Reading for HIV, HBV, and HCV Postexposure Management

HIV Exposure

- National HIV/AIDS Clinicians' Consultation Center. Available from: http://www.nccc.ucsf.edu/about_nccc/pepline/ (PEPline Hotline 1-888-448-4911)

- HIV/AIDS Prevention at CDC. Atlanta (GA): Centers for Disease Control and Prevention. [cited 2010 Nov 20]. Available from: http://www.cdc.gov/hiv/aboutDHAP.htm
- AIDSinfo. Rockville (MD): AIDSinfo. [cited 2010 Nov 20]. Available from: http://aidsinfo.nih.gov/
- Landovitz RJ, Currier JS. N Engl J Med. 2009 Oct 29;361(18):1768-75

HBV and HCV Exposure

- National Center for HIV/AIDS, Viral Hepatitis, STD, and TB Prevention. Atlanta (GA): Centers for Disease Control and Prevention. [cited 2010 Nov 20]. Available from: http://www.cdc.gov/ncidod/diseases/hepatitis/index.htm

Tick-Borne Infections

Tick Vectors

Numerous species of ticks have been associated with transmission of infectious diseases to humans. Recognizing the type of tick and its geographic distribution can aid identification of select bacterial, viral, and protozoan infection risk assessment.

Table 97 Tick Vectors

Family	Genus/Species	Common Name	Distribution
Hard ticks (Ixodidae)	*Amblyomma americanum*	Lone Star tick	Southern and eastern US
	Dermacentor andersoni	Rocky Mountain wood tick	Southern and western US
	D variabilis	American dog tick	Southern and eastern US
	Ixodes holocyclus	Australian paralysis tick	Australia
	I pacificus	Western black-legged tick	Western US
	I ricinus	Sheep tick, deer tick	Europe
	I scapularis	Black-legged tick, deer tick	Northeastern and eastern US
	Rhipicephalus sanguineus	Deer tick, brown dog tick	US, Australia, Europe
Soft ticks (Argasidae)	*Ornithodoros hermsii, O turicata, O parkeri, O coriaceus*	NA	Western half of US, British Columbia, Mexico
	O moubata	African hut tampan	Eastern and southern Africa

Ixodidae Family

General Information

- Consists of the hard ticks that transmit nearly all tick-borne human diseases; 2-30 mm
- Ixodids do not cause pain while feeding; immature stages are frequently not detected because of their small size

Types of Ticks
- **Ixodes:** *I scapularis, I pacificus, I ricinus*
  - Black; female has red dorsal posterior
  - Can attach to humans during all 3 stages of development: Larva, nymph, adult (3-host life cycle)
- **D variabilis:** American dog tick
  - Brown and white; larger than deer tick (*Ixodes*)
  - Attaches to humans predominantly in adult stage
- **A americanum:** Lone Star tick
  - Oval and black with white spot near center
  - Can attach to humans during all 3 stages of development

Argasidae Family

General Information
- Soft ticks; predominantly found in arid environments
- Transmits tick-borne relapsing fever, also called endemic relapsing fever; caused by *Borrelia hermsii, B duttonii, B parkeri*

Types of Infections Spread by Tick Bites

Lyme Disease (*Borrelia burgdorferi*)

Geographic Distribution
- Southern New England, eastern Mid-Atlantic states, upper Midwest, northern Pacific Coast

Tick Vectors
- In the northeastern and north-central US, the black-legged tick (*I scapularis*) transmits Lyme disease. In the Pacific coastal US, the disease is spread by the western black-legged tick (*I pacificus*).
- Tick must feed for about 36-48 hours (to become engorged) before transmission of *B burgdorferi* can occur

Clinical Signs and Symptoms
- Erythema chronicum migrans (ECM): Circular erythematous skin lesion, often with central clearing; usually appears 7 days after tick bite (range, 3-10 days); relatively rapid expansion of outer margins, if untreated (erythematous margin contains organisms seen on biopsy)
- Early disseminated Lyme disease
  - Multiple ECM lesions
  - Migratory arthralgia
  - Cranial nerve palsy (especially facial nerve palsy or Bell palsy)
  - Meningitis, transverse myelitis, mononeuritis multiplex
  - Carditis with variable degrees of atrioventricular nodal block
- Late Lyme disease
  - Oligoarticular arthritis, usually in large joints (eg, hips, knees); can be relapsing
  - Encephalitis, encephalopathy, axonal polyneuropathy
  - Acrodermatitis chronica atrophicans

Diagnosis

- Skin biopsy and culture or polymerase chain reaction (PCR) of edge of ECM lesion
- Serum enzyme-linked immunosorbent assay (ELISA) for initial screening; Western blot assay to confirm positive ELISA
  - ELISA can be false-negative during early infection (eg, during appearance of ECM lesion)
- If ELISA or immunofluorescence assay is negative and symptoms have been present for >1 month, it is highly unlikely that the person has Lyme disease; no further testing for Lyme disease recommended

Treatment (see Table 98 on "Treatment of Lyme Disease" below)

Table 98 Treatment of Lyme Disease[a,b]

Disease Category	Antimicrobial Therapy
Recognized tick bite	doxycycline 200-mg single dose for high-risk criteria[c]
Early localized disease	
Adults and children ≥8 y	First-line treatment: doxycycline 100 mg oral bid daily for 14-21 days
	Alternate treatment: amoxicillin 500 mg oral tid for 14-21 days, or cefuroxime 500 mg oral bid for 14-21 days
Children <8 y	amoxicillin oral 50 mg/kg daily in 3 divided doses (max 1.5 mg daily) for 14-21 days, or cefuroxime 30 mg/kg daily in 2 divided doses (max 1 g/day) or 1 g daily for 14-21 days
Early disseminated disease	
Multiple ECM	Same as above for early localized disease
Isolated facial nerve palsy	Same as above for early localized disease
Facial nerve palsy with CNS involvement[d,e]	Same as below for meningitis
Carditis	
Mild	Same as above for early localized disease
Severe	Same as below for meningitis
Meningitis[e]	
Adults	First-line treatment: ceftriaxone 2 g IV daily for 14-28 days
	Alternate treatment: cefotaxime 2 g IV q8h, or penicillin G 18-24 million units IV in divided doses q4h for 14-28 days

(Continues)

Table 98 Treatment of Lyme Disease[a,b] (Cont'd.)

Disease Category	Antimicrobial Therapy
Children	First-line treatment: ceftriaxone 75-100 mg/kg IV daily (max 2 g once daily) for 14-28 days
	Alternate treatment: penicillin 300,000 units/kg/24h divided doses q4h (max 20 million units per day) for 14-28 days
Late disease	
Arthritis	Same as above for early localized disease but treat for 28 days
Persistent or recurrent arthritis	Same as above for meningitis
Neurologic disease (eg, encephalitis,[e] polyneuropathy)	Same as above for meningitis

[a] Jarisch-Herxheimer reaction (eg, elevated temperature, myalgia) occurs occasionally; treat with nonsteroidal anti-inflammatory drugs; reaction usually lasts 1-2 days.

[b] Prolonged antimicrobial therapy demonstrates no clinical benefit for any manifestation of Lyme disease.

[c] A single preventive dose of doxycycline after a tick bite may be given when all criteria are met: 1) identified tick is a nymphal or an adult Ixodes tick that has been attached for >36 hours (based on tick engorgement and time of exposure); 2) doxycycline dose can be given within 72 hours of tick removal; 3) geographic endemic prevalence of Ixodes tick infection with B burgdorferi is at least 20%; and 4) doxycycline treatment is not contraindicated (eg, by pregnancy or age <8 years).

[d] Perform cerebrospinal fluid (CSF) evaluation if there is facial palsy accompanied by other abnormal neurologic findings (eg, severe headache, nuchal rigidity). With CSF pleocytosis, consider IV antibiotic therapy.

[e] Oral doxycycline can be a safe, effective treatment for Lyme disease meningitis, cranial neuritis, and radiculitis, with IV therapy reserved for patients with parenchymal CNS Lyme disease or with severe or unresponsive neurologic disease.

Data from Halperin JJ, et al. Neurology. 2007 Jul 3;69(1):91-102. Epub 2007 May 23. Erratum in: Neurology. 2008 Apr 1;70(14):1223.

Ehrlichiosis and Anaplasmosis

Types of Infection

Ehrlichiosis is caused by organisms in the genus *Ehrlichia*. *E chaffeensis* causes human ehrlichiosis, which is also called human monocytotropic ehrlichiosis (HME). In addition, human infections with *E ewingii* and *E canis* (both more common in dogs) have been described. Anaplasmosis (also called human granulocytotropic anaplasmosis [HGA]) is caused by a genetically distinct organism, *Anaplasma phagocytophilum* (formerly known as *Ehrlichia phagocytophila*).

- *E chaffeensis* causes HME
  - Geographic distribution: Southern, eastern, and south-central United States

- Tick vector: *A americanum* (Lone Star tick), the primary vector of *E chaffeensis* in the US
  - Morulae of *E chaffeensis* predominantly invade and can be seen in macrophages and monocytes
- *A phagocytophilum* causes anaplasmosis (or HGA)
  - Geographic distribution: South-central and southeastern US
  - Tick vectors: Anaplasmosis is transmitted to humans by tick bites primarily from the black-legged tick (*I scapularis*) in the eastern US and from the western black-legged tick (*I pacificus*) in the western US
  - Coinfection with *B burgdorferi* (Lyme disease) and *Babesia* may occur by similar tick vector
  - Morulae of *A phagocytophilum* predominantly invade and can be seen in neutrophils
- Human *E ewingii*
  - Predominantly a canine pathogen; occasional infection in humans
  - Geographic distribution: Most cases reported in Tennessee, Missouri, Oklahoma
  - Multiplies in neutrophils (like *A phagocytophilum*)
  - Tick vector: *A americanum* (Lone Star tick)
- *E muris*–like agent
  - Discovered summer 2009
  - Geographic distribution: Minnesota and Wisconsin
  - Tick vector: *I scapularis*

Clinical Symptoms and Laboratory Findings

- Nonspecific; range from mild to severe: Fever, myalgia, headache, arthralgia, nausea, cough; skin rash uncommon; respiratory insufficiency and neurologic symptoms may occur
- Laboratory findings commonly include leukopenia, thrombocytopenia; elevated alanine aminotransferase or aspartate aminotransferase

Diagnosis

- Intracytoplasmic morulae (more common in anaplasmosis) on peripheral blood smear; morulae within neutrophils in anaplasmosis and within monocytes in HME
- Serology (symptoms may precede seroconversion)
- PCR

Treatment

- First-line treatment: doxycycline 100 mg bid for 7-14 days
- Alternate treatment: rifampin

Babesiosis

Geographic Distribution

- *Babesia microti*: Northeastern US, upper midwestern US, Washington state
- *B divergens*: Europe (especially Great Britain, France, and Ireland)

Tick Vectors

- *I scapularis* (possible coinfection with *B burgdorferi* [Lyme disease] or *A phagocytophilum* [anaplasmosis])

Clinical Symptoms
- Nonspecific; can be severe in asplenic patient: Fever, arthralgia, nausea, vomiting, headache, weakness
- More severe cases involve hepatosplenomegaly, jaundice, renal failure, respiratory insufficiency
- Mild-to-severe hemolytic anemia may be present

Diagnosis
- Peripheral blood smear (Wright-Giemsa stain): Intraerythrocytic parasites (ring-shaped forms); distinguishing features of *Babesia* infection compared with *Plasmodium* (malaria) smear include:
  - *Babesia* organisms usually form tetrads ("Maltese cross") of merozoites
  - No hemoglobin-derived pigments within infected red blood cells
  - Larger ring-shaped forms contain central white vacuoles
  - Presence of extracellular merozoites
- Serology: Immunofluorescence assay
- PCR

Treatment
- B microti: Treat 7-10 days with atovaquone (750 mg twice daily) plus azithromycin (500 mg to 1 g on day 1, then 250 mg daily thereafter); or clindamycin (600 mg every 6-8 hours IV) plus quinine (650 mg oral 3 times daily) for severe cases
- B divergens: clindamycin IV plus quinine
- Exchange transfusion in severe cases

Rocky Mountain Spotted Fever (*Rickettsia rickettsii*)

Geographic Distribution
- Atlantic and south-central US; also Idaho and Montana; Canada, Central America, and parts of South America

Tick Vectors
- D variabilis (dog tick) predominantly in eastern and southeastern US
- D andersoni (wood tick) in western US; A americanum

Clinical Symptoms
- *Rickettsia* infects the endothelial lining of small blood vessels, producing vasculitis
- Typically abrupt onset of fever, headache, and rash (classic triad)
- 90% of patients have rash that typically involves ankles, wrists, palms, and soles (10% of patients have no rash; called Rocky Mountain spotless fever); digital gangrene may occur
- More severe cases result in renal failure, pulmonary infiltrate, hypotension, hepatic insufficiency, splenomegaly, neurologic symptoms, and disseminated intravascular coagulation with thrombocytopenia

Diagnosis
Acute illness is best detected by PCR and immunohistochemical examination of skin biopsy specimens. Serologic tests can also aid detection; however, an antibody response may not be detectable in initial samples, and paired acute and convalescent samples are essential for confirmation.

Treatment

- Usually started empirically before laboratory testing confirmation
- First-line treatment: doxycycline 100 mg twice daily for 7-10 days
- Alternate treatment: chloramphenicol

Other Rickettsial Infections Transmitted by Ticks or Other Vectors

- *R prowazekii* (epidemic or louse-born typhus) from body louse (*Pediculus humanus* var *corporis*) and via flying squirrel; found worldwide
- *R conorii* (Boutonneuse fever; Mediterranean spotted fever); found in various hard ticks; common in Africa, the Middle East, India, and the Mediterranean basin; infection is common in travelers
- *R africae* (African tick-bite fever; tick typhus); endemic to regions of Africa and the eastern Caribbean
- *R slovaca* (tick-borne lymphadenopathy); found in Europe

Tularemia (*Francisella tularensis*)

Geographic Distribution

- Western, central, and southern US

Tick Vectors

- *A americanum* (Lone Star tick)
- *D andersoni* (Rocky Mountain wood tick)
- *D variabilis* (American dog tick)
- Note: *F tularensis* is also transmitted by deer flies, other biting insects, and animals (eg, rabbits, deer, cats, squirrels, muskrats)

Clinical Symptoms: Six Well-Described Clinical Presentations

- Ulceroglandular: Most common form; 80% of cases; tender ulcer with painful regional adenopathy
- Glandular: Tender regional adenopathy without (or with minimal) skin lesions
- Oculoglandular: Painful conjunctivitis
- Pharyngeal: Exudative pharyngitis
- Typhoidal: More systemic symptoms (eg, fever, abdominal pain)
- Pneumonic: Pulmonary infiltrate, hilar adenopathy, pleural effusion; potential bioterrorism agent

Diagnosis

Serology (ie, tube agglutination or ELISA), PCR, and culture in reference laboratory; *F tularensis* may be identified through direct examination of secretions, Gram stain of exudates or biopsy specimens, direct fluorescent antibody, immunostains, or PCR

Treatment

- First-line treatment: streptomycin 10 mg/kg every 12 hours (up to 2 g/daily) for 7-10 days
- Alternate treatment: gentamicin 5 mg/kg divided every 8 hours; tetracycline, doxycycline, or chloramphenicol

Other Tick-Borne Infections

Tick-Borne Encephalitis (TBE)

- Etiology: TBE is caused by tick-borne encephalitis virus (TBEV), a member of the family Flaviviridae

- Vectors: Transmitted by *Ixodes* ticks
- Clinical symptoms: Biphasic course (20-30% cases), initially with fever and myalgia, followed later by CNS symptoms
- Treatment: No specific drug therapy for TBE

Colorado Tick Fever

- Etiology: Caused by infection with the Colorado tick fever virus
- Vector: Transmitted by *D andersoni* (Rocky Mountain wood tick)
- Clinical symptoms: High fever, retro-orbital pain, abdominal pain, biphasic illness in 50% of patients; leukopenia (common)
- Treatment: No specific treatment

Tick Paralysis

- Etiology: Caused by salivary toxins and produced by various ticks; affects humans and animals, often after prolonged tick attachment or feeding
- Vectors: *D andersoni* (Rocky Mountain wood tick) is most common tick in US and Canada; other ticks include *D variabilis, A americanum, I scapularis,* and *I pacificus*
- Clinical symptoms: Symmetric paralysis in lower extremities with ascending progression; typically no fever
- Treatment: Removal of tick, which typically leads to rapid resolution

Southern Tick-Associated Illness (STARI)

- Etiology: The cause of STARI is unknown
- Vector: STARI is specifically associated with bites of *A americanum*, known commonly as the Lone Star tick
- Clinical symptoms: STARI-associated rash is a red, expanding "bull's eye" lesion that develops around the site of a Lone Star tick bite; unlike Lyme disease, STARI has not been linked to any arthritic, neurologic, or chronic symptoms
- Treatment: In cases of STARI studied to date, oral antibiotics promptly resolved the rash and accompanying symptoms

Zoonotic (Animal-Associated) Infections

Table 99 Select Zoonotic (Animal-Associated) Infections

Transmission Route	Pathogen	Disease
Direct animal contact	*Brucella*	Brucellosis
	Coxiella burnetii	Q fever
	Francisella tularensis	Tularemia
	Bacillus anthracis	Anthrax
	Leptospira interrogans	Leptospirosis
	Yersinia pestis	Plague
	Rhodococcus equi	Respiratory tract infection
	Erysipelothrix insidiosa	Erysipeloid; soft tissue infection
	Echinococcus	Hydatid cyst; alveolar cyst
	Toxoplasma gondii	Toxoplasmosis
Animal bite	Rabies virus	Rabies
	Capnocytophaga canimorsus	Soft tissue infection
	Pasteurella	Soft tissue infection
	Bartonella henselae	Cat-scratch disease

Infections Contracted Through Direct Animal Contact

Brucellosis (*B abortus, B canis, B melitensis, B suis*)
- **General information:** Four species are known to cause disease in humans: *B abortus* (cattle), *B canis* (kennel-raised dogs), *B melitensis* (goats and sheep), and *B suis* (swine)
- **Geographic distribution:** Mediterranean (eg, Spain, Italy, Greece), Latin America, Middle East (eg, Saudi Arabia, Syria, Iraq, Kuwait)
- **Human infection routes**
  - **Direct animal contact:** Skin abrasions, wound contact, eye inoculation
  - **Inhalation:** Risk for abattoir workers
  - **Ingestion:** Contaminated dairy products, unpasteurized milk and cheese, raw meat

- **Clinical disease**
  - **Acute brucellosis (Malta fever):** Fever, chills, sweats, headache, back pain, splenomegaly (20-30%), adenopathy (10-20%), hepatomegaly (20-30%)
  - **Subacute and chronic brucellosis:** Indolent, intermittent fever (undulant fever); sacroiliitis and arthritis, granulomatous hepatitis and hepatic abscesses, endocarditis, meningitis, bone marrow suppression (ie, anemia, leukopenia, thrombocytopenia); diffuse adenopathy; can involve any organ system
- **Diagnosis:** Serology, culture, polymerase chain reaction (PCR)
- **Treatment (duration varies by syndrome from weeks to months):** Combination drug therapy with doxycycline plus rifampin, doxycycline plus gentamicin or streptomycin; trimethoprim-sulfamethoxazole (TMP-SMX) plus rifampin

Q Fever (*Coxiella burnetii*)

- **General information:** Commonly found in urine, stool, birth products, and milk from infected farm animals (eg, cattle, sheep, goats); also found in other animals (eg, dogs, cats, rabbits, pigeons, rats)
- **Geographic distribution:** Worldwide, common in Nova Scotia, Israel, and southern France
- **Human infection routes**
  - Inhalation of contaminated aerosol
  - Contact with body fluids of infected animals; exposure to skin or placenta of infected animals
  - Consumption of unpasteurized milk
- **Clinical disease:** Highly variable
  - **Acute Q fever:** Can manifest as self-limiting febrile or flulike illness, pneumonia, or hepatitis
    - **Flulike illness:** Abrupt onset, high-grade fever, myalgia, headache, fatigue
    - **Pneumonia:** Typically nonproductive cough; can be mild or progressive; multiple round opacities on chest radiographs are highly suggestive after likely exposure to infected animal
    - **Other:** Rash, pericarditis, myocarditis, aseptic meningitis
  - **Chronic Q fever:** Symptoms typically persist beyond 6 months
    - **Endocarditis:** Most common syndrome in chronic Q fever; valvular vegetations can be small and difficult to identify with echocardiography
    - **Infected aneurysms and vascular grafts**
    - **Hepatitis:** Elevated transaminases; liver biopsy may show classic doughnut-shaped granulomas (lipid vacuole surrounded by fibrinoid ring); hepatic fibrosis, cirrhosis
    - **Osteomyelitis, osteoarthritis**
- **Diagnosis:** Serology (immunofluorescence assay) with antibody titers >1:200 for antiphase II IgG (immunoglobulin G) and >1:50 for antiphase II IgM (immunoglobulin M) indicates acute infection; single antiphase I IgG titer >1:800 and IgA (immunoglobulin A) titer >1:100 indicate evidence of chronic infection
- **Treatment:** Treat symptomatic patients and patients who have chronic disease

- **Acute or chronic Q fever:** doxycycline or tetracycline; alternate treatments include TMP-SMX, rifampin, fluoroquinolones
- **Q fever endocarditis:** Treat symptomatic patients and patients who have chronic disease; doxycycline plus hydroxychloroquine; alternate treatments include doxycycline plus rifampin, doxycycline plus a fluoroquinolone, or doxycycline plus TMP-SMX; prolonged duration of combination therapy recommended; valve replacement (common)

Tularemia (*F tularensis*)

(See information on tularemia in text after Table 98 in the section on "Tick-Borne Infections")

Anthrax (*B anthracis*)

- **General information:** Found in soil and herbivores (eg, cattle, goats); zoonotic transmission is more likely in Iran, Iraq, Turkey, Pakistan, and sub-Saharan Africa; spores in soil can survive for long periods
- **Human infection routes:** Direct contact with abraded skin; inhalation; enteric exposure
- **Clinical disease**
  - **Cutaneous anthrax:** Most common form; infection by direct contact with infected animals, hides or wool from infected animals, or infected soil; painless papules develop into vesicles, which lead to ulcers, which then lead to black eschars surrounded by gelatinous haloes and nonpitting edema; painful regional adenopathy
  - **Respiratory anthrax:** Infection by inhalation of spores (ie, woolsorter's disease; can be used as a bioterrorism agent); typically biphasic clinical pattern with hemorrhagic mediastinitis, hemoptysis, and respiratory distress; high mortality; respiratory anthrax is not contagious, thus respiratory isolation is not necessary
  - **Gastrointestinal anthrax:** Hemorrhagic enteritis, acute abdominal pain, bloody diarrhea; ileocecal ulcerations (common)
  - **Oropharyngeal anthrax:** Cellulitis of the neck; oropharyngeal ulcers
- **Diagnosis:** Gram stain of large gram-positive bacillus from infected tissue; culture; serology
- **Treatment (depends on presentation):** Use ciprofloxacin (or doxycycline) plus rifampin; consider adding clindamycin or vancomycin for respiratory or severe disease; other agents active against *B anthracis* include penicillin (although some isolates may produce β-lactamase), ampicillin, meropenem; consult public health department if respiratory anthrax is suspected or confirmed

Leptospirosis (*L interrogans*)

- **General information:** Worldwide presence with higher prevalence in rural areas; warmer climates (tropical and subtropical regions); animal sources of infection (eg, rodents, cattle, swine, dogs, horses, sheep, goats)
- **Human infection routes:** Primarily by direct exposure to water or soil contaminated by urine from infected animals, such as during recreational (eg, triathlons, swimming) and occupational (eg, dairy farmers, sewer workers) activities

- *Leptospira* can penetrate abraded skin and intact mucous membranes (eg, conjunctiva; nasopharyngeal and genital epithelium) and can progress to hematologic dissemination
- **Clinical disease:** Ranges from subclinical to life-threatening; infections produce small-vessel vasculitis with multisystem disease; distinct biphasic course
  - **Acute septicemic phase**
    - Sudden headache, retro-ocular pain, myalgia, fever, nausea and vomiting, conjunctival suffusion, occasional rash
    - Patients may improve for a few days, then have recurring fever with immunologic sequelae
  - **Immunologic phase:** Organisms generally are cleared from blood and cerebrospinal fluid (CSF)
    - Aseptic meningitis
    - Myositis (elevated creatine kinase)
    - Respiratory insufficiency (eg, pulmonary edema, acute respiratory distress syndrome, hemoptysis) may develop
    - Cardiomyopathy, myocarditis
    - Thrombocytopenia leading to coagulopathy
    - Exanthematous rash
    - Weil syndrome: More severe disease with hepatic insufficiency (with jaundice) and renal insufficiency (nonoliguric)
- **Diagnosis:** Bacterial culture of blood (early) or urine (later); serology; PCR (investigational)
- **Treatment**
  - Mild disease (often self-limiting): Oral amoxicillin or doxycycline (doxycycline is also effective against *Rickettsia*, which can have a similar clinical presentation)
  - More severe disease: Intravenous (IV) penicillin, ampicillin, doxycycline, ceftriaxone, cefotaxime; monitor for Jarisch-Herxheimer reaction in patients receiving penicillin

Plague (*Y pestis*)

- **General information:** Sources of infection include rodents (eg, squirrels, prairie dogs) and the fleas that feed on them
- **Human infection routes:** Direct contact by handling animal tissue; from animal bites or scratches or from bites of fleas; human-to-human transmission by pneumonic plague; aerosol inhalation (bioterrorism hazard)
- **Clinical disease**
  - **Bubonic plague (febrile lymphadenitis):** Most common form
    - Rapidly tender, enlarged, infected lymph node (bubo) with fever
    - Inguinal and femoral lymph nodes most commonly involved; cervical and axillary less common; buboes may further suppurate and drain
  - **Septicemic plague**
    - Disseminated infection; can affect any organ; no buboes
    - Hemorrhagic tissue necrosis ("red death") and gangrenous lesions of skin and digits ("black death")
  - **Pneumonic plague**
    - Inhalation or hematogenous seeding to lungs

- High mortality and highly contagious to other humans (aerosolized droplets)
- **Diagnosis:** Watson or Gram stain of infected tissue shows classic bipolar "safety-pin" morphology; culture and serology; PCR (investigational)
- **Treatment:** Streptomycin or gentamicin for 10 days; alternates include doxycycline, chloramphenicol, TMP-SMX

Rhodococcus Infection (*R equi*)

- **General information:** Found in intestinal tracts of herbivores and in contaminated soil of horse farms; organism is gram positive and also partially acid-fast staining
- **Clinical disease:** Typically affects immunocompromised patients (eg, patients with human immunodeficiency virus [HIV] infection; patients with low cell-mediated immunity)
  - **Pulmonary infection (most common):** Subacute onset, necrotizing cavitation in >50% of cases, consolidation; pleural effusions and empyema
  - **Central nervous system infection:** Brain abscess, meningitis, encephalopathy
  - **Skin and soft tissue infection**
  - **Bloodstream infection:** Secondary hematogenous seeding of multiple organs and joints
  - **Enteric infection:** Localized and mesenteric adenitis
- **Diagnosis:** Organism grows well in culture; blood cultures are commonly positive
- **Treatment (combination therapy recommended; variable duration based on syndrome and severity [eg, 2-6 months]):** azithromycin or clarithromycin, fluoroquinolones, rifampin, vancomycin, imipenem, gentamicin or amikacin

Erysipeloid (*E rhusiopathiae*)

- **General information:** Infects domestic animals such as swine (major reservoir) but also found in sheep, horses, cattle, chickens, crabs, fish, dogs, and cats; occupational exposure in abattoir workers, butchers, fishermen, farmers, and veterinarians
- **Clinical disease**
  - **Localized infection (erysipeloid):** Localized cellulitis; fingers most commonly involved, violaceous skin infection; highly painful; localized lymphangitis and adenitis in about 30% of cases
  - **Diffuse cutaneous disease:** Less common; fever and arthralgia (common)
  - **Bacteremia:** Usually associated with severe illness; often complicated by endocarditis with extensive valve destruction; more common with alcoholism and chronic liver disease
- **Treatment:** Localized disease often resolves without specific treatment but treatment with penicillins, carbapenems, cephalosporins, clindamycin, doxycycline, or macrolides quickens healing; note resistance to vancomycin, sulfonamides, and aminoglycosides

Hydatid and Alveolar Cyst Disease (*Echinococcus granulosus, E vogeli,* and *E multilocularis*)

- **General information:** Cestode (tapeworm) infections produce notable disease of expanding cysts in organs. *E granulosis* is found worldwide (including southwestern US, Africa, southern Europe, Latin America, the Mediterranean, North and East Africa, Australia, New Zealand, western China); *E multilocularis* is predominant in forested regions of northern Europe, North America, Asia, and Arctic regions; *E vogeli* is found in the highlands of South America.
- **Human infection routes:** Humans ingest food contaminated with Echinococcus eggs; oncospheres penetrate gut wall and travel by blood and lymphatics to liver (80%), lungs (18%), or (less commonly) kidneys, bones, brain, eyes
- **Clinical disease**
  - *E granulosus* (dogs and sheep; wolves and moose); associated with livestock and working dogs that are fed slaughtered animals
    - **Cystic hydatidosis, or unilocular hydatid cyst:** Expands as a discrete fluid-filled mass within a fibrous capsule; daughter parasitic cysts develop within the primary cyst
    - **Hydatid cysts:** Found in almost any site; liver is affected in about two-thirds of patients, lungs in 25%; less common in brain, muscles, kidneys, bones, heart, pancreas
    - **Appearance:** Cysts are fluid filled with characteristic internal septa surrounded by a fibrous capsule. Hooklets may be seen upon examination of cyst fluid.
  - *E multilocularis* (foxes and rodents)
    - Alveolar cyst disease; does not form a discrete capsule
    - Liver and other tissue lesions can be extensive and characterized by the alveolar-like structure of aggregations of parasitic cysts
    - Tumor-like cysts develop into multiple fluid-filled vesicles that can invade adjacent tissue or metastasize to other parts of the body
  - *E vogeli* produces a polycystic hydatid disease
- **Treatment**
  - **Surgical resection:** With preoperative and postoperative medical therapy (albendazole or mebendazole, possibly in combination with praziquantel)
  - **Percutaneous aspiration:** With scolicidal agent and reaspiration (PAIR) with pre- and postprocedure medical therapy
  - **Medical therapy alone (albendazole, mebendazole):** For inoperative, multiple, or very small cysts

Toxoplasmosis (*T gondii*)

- **General information:** Domestic cats are primary reservoir; also found in sheep and swine, and in bears and other carnivores
- **Human infection routes**
  - Ingestion of raw or undercooked meat containing tissue cysts; ingestion of food, water, or soil contaminated with cat feces containing infective oocysts
  - Transplacental passage of infective tachyzoites (in mothers with primary infection)

- Transfusion of infected white blood cells or transplantation of an infected organ
- **Clinical disease in immunocompetent patients**
  - **Acute toxoplasmosis:** Resembles mononucleosis syndrome in immunocompetent patient (eg, cervical adenopathy, atypical lymphocytes); heterophil antibody (monospot) test is negative
  - **Congenital toxoplasmosis:** Classic triad of hydrocephalus, cerebral calcification, and chorioretinitis; most infants with congenital toxoplasmosis appear healthy at birth but have a high incidence of serious ophthalmologic and neurologic sequelae that develop over the next 20 years
  - **Toxoplasmic chorioretinitis:** Retinitis with yellowish cotton-wool spots and atrophic black pigmentation
- **Clinical disease in immunosuppressed patients**
  - **Encephalitis:** Multiple small, ring-enhancing lesions at corticomedullary junction and basal ganglia; especially common in patients with advanced HIV infection or AIDS; reactivated (nonprimary) disease
  - **Pneumonitis (severe):** Fever, nonproductive cough; chest radiograph typically shows interstitial infiltrate
  - **Visceral organ disease:** Transplant recipients
  - **Chorioretinitis**
- **Diagnosis**
  - **Serology:** Variable interpretation based on specific assays (often more helpful when applied with head imaging for suspicion of toxoplasmic encephalitis, such as in AIDS patients)
  - **Direct tissue examination:** Tachyzoites; immunoperoxidase stain
  - **Tissue culture**
  - **PCR:** CSF or other body fluid or tissue
- **Treatment**
  - **Immunocompetent patients (eg, generalized adenopathy, fever, malaise):** Treatment is rarely needed unless illness is severe or prolonged; most clinical illness responds spontaneously
  - **Toxoplasmic encephalitis:** See section on "Select Opportunistic Infections in Adult Patients With HIV" (Tables 87-93)
  - **Visceral organ disease (eg, transplant patients):** Combination pyrimethamine and sulfadiazine (or combination pyrimethamine and clindamycin) 4-6 weeks after resolution of symptoms; secondary therapy based on degree and duration of immunosuppression
  - **Toxoplasmic chorioretinitis:** Treat in consultation with an ophthalmologist; use combination pyrimethamine and sulfadiazine (or combination pyrimethamine and clindamycin) for more severe vitreous inflammation
  - **Primary infection during pregnancy:** When infection occurs before 18 weeks' gestation, treat with spiramycin 1 g oral every 8 hours until delivery

Infections Through Animal Bites

Rabies
- **General information:** Transmission can be significantly reduced by preemptive measures
  - Good wound care (immediate soap and water) can reduce rabies risk by 90%
  - Postexposure immunization during incubation period before virus enters central nervous system (CNS) (before onset of neurologic symptoms)
- **Animal vectors**
  - **US:** Bats (most common), skunks, raccoons, some foxes; dogs (rarely)
  - **Third-world or developing nations:** Dogs (most common); wild animals
- **Clinical disease:** Highly neurotropic virus
  - Infection by animal bite eventually enters peripheral nerves (sensory and motor); viral replication occurs with retrograde axoplasmic flow transport to CNS; after spread throughout CNS, virus moves anterograde down peripheral nerves
  - Once symptoms start (eg, pain and paresthesias at wound site), virus has reached spinal ganglion and progressive or rapid encephalitis follows, with mortality approaching 100%
  - **Stages of infection**
    - **Incubation period (variable):** Typically 1-3 months (range, 10 days to several years); 75% of untreated patients become ill within 3 months, 95% within 1 year
    - **Prodrome:** Pain or paresthesia at site of inoculation; early anxiety, apprehension, or irritability
    - **Acute neurologic period:** Autonomic dysfunction (eg, increased salivation and fever): 2 types
      - **Furious rabies (encephalitic rabies):** Hyperreaction, disorientation, hydrophobia (pharyngeal spasms), aerophobia
      - **Paralytic rabies (dumb rabies):** Paralysis; salivary drooling due to paralysis of swallowing muscles
    - **Coma:** Usually occurs within 2 weeks of onset of symptoms; respiratory arrest
- **Diagnosis**
  - **Testing from multiple sources (direct fluorescent antibody staining, PCR, culture):** Skin biopsy from nape of neck, saliva, serum, CSF, and cornea (consult state health department and Centers for Disease Control and Prevention for specific tests)
  - **Brain biopsy (often postmortem):** For Negri bodies (eosinophilic cytoplasmic inclusions)
- **Treatment:** Wash wound and administer postexposure prophylaxis (PEP)
  - **Evaluate for rabies PEP:** See Table 100 below on PEP
  - **Rabies PEP:** Vigorously clean wound in all cases
    - **Patient previously vaccinated:** Vaccinate with 2 doses (on days 0 and 3) with HDCV (human diploid cell vaccine) or PCECV

(purified chick embryo cell vaccine); no rabies immunoglobulin needed
- **Patient not previously vaccinated**
  - Give rabies immunoglobulin 20 IU/kg once (one-half in wound, one-half deep in intramuscular [IM] site)
  - IM vaccination with either HDCV or PCECV in 4 doses (days 0, 3, 7, and 14); for immunosuppressed patients, add a 5th vaccine dose on day 28

Table 100 Recommended PEP for Rabies (in US)

Animal	Condition of Animal	PEP Recommendations
Dogs, cats, ferrets	Healthy and available for 10-day observation	Do not begin PEP unless quarantined animal develops signs or symptoms of rabies[a]
	Known or suspected rabid	Immediate PEP
	Unknown (escaped or animal not available)	Consult local public health officials
Bats, skunks, raccoons, foxes, most other carnivores	Regard as rabid unless geographic area is known to be free of rabies or the animal tests negative for rabies	Immediate PEP[b]
Livestock, rodents, rabbits	Consider each case individually	Consult local public health officials

[a] If animal shows signs of rabies during 10-day holding period, begin PEP immediately. Exception for bites to head and neck: Begin PEP immediately, as rabies incubation period can be <10 days, but stop PEP if animal is healthy after 10 days.

[b] Wild animals such as skunks, raccoons, and bats should be captured, if possible, and killed and tested immediately for rabies rather than being held for observation.

For more information see Rupprecht CE, et al. MMWR Recomm Rep. 2010 Mar 19;59(RR-2): 1–9. Erratum in: MMWR Recomm Rep. 2010 Apr 30;59(16):493.

C canimorsus

- **General information:** Infections typically occur by dog bites (canine oral flora) or scratches
- **Clinical disease:** More severe disease in immunosuppressed patients
  - Soft tissue infection; wide spectrum of disease from mild to fulminant; can be rapid and severe in asplenic patients; digital gangrene may occur
  - Bacteremia and multiorgan involvement (eg, meningitis, endocarditis, pneumonia, cellulitis, bone and joint infections)
- **Treatment:** Use penicillins, carbapenems, clindamycin, 3rd-gen cephalosporins, doxycycline, fluoroquinolones

Pasteurella

- **General information:** *Pasteurella* are part of normal oral flora of many animals (eg, cats [*P multocida*], dogs [*P canis*], rats, cattle, horses, swine, sheep)
- **Clinical disease:** Typically by animal bites
  - **Soft tissue infection:** Very rapid onset (within 24 hours); pain and swelling prominent; purulent drainage in 40% of patients, lymphangitis in 20%, and regional adenopathy in 10%
  - **Bone, joint, and tendon infections**
  - **Respiratory tract infection:** Patients usually have underlying chronic lung disease
  - **Disseminated infection:** Hematogenous spread (usually from wound)
- **Treatment (wounds commonly polymicrobial):** Use penicillins, amoxicillin/clavulanate, β-lactam/β-lactamase inhibitors, carbapenems, doxycycline, most 2nd- and 3rd-gen cephalosporins

Cat-Scratch Disease (B henselae)

- **General information:** Domestic cat is primary carrier and vector; transmission by cat bite or scratch (or flea bite)
- **Clinical disease**
  - **Primary cutaneous lesion:** Develops in 3-10 days at site of bite or scratch
  - **Regional adenopathy:** Tender initially; solitary adenopathy more common but multifocal adenitis can occur
    - **Most common sites:** Axillary, epitrochlear, cervical, supraclavicular, and submandibular lymph nodes
    - **Course:** Persists for several weeks or months, then spontaneously resolves
  - **Parinaud oculoglandular syndrome:** Conjunctivitis, conjunctival granuloma, and adjacent ipsilateral preauricular lymphadenopathy
  - **Other sites (less common) and complications:**
    - Fever of unknown origin
    - Hepatic (granulomatous hepatitis) and splenic involvement
    - Painful arthropathy
    - Osteolytic lesions
    - Neuroretinitis, encephalopathy
- **Diagnosis:** Serology, Warthin-Starry silver staining of node or infected tissue, culture, and PCR
- **Treatment:** Usually not required for isolated cutaneous disease or limited adenopathy; treat persistent or severe symptoms or visceral disease with azithromycin, clarithromycin, TMP-SMX, rifampin, ciprofloxacin, gentamicin, or doxycycline; avoid localized debridement of suppurative lesions, which can cause chronic sinus tract formation

Vaccination Schedules

Recommended Immunization Schedule for Persons Aged 0 Through 6 Years: United States (2011)

The recommended immunization schedule for those 0-6 years is presented in Figure 5. For those who fall behind in the immunization schedule or start late, see the catch-up schedule available on the CDC Web site: http://www.cdc.gov/vaccines/recs/schedules/downloads/child/catchup-schedule-pr

Vaccine	Birth	1 mo	2 mo	4 mo	6 mo	12 mo	15 mo	18 mo	19-23 mo	2-3 y	4-6 y
Hepatitis B[a]	HepB	HepB			HepB						
Rotavirus[b]			RV	RV	RV[b]						
Diphtheria, tetanus, pertussis[c]			DTaP	DTaP	DTaP		DTaP				DTaP
Haemophilus influenzae type b[d]			Hib	Hib[d]	Hib	Hib					
Pneumococcal[e]			PCV	PCV	PCV	PCV				PPSV	PPSV
Inactivated poliovirus[f]			IPV	IPV	IPV						IPV
Influenza[g]					Influenza (yearly)						
Measles, mumps, rubella[h]						MMR		See footnote[h]			MMR
Varicella[i]						Varicella		See footnote[i]			Varicella
Hepatitis A[j]						HepA (2 doses)				HepA series	HepA series
Meningococcal[k]										MCV4	MCV4

Range of recommended ages for all children

Range of recommended ages for certain high-risk groups

Figure 5 Recommended Immunization Schedule for Persons Aged 0 Through 6 Years: United States (2011). (Adapted from Department of Health and Human Services. Centers for Disease Control and Prevention. Available from: http://www.cdc.gov/vaccines/recs/schedules/downloads/child/0-6yrs-schedule-pr.pdf.)

[a] **Hepatitis B (HepB) vaccine.** (Minimum age: Birth.)

- At birth:
  - Administer monovalent HepB to all newborns before hospital discharge.
  - If mother is hepatitis B surface antigen (HBsAg)-positive, administer HepB and 0.5 mL of hepatitis B immune globulin (HBIG) within 12 hours of birth.
  - If mother's HBsAg status is unknown, administer HepB within 12 hours of birth. Determine mother's HBsAg status as soon as possible and, if HBsAg-positive, administer HBIG (no later than age 1 week).
- Doses following the birth dose:
  - The 2nd dose should be administered at age 1 or 2 months. Monovalent HepB vaccine should be used for doses administered before age 6 weeks.
  - Infants born to HBsAg-positive mothers should be tested for HBsAg and antibody to HBsAg 1 to 2 months after completion of at least 3 doses of the HepB series, at age 9 through 18 months (generally at the next well-child visit).
  - Administration of 4 doses of HepB to infants is permissible when a combination vaccine containing HepB is administered after the birth dose.
  - Infants who did not receive a birth dose should receive 3 doses of HepB on a schedule of 0, 1, and 6 months.
  - The final (3rd or 4th) dose in the HepB series should be administered no earlier than age 24 weeks.

[b] **Rotavirus (RV) vaccine.** (Minimum age: 6 weeks.)

- Administer 1st dose at age 6 through 14 weeks (maximum age: 14 weeks and 6 days). Vaccination should not be initiated for infants aged 15 weeks and 0 days or older.
- Maximum age for final dose in RV series is 8 months and 0 days.
- If Rotarix is administered at ages 2 and 4 months, a dose at 6 months is not indicated.

[c] **Diphtheria and tetanus toxoids and acellular pertussis (DTaP) vaccine.** (Minimum age: 6 weeks.)

- The 4th dose may be administered as early as age 12 months, provided at least 6 months have elapsed since the 3rd dose.
- Administer final dose in series at age 4 through 6 years.

[d] **Haemophilus influenzae type b (Hib) conjugate vaccine.** (Minimum age: 6 weeks.)

- If PRP-OMP (PedvaxHIB or Comvax [HepB-Hib]) is administered at ages 2 and 4 months, a dose at age 6 months is not indicated.
- Hiberix should not be used for doses at age 2, 4, or 6 months for the primary series but can be used as the final dose in children aged 12 months through 4 years.

[e] **Pneumococcal vaccine.** (Minimum age: 6 weeks for pneumococcal conjugate vaccine [PCV]; 2 years for pneumococcal polysaccharide vaccine [PPSV].)

- PCV is recommended for all children aged <5 years. Administer 1 dose to all healthy children aged 24 through 59 months who are not completely vaccinated for their age.
- A PCV series begun with 7-valent PCV (PCV7) should be completed with 13-valent PCV (PCV13).
- A single supplemental dose of PCV13 is recommended for all children aged 14 through 59 months who have received an age-appropriate series of PCV7.
- A single supplemental dose of PCV13 is recommended for all children aged 60 through 71 months with underlying medical conditions who have received an age-appropriate series of PCV7.
- The supplemental dose of PCV13 should be administered at least 8 weeks after the previous dose of PCV7. See MMWR Recomm Rep. 2010 Dec 10;59(RR-11):1-18.
- Administer PPSV at least 8 weeks after last dose of PCV to children aged ≥2 years with certain underlying medical conditions, including a cochlear implant.

[f] **Inactivated poliovirus (IPV) vaccine.** (Minimum age: 6 weeks.)

- If ≥4 doses are administered before age 4 years, an additional dose should be administered at ages 4 through 6 years.
- Final dose in IPV series should be administered on or after 4th birthday and at least 6 months after previous dose.

[g] **Influenza vaccine (seasonal).** (Minimum age: 6 months for trivalent inactivated influenza vaccine [TIV]; 2 years for live, attenuated influenza vaccine [LAIV].)

- For healthy children aged ≥2 years (ie, those who do not have underlying medical conditions that predispose them to influenza complications), use either TIV or LAIV, except LAIV should not be given to children aged 2 through 4 years who have had wheezing in the past 12 months.
- Administer 2 doses (separated by at least 4 weeks) to children aged 6 months through 8 years who are receiving influenza vaccine for the 1st time or who were vaccinated for the 1st time during the previous influenza season but received only 1 dose.

- Children aged 6 months through 8 years who received no doses of monovalent 2009 H1N1 vaccine should receive 2 doses of 2010-2011 seasonal influenza vaccine. See MMWR Recomm Rep. 2010 Aug 6;59(RR-8):1-62. Update in: MMWR Recomm Rep. 2010 Aug 13;59(31):989-92. Errata in: MMWR Recomm Rep. 2010 Aug 13;59(31):993, and MMWR Recomm Rep. 2010 Sep 10;59(35):1147.

[h] **Measles, mumps, and rubella (MMR) vaccine.** (Minimum age: 12 months.)

- Second dose may be administered before age 4 years, provided at least 4 weeks have elapsed since 1st dose.

[i] **Varicella vaccine.** (Minimum age: 12 months.)

- Second dose may be administered before age 4 years, provided at least 3 months have elapsed since 1st dose.
- For children aged 1 through 12 years, the recommended minimum interval between doses is 3 months. However, if 2nd dose was administered at least 4 weeks after 1st dose, it can be accepted as valid.

[j] **Hepatitis A (HepA) vaccine.** (Minimum age: 12 months.)

- Administer 2 doses at least 6 months apart.
- HepA is recommended for children older than 23 months who live in areas where vaccination programs target older children, who are at increased risk for infection, or for whom immunity against hepatitis A virus (HAV) is desired.

[k] **Meningococcal conjugate vaccine, quadrivalent (MCV4).** (Minimum age: 2 years.)

- Administer 2 doses of MCV4 at least 8 weeks apart to children aged 2 through 10 years with persistent complement component deficiency and anatomical or functional asplenia, and administer 1 dose every 5 years thereafter.
- Persons with human immunodeficiency virus (HIV) infection who are vaccinated with MCV4 should receive 2 doses at least 8 weeks apart.
- Administer 1 dose of MCV4 to children aged 2 through 10 years who travel to countries with highly endemic or epidemic disease and during outbreaks caused by a vaccine serogroup.
- Administer MCV4 to children at continued risk for meningococcal disease who were previously vaccinated with MCV4 or meningococcal polysaccharide vaccine after 3 years if the 1st dose was administered at ages 2 through 6 years.

This schedule includes recommendations in effect as of December 21, 2010. Any dose not administered at the recommended age should be administered at a subsequent visit, when indicated and feasible. The use of a combination vaccine generally is preferred over separate injections of its equivalent component vaccines. Considerations should include provider assessment, patient preference, and the potential for adverse events. Providers should consult the relevant Advisory Committee on Immunization Practices (ACIP) statement on the Centers for Disease Control and Prevention (CDC) Web site for detailed recommendations (http://www.cdc.gov/vaccines/pubs/acip-list.htm). Clinically significant adverse events that follow immunization should be reported to the Vaccine Adverse Event Reporting System (VAERS) (http://www.vaers.hhs. gov [telephone: 800-822-7967]).

Recommended Immunization Schedule for Persons Aged 7 Through 18 Years: United States (2011)

For those 4 months through 18 years who fall behind the immunization schedule or start late (Figure 6), see the catch-up schedule at http://www.cdc.gov/vaccines/recs/schedules/downloads/child/catchup-schedule-pr.pdf.

Vaccine	Age			
	7-10 y	11-12 y	13-18 y	
Tetanus, diphtheria, pertussis[a]		Tdap	Tdap	
Human papillomavirus[b]	See footnote[b]	HPV (3 doses) (females)	HPV series	
Meningococcal[c]	MCV4	MCV4	MCV4	
Influenza[d]	Influenza (yearly)			
Pneumococcal[e]	Pneumococcal			
Hepatitis A[f]	HepA series			
Hepatitis B[g]	HepB series			
Inactivated poliovirus[h]	IPV series			
Measles, mumps, rubella[i]	MMR series			
Varicella[j]	Varicella series			

Range of recommended ages for all children

Range of recommended ages for catch-up immunization

Range of recommended ages for certain high-risk groups

Figure 6 Recommended Immunization Schedule for Persons Aged 7 Through 18 Years: United States (2011). (Adapted from Department of Health and Human Services. Centers for Disease Control and Prevention. Available from: http://www.cdc.gov/vaccines/recs/schedules/downloads/child/7-18yrs-schedule-pr.pdf.)

[a] **Tetanus and diphtheria toxoids and acellular pertussis (Tdap) vaccine.** (Minimum age: 10 years for Boostrix and 11 years for Adacel.)
- Persons aged 11 through 18 years who have not received Tdap should receive a dose followed by diphtheria toxoid (Td) booster doses every 10 years thereafter.
- Persons aged 7 through 10 years who are not fully immunized against pertussis (including those never vaccinated or with unknown pertussis vaccination status) should receive a single dose of Tdap. Refer to the catch-up schedule if additional doses of tetanus and diphtheria toxoid-containing vaccine are needed.
- Tdap can be administered regardless of the interval since the last tetanus and diptheria toxoid-containing vaccine.

[b] **Human papillomavirus (HPV) vaccine.** (Minimum age: 9 years.)
- Quadrivalent HPV vaccine (HPV4) or bivalent HPV vaccine (HPV2) is recommended for prevention of cervical precancers and cancers in females.
- HPV4 is recommended for prevention of cervical precancers, cancers, and genital warts in females.
- HPV4 may be administered in a 3-dose series to males aged 9 through 18 years to reduce their likelihood of acquiring genital warts.
- Administer 2nd dose 1 to 2 months after 1st dose, and 3rd dose 6 months after 1st dose (at least 24 weeks after 1st dose).

[c] **Meningococcal conjugate vaccine, quadrivalent (MCV4).** (Minimum age: 2 years.)
- Administer at ages 11 through 12 years with a booster dose at age 16 years.
- Administer 1 dose at ages 13 through 18 years if not previously vaccinated.
- Persons who received their first dose at ages 13 through 15 years should receive a booster dose at ages 16 through 18 years.
- Administer 1 dose to previously unvaccinated college freshmen living in a dormitory.
- Administer 2 doses at least 8 weeks apart to children aged 2 through 10 years with persistent complement component deficiency and anatomical or functional asplenia, and 1 dose every 5 years thereafter.
- Persons with HIV infection who are vaccinated with MCV4 should receive 2 doses at least 8 weeks apart.
- Administer 1 dose to children aged 2 through 10 years who travel to countries with highly endemic or epidemic disease and during outbreaks caused by a vaccine serogroup.
- Administer to children at continued risk for meningococcal disease who were previously vaccinated with MCV4 or meningococcal polysaccharide vaccine after 3 years (if 1st dose was administered at age 2 through 6 years) or after 5 years (if 1st dose was administered at age ≥7 years).

[d] **Influenza vaccine (seasonal).**
- For healthy nonpregnant persons aged 7 through 18 years (ie, those who do not have underlying medical conditions that predispose them to influenza complications), either TIV or LAIV may be used.
- Administer 2 doses (separated by at least 4 weeks) to children aged 6 months through 8 years who are receiving seasonal influenza vaccine for the 1st time or who were vaccinated for the 1st time during the previous influenza season but received only 1 dose.
- Children 6 months through 8 years of age who received no doses of monovalent 2009 H1N1 vaccine should receive 2 doses of 2010-2011 seasonal influenza vaccine. See MMWR Recomm Rep. 2010 Aug 6;59(RR-8):1-62. Update in: MMWR Recomm Rep. 2010 Aug 13;59(31):989-92. Errata in: MMWR Recomm Rep. 2010 Aug 13;59(31):993, and MMWR Recomm Rep. 2010 Sep 10;59(35):1147.

[e] **Pneumococcal vaccine.**
- A single dose of 13-valent pneumococcal conjugate vaccine (PCV13) may be administered to children aged 6 through 18 years who have functional or anatomical asplenia, HIV infection or other immunocompromising condition, cochlear implant, or cerebrospinal fluid leak. See MMWR Recomm Rep. 2010 Dec 10;59(RR-11):1-18.
- The dose of PCV13 should be administered at least 8 weeks after the previous dose of PCV7.
- Administer pneumococcal polysaccharide vaccine (PPSV) at least 8 weeks after the last dose of PCV to children with certain underlying medical conditions, including a cochlear implant. A single revaccination should be administered after 5 years to children with functional or anatomical asplenia or an immunocompromising condition.

[f] **Hepatitis A (HepA) vaccine.**
- Administer 2 doses at least 6 months apart.

- HepA is recommended for children aged >23 months who live in areas where vaccination programs target older children, who are at increased risk for infection, or for whom immunity against hepatitis A (HAV) is desired.

ᵍ **Hepatitis B (HepB) vaccine.**

- Administer the 3-dose series to those not previously vaccinated. For those with incomplete vaccination, follow the catch-up schedule.
- A 2-dose series (separated by at least 4 months) of adult formulation Recombivax HB is licensed for children aged 11 through 15 years.

ʰ **Inactivated poliovirus (IPV) vaccine.**

- The final dose in the series should be administered on or after the 4th birthday and at least 6 months after the previous dose.
- If both OPV and IPV were administered as part of a series, a total of 4 doses should be administered, regardless of the child's current age.

ⁱ **Measles, mumps, and rubella (MMR) vaccine.**

- The minimum interval between the 2 doses is 4 weeks.

ʲ **Varicella vaccine.**

- For persons aged 7 through 18 years without evidence of immunity (see MMWR Recomm Rep. 2007 Jun 22;56[RR-4]:1-40), administer 2 doses if not previously vaccinated or 2nd dose if only 1 dose has been administered.
- For persons aged 7 through 12 years, the recommended minimum interval between doses is 3 months. However, if 2nd dose was administered at least 4 weeks after 1st dose, it can be accepted as valid.
- For persons aged ≥13 years, the minimum interval between doses is 4 weeks.

This schedule includes recommendations in effect as of December 15, 2010. Any dose not administered at the recommended age should be administered at a subsequent visit, when indicated and feasible. The use of a combination vaccine generally is preferred over separate injections its equivalent component vaccines. Considerations should include provider assessment, patient preference, and the potential for adverse events. Providers should consult the relevant ACIP statement for detailed recommendations (http://www.cdc.gov/vaccines/pubs/acip-list.htm).

Recommended Adult Immunization Schedule by Vaccine and Age Groups and Vaccines That Might Be Indicated for Adults, Based on Medical and Other Indications: United States (2011)

Note: These recommendations (Figure 7 and Figure 8) **MUST** be read along with the footnotes that follow containing number of doses, intervals between doses, and other important information.

Vaccine	Age Group				
	19-26 y	27-49 y	50-59 y	60-64 y	≥65 y
Influenza[a]	1 dose annually				
Tetanus, diphtheria, pertussis (Td/Tdap)[b]	Substitute 1-time dose of Tdap for Td booster; then boost with Td every 10 y				Td booster every 10 y
Varicella[c]	2 doses				
Human papillomavirus (HPV)[d]	3 doses (females)				
Zoster[e]				1 dose	
Measles, mumps, rubella (MMR)[f]	1 or 2 doses			1 dose	
Pneumococcal (polysaccharide)[g, h]		1 or 2 doses			1 dose
Meningococcal[i]	1 or more doses				
Hepatitis A[j]	2 doses				
Hepatitis B[k]	3 doses				

For all persons in this category who meet age requirements and lack evidence of immunity (eg, no documentation of vaccination or evidence of prior infection)

Recommended if some other risk factor is present (eg, on basis of medical, occupational, lifestyle, or other indications)

No recommendation

Figure 7 Recommended Adult Immunization Schedule by Vaccine and Age Groups: United States (2011). (Adapted from Department of Health and Human Services. Centers for Disease Control and Prevention. Available from: http://www.cdc.gov/vaccines/recs/schedules/downloads/adult/mmwr-adult-schedule.pdf.) For explanation of Figure 7 footnotes, see pages 352-355.

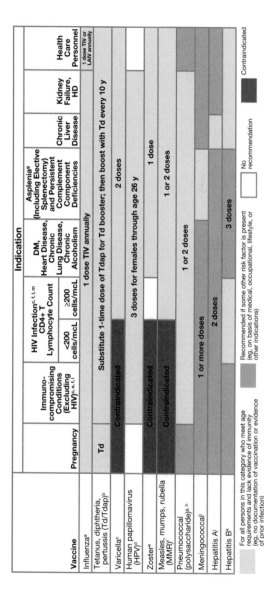

Figure 8 Vaccines That Might Be Indicated for Adults, Based on Medical and Other Indications: United States (2011). (Adapted from Department of Health and Human Services. Centers for Disease Control and Prevention. Available from: http://www.cdc.gov/vaccines/recs/schedules/downloads/adult/mmwr-adult-schedule.pdf.) For explanation of Figure 8 footnotes, see pages 352-355.

[a] **Influenza vaccine.**

- Annual vaccination against influenza is recommended for all persons aged ≥6 months, including all adults. Healthy, nonpregnant adults aged <50 years without high-risk medical conditions can receive either intranasally administered live, attenuated influenza vaccine (FluMist) or inactivated influenza vaccine. Other persons should receive the inactivated vaccine. Adults aged ≥65 years can receive the standard influenza vaccine or the high-dose (Fluzone) influenza vaccine. Additional information about influenza vaccination is available at http://www.cdc.gov/flu/protect/vaccine/.

[b] **Tetanus and diphtheria toxoids (Td) vaccine; tetanus and diphtheria toxoids and acellular pertussis (Tdap) vaccine.**

- Administer a 1-time dose of Tdap to adults aged <65 years who have not received Tdap previously or for whom vaccine status is unknown to replace 1 of the 10-year Td boosters, and as soon as feasible to all 1) postpartum women, 2) close contacts of infants aged <12 months (eg, grandparents and child-care providers), and 3) health care personnel with direct patient contact. Adults aged ≥65 years who have not previously received Tdap and who have close contact with an infant aged <12 months also should be vaccinated. Other adults aged ≥65 years may receive Tdap. Tdap can be administered regardless of interval after the most recent tetanus or diphtheria-containing vaccine.

- Adults with uncertain or incomplete history of completing a 3-dose primary vaccination series with Td-containing vaccines should begin or complete a primary vaccination series. For unvaccinated adults, administer the 1st 2 doses at least 4 weeks apart and the 3rd dose 6-12 months after the 2nd dose. If incompletely vaccinated (ie, <3 doses), administer remaining doses. Substitute a 1-time dose of Tdap for 1 dose of Td, either in the primary series or for the routine booster, whichever comes first.

- If a pregnant woman received the most recent Td vaccination ≥10 years previously, administer Td during the 2nd or 3rd trimester. If the woman received the most recent Td vaccination <10 years previously, administer Tdap during the immediate postpartum period. At the clinician's discretion, Td may be deferred during pregnancy, and Tdap may be substituted in the immediate postpartum period; or Tdap may be administered instead of Td to a pregnant woman after an informed consent discussion.

- Consult the ACIP statement for recommendations for administering Td as prophylaxis in wound management (http://www.cdc.gov/vaccines/pubs/acip-list.htm).

[c] **Varicella vaccine.**

- All adults without evidence of immunity to varicella should receive 2 doses of single-antigen varicella vaccine if not previously vaccinated or the 2nd dose if they have received only 1 dose, unless they have a medical contraindication. Special consideration should be given to those who 1) have close contact with persons at high risk for severe disease (eg, health care personnel and family contacts of persons with immunocompromising conditions), or 2) are at high risk for exposure or transmission (eg, teachers; child-care employees; residents and staff members of institutional settings, including correctional institutions; college students; military personnel; adolescents and adults living in households with children; nonpregnant women of childbearing age; and international travelers).

- Evidence of immunity to varicella in adults includes any of the following: 1) documentation of 2 doses of varicella vaccine at least 4 weeks apart; 2) US-born before 1980 (although for health care personnel and pregnant women, birth before 1980 should not be considered evidence of immunity); 3) history of varicella based on diagnosis or verification of varicella by a health care provider (for a patient reporting a history of or having an atypical case, a mild case, or both, health care providers should seek either an epidemiologic link to a typical varicella case or to a laboratory-confirmed case or evidence of laboratory confirmation, if testing was performed at the time of acute disease); 4) history of herpes zoster based on diagnosis or verification of herpes zoster by a health care provider; or 5) laboratory evidence of immunity or laboratory confirmation of disease.

- Pregnant women should be assessed for evidence of varicella immunity. Women who do not have evidence of immunity should receive the 1st dose of varicella vaccine upon completion or termination of pregnancy and before discharge from the health care facility. The 2nd dose should be administered 4-8 weeks after the 1st dose.

[d] **Human papillomavirus (HPV) vaccine.**

- HPV vaccination with either HPV4 or HPV2 is recommended for females at age 11 or 12 years with catch-up vaccination for females aged 13 through 26 years.

- Ideally, vaccine should be administered before potential exposure to HPV through sexual activity; however, females who are sexually active should still be vaccinated consistent with age-based recommendations. Sexually active females who have not been infected with any of the 4 HPV vaccine types (types 6, 11, 16, and 18, all of which HPV4 prevents) or with any of the 2 HPV vaccine types (types 16 and 18, both of which HPV2 prevents) receive the full benefit of the vaccination. Vaccination is less beneficial for females who have already been infected with 1 or more of the HPV vaccine types. HPV4 or HPV2 can be administered to persons with a history of genital warts, abnormal Papanicolaou test, or positive HPV DNA test, because these conditions are not evidence of previous infection with all vaccine HPV types.

- HPV4 may be administered to males aged 9 through 26 years to reduce their likelihood of contracting genital warts. HPV4 would be most effective when administered before exposure to HPV through sexual contact.
- A complete series for either HPV4 or HPV2 consists of 3 doses. The 2nd dose should be administered 1-2 months after the 1st dose; the 3rd dose should be administered 6 months after the 1st dose.
- Although HPV vaccination is not specifically recommended for persons with the medical indications described in Figure 8 ("Vaccines That Might Be Indicated for Adults, Based on Medical and Other Indications [2011]"), it may be administered to these persons because the HPV vaccine is not a live-virus vaccine. However, the immune response and vaccine efficacy might be more reduced for persons with the medical indications described in Figure 8 than for persons who are immunocompetent or who do not have the medical indications described. Health care personnel are not at increased risk because of occupational exposure, and should be vaccinated consistent with age-based recommendations.

^e Herpes zoster vaccine.

- A single dose of zoster vaccine is recommended for adults aged ≥60 years regardless of whether they report a previous episode of herpes zoster. Persons with chronic medical conditions may be vaccinated unless their condition constitutes a contraindication.

^f Measles, mumps, and rubella (MMR) vaccine.

- Adults born before 1957 generally are considered immune to measles and mumps. All adults born in 1957 or later should have documentation of 1 or more doses of MMR vaccine unless they have 1) a medical contraindication to the vaccine; 2) laboratory evidence of immunity to each of the 3 diseases; or 3) documentation of provider-diagnosed measles or mumps disease. For rubella, documentation of provider-diagnosed disease is not considered acceptable evidence of immunity.
- **Measles component:** A 2nd dose of MMR vaccine, administered a minimum of 28 days after the 1st dose, is recommended for adults who 1) have been exposed recently to measles or are in an outbreak setting; 2) are students in postsecondary educational institutions; 3) work in a health care facility; or 4) plan to travel internationally. Persons who received inactivated (killed) measles vaccine or measles vaccine of unknown type during 1963-1967 should be revaccinated with 2 doses of MMR vaccine.
- **Mumps component:** A 2nd dose of MMR vaccine, administered a minimum of 28 days after the 1st dose, is recommended for adults who 1) live in a community experiencing a mumps outbreak and are in an affected age group; 2) are students in postsecondary educational institutions; 3) work in a health care facility; or 4) plan to travel internationally. Persons vaccinated before 1979 with either killed mumps vaccine or mumps vaccine of unknown type who are at high risk for mumps infection (eg, persons who are working in a health care facility) should be revaccinated with 2 doses of MMR vaccine.
- **Rubella component:** For women of childbearing age, regardless of birth year, rubella immunity should be determined. If there is no evidence of immunity, women who are not pregnant should be vaccinated. Pregnant women who do not have evidence of immunity should receive MMR vaccine upon completion or termination of pregnancy and before discharge from the health care facility.
- **Health care personnel born before 1957:** For unvaccinated health care personnel born before 1957 who lack laboratory evidence of measles, mumps, and/or rubella immunity or laboratory confirmation of disease, health care facilities should 1) consider routinely vaccinating personnel with 2 doses of MMR vaccine at the appropriate interval (for measles and mumps) and 1 dose of MMR vaccine (for rubella), and 2) recommend 2 doses of MMR vaccine at the appropriate interval during an outbreak of measles or mumps, and 1 dose during an outbreak of rubella. Complete information about evidence of immunity is available at http://www.cdc.gov/vaccines/recs/provisional/downloads/mmr-evidence-immunity-Aug2009-508.pdf.

ᵍ Pneumococcal polysaccharide (PPSV) vaccine.

- Vaccinate all persons with the following indications:
  - **Medical:** Chronic lung disease (including asthma); chronic cardiovascular diseases; diabetes mellitus; chronic liver diseases, cirrhosis; chronic alcoholism; functional or anatomical asplenia (eg, sickle cell disease or splenectomy [if elective splenectomy is planned, vaccinate at least 2 weeks before surgery]); immunocompromising conditions (including chronic renal failure or nephrotic syndrome); and cochlear implants and cerebrospinal fluid leaks. Vaccinate as close to HIV diagnosis as possible.
  - **Other:** Residents of nursing homes or long-term care facilities and persons who smoke cigarettes. Routine use of PPSV is not recommended for American Indians or Alaska Natives or persons aged <65 years unless they have underlying medical conditions that are PPSV indications. However, public health authorities may consider recommending PPSV for American Indians or Alaska Natives and persons aged 50 through 64 years who are living in areas where the risk for invasive pneumococcal disease is increased.

ʰ Revaccination with PPSV.

- One-time revaccination after 5 years is recommended for persons aged 19 through 64 years with chronic renal failure or nephrotic syndrome; functional or anatomical asplenia (eg, sickle cell disease or splenectomy); and for persons with immunocompromising conditions. For persons aged ≥65 years, 1-time revaccination is recommended if they were vaccinated ≥5 years previously and were aged <65 years at the time of primary vaccination.

ⁱ Meningococcal vaccine.

- Meningococcal vaccine should be administered to persons with the following indications:
  - **Medical:** A 2-dose series of meningococcal conjugate vaccine is recommended for adults with anatomical or functional asplenia, or with persistent complement component deficiencies. Adults with HIV infection who are vaccinated should also receive a routine 2-dose series. The 2 doses should be administered at 0 and 2 months.
  - **Other:** A single dose of meningococcal vaccine is recommended for unvaccinated first-year college students living in dormitories; microbiologists routinely exposed to isolates of *Neisseria meningitidis*; military recruits; and persons who travel to or live in countries where meningococcal disease is hyperendemic or epidemic (eg, the "meningitis belt" of sub-Saharan Africa during the dry season [December through June]), particularly if their contact with local populations will be prolonged. Vaccination is required by the government of Saudi Arabia for all travelers to Mecca during the annual hajj.
- MCV4 is preferred for adults with any of the preceding indications who are aged ≤55 years; MPSV4 is preferred for adults aged ≥56 years. Revaccination with MCV4 after 5 years is recommended for adults previously vaccinated with MCV4 or MPSV4 who remain at increased risk for infection (eg, adults with anatomical or functional asplenia, or with persistent complement component deficiencies).

ʲ Hepatitis A vaccine.

- Vaccinate persons with any of the following indications and any person seeking protection from HAV infection:
  - **Behavioral:** Men who have sex with men and persons who use injection drugs.
  - **Occupational:** Persons working with HAV-infected primates or with HAV in a research laboratory setting.
  - **Medical:** Persons with chronic liver disease and persons who receive clotting factor concentrates.
  - **Other:** Persons traveling to or working in countries that have high or intermediate endemicity of HAV (a list of such countries is available at http://wwwnc.cdc.gov/travel/yellowbook/2012/chapter-3-infectious-diseases-related-to-travel/hepatitis-a.htm).
- Unvaccinated persons who anticipate close personal contact (eg, household contact or regular babysitting) with an international adoptee from a country of high or intermediate endemicity during the 1st 60 days after arrival of the adoptee in the US should be vaccinated. The 1st dose of the 2-dose HAV series should be administered as soon as adoption is planned, ideally ≥2 weeks before the arrival of the adoptee.
- Single-antigen vaccine formulations should be administered in a 2-dose schedule at either 0 and 6-12 months (Havrix) or at 0 and 6-18 months (Vaqta). If the combined HAV and hepatitis B vaccine (Twinrix) is used, administer 3 doses at 0, 1, and 6 months; alternatively, a 4-dose schedule may be administered on days 0, 7, and 21-30, followed by a booster dose at month 12.

ᵏ **Hepatitis B vaccine.**
- Vaccinate persons with any of the following indications and any person seeking protection from hepatitis B virus (HBV) infection:
  - **Behavioral:** Sexually active persons who are not in a long-term, mutually monogamous relationship (eg, persons with more than 1 sex partner during the previous 6 months); persons seeking evaluation or treatment for a sexually transmitted disease (STD); current or recent injection-drug users; and men who have sex with other men.
  - **Occupational:** Health care personnel and public safety workers who are exposed to blood or other potentially infectious body fluids.
  - **Medical:** Persons with end-stage renal disease, including patients receiving hemodialysis; persons with HIV infection; and persons with chronic liver disease.
  - **Other:** Household contacts and sex partners of persons with chronic HBV infection; clients and staff members of institutions for persons with developmental disabilities; and international travelers to countries with high or intermediate prevalence of chronic HBV infection (a list of countries is available at wwwnc.cdc.gov/travel/yellowbook/2012/chapter-3-infectious-diseases-related-to-travel/hepatitis-b.htm).
- HBV vaccination is recommended for all adults in the following settings: STD treatment facilities; HIV testing and treatment facilities; facilities providing drug-abuse treatment and prevention services; health care settings targeting services to injection-drug users or men who have sex with other men; correctional facilities; end-stage renal disease programs and facilities for chronic hemodialysis patients; and institutions and nonresidential day care facilities for persons with developmental disabilities.
- Administer missing doses to complete a 3-dose series of HepB to those persons not previously vaccinated or not completely vaccinated. The 2nd dose should be administered 1 month after the 1st dose; the 3rd dose should be administered at least 2 months after the 2nd dose (and at least 4 months after the 1st dose). If the combined HAV and HBV vaccine (Twinrix) is used, administer 3 doses at 0, 1, and 6 months; alternatively, a 4-dose Twinrix schedule may be used, administered on days 0, 7, and 21-30, followed by a booster dose at month 12.
- Adult patients receiving hemodialysis or who have other immunocompromising conditions should receive 1 dose of 40 mcg/mL (Recombivax HB) administered on a 3-dose schedule or 2 doses of 20 mcg/mL (Engerix-B) administered simultaneously on a 4-dose schedule at 0, 1, 2, and 6 months.

ˡ **Immunocompromising conditions (Figure 8 only).**
- Inactivated vaccines generally are acceptable (eg, pneumococcal, meningococcal, influenza [inactivated influenza vaccine]) and live vaccines generally are avoided in persons with immune deficiencies or immunocompromising conditions. Information on specific conditions is available at http://www.cdc.gov/vaccines/pubs/acip-list.htm.

ᵐ **Select conditions for which Hib vaccine may be used (Figure 8 only).**
- One dose of Hib vaccine should be considered for persons who have sickle cell disease, leukemia, or HIV infection, or who have had a splenectomy, if they have not previously received Hib vaccine.

Additional information about the vaccines in this schedule (Figures 7 and 8), extent of available data, and contraindications for their use is also available at http://www.cdc.gov/vaccines/ or from the CDC-INFO Contact Center at 800-CDC-INFO (800-232-4636) in English and Spanish, 24 hours a day, 7 days a week.

Use of trade names and commercial sources is for identification only and does not imply endorsement by the US Department of Health and Human Services or Mayo Clinic.

The schedules in Figure 8 indicate the recommended age groups and medical indications for which administration of currently licensed vaccines is commonly indicated for adults aged ≥19 years as of January 1, 2010. Licensed combination vaccines may be used whenever any components of the combination are indicated and when the vaccine's other components are not contraindicated. For detailed recommendations on all vaccines, including those used primarily for travelers or that are issued during specific times of the year, consult the manufacturers' package inserts and the complete statements from the ACIP (http://www.cdc.gov/vaccines/pubs/acip-list.htm).

For complete immunization statements by the ACIP, see http://www.cdc.gov/vaccines/pubs/acip-list.htm.

Travel Medicine/Prophylaxis

Travel Prophylaxis

Insect Bite Precautions and Prevention of Insect-Transmitted Diseases

- Insect bite precautions are essential.
  - **DEET (N,N-diethyl-meta-toluamide)** or picaridin-containing insect repellents
    - Concentration: A DEET concentration of 20-50% is safe for both adults and children >2 months of age. A DEET concentration of >50% is **NOT** recommended because it affords no additional benefit.
  - Long sleeves and long pants
  - The insecticide permethrin can be applied to clothing, shoes, tents, mosquito nets, and other gear for additional protection. It is **NOT** intended for use directly on skin. Properly treated permethrin-soaked clothing is effective for up to 5-6 washes and 4 weeks.

Malaria Prevention

- The risk of contracting malaria varies from country to country.
  - Countries with malaria transmission are located in Africa, Asia, Southeast Asia, Central and South America, the Middle East, and the Caribbean.
- Prophylaxis choice depends on the itinerary, geographic area, duration of travel, and the patient's medical history and ability to pay for medications. Common options include:
  - chloroquine
  - atovaquone/proguanil (Malarone)
  - doxycycline
  - mefloquine
- Patients should be told to seek immediate medical attention if a febrile illness develops after they travel to a malaria-endemic country. They should inform any health care providers evaluating them that they have traveled to a malaria-endemic country.
- Standby malaria treatment doses should rarely be carried by patients traveling for a prolonged period in high-risk countries or regions of the world. Standby treatment is either with the combination pill atovaquone/proguanil or with the combination pill artemether/lumefantrine (Coartem).

Table 101 Common Malaria Chemoprophylaxis Medications

	Medication	
Characteristic	**mefloquine**	**atovaquone/proguanil**
Formulation	Tab	Tab
Effectiveness	90-100%	90-95%
Dosing	1 tab weekly	1 tab daily
Schedule	2 wk before travel, weekly while there, and for 4 wk after return	2 days before travel, daily while there, and for 1 wk after return
Advantages	Weekly	Minimal side effects
Disadvantages or side effects	Dreams, insomnia, and (in 1% of patients) acute neuropsychotic reaction	Occasional diarrhea, insomnia
Pregnancy use	Generally do not use unless absolutely necessary (mefloquine is the only chemoprophylaxis option for pregnant patients who must travel to CQ-resistant areas; minimal to no risk in 2nd or 3rd trimester; can also be given cautiously in 1st trimester if no other options are available; see CDC guidelines at http://wwwnc.cdc.gov/travel/yellowbook/2010/chapter-2/malaria.aspx)	No
Approximate cost	$10/wk	$5/day

Medication	
doxycycline	**chloroquine (for CQ-Sensitive Areas Only)**
Tab	Tab or suspension
90-95%	90-100%
1 tab daily	1 tab weekly
2 days before travel, daily while there, and for 4 wk after return	1-2 wk before travel, weekly while there, and for 4 wk after return
Results in possible decrease in diarrhea	Weekly
Can cause GI symptoms, including esophageal ulcers (take with a full glass of water), increased skin sensitivity to sun, yeast infections (female patients); risk of *Clostridium difficile* colitis	Bitter taste; ear effects (tinnitus, hearing loss) or eye effects (blurred vision, retinopathy) with prolonged use (months to years)
No	Yes
$0.25/day	$10/wk

Recommendations for Prevention of Vaccine-Preventable Diseases While Traveling

- Ideally, vaccinations prior to travel should be completed at least 4 weeks before departure
- Individual risk–benefit discussion should be undertaken before vaccination
- Specific vaccine contraindications should be reviewed before vaccination
- Prolonged travel of months to years, such as expatriation, may require vaccination many months before departure (eg, hepatitis B vaccine series can take up to 6 months to complete)

Table 102 General Geography-Based Vaccine Recommendations for Adults Traveling Internationally[a,b]

Routine Vaccines Appropriate for All Adults Prior to Travel	Travel Only to Western Europe, Japan, Australia, or New Zealand
Hepatitis A vaccine: Series: 2 doses Immunity: About 20-25 y after 2nd dose	No additional special vaccines; update routine adult vaccinations; give annual influenza vaccine
Influenza vaccine: Annually for persons aged ≥50 y or for patients with underlying medical problems such as asthma; 2 types of vaccines (inactivated injectable or live attenuated nasal vaccine, the latter not recommended for patients who are immunocompromised, >50 y old, or asthmatic)	**Tick-borne encephalitis vaccine:** May be needed in some areas of Europe (not available in US) for prolonged stays (especially those with extensive outdoor exposure); insect precautions advised
Td or Tdap: Administer per ACIP guidelines; vaccine booster in adults required every 10 y	**Japanese encephalitis vaccine:** Recommended before prolonged travel to Japan (see last entry in hepatitis A vaccine row above)

Travel to Countries in South America, Africa, or the Middle East	Travel to Eastern Europe, the Former USSR, or Asia
Meningococcal vaccine:	**Japanese encephalitis vaccine inactivated, adsorbed (Ixiaro)** (for Asia only):
Give before travel to some countries in Africa and the Middle East	Series: 2 doses 28 days apart or 3 doses over 30 days (JE-VAX for persons aged <17 y) for prolonged (>4 wk) or extensive rural travel
Immunity: Depends on type of vaccine; 3 y (older polysaccharide vaccine) to 10 y (conjugated vaccine)	Immunity: 3 y
Yellow fever vaccine:	**Yellow fever vaccine:**
Required **10 days before** entry to a country where yellow fever is endemic; live viral vaccine not recommended for patients who are immunocompromised, affected by thymic dysfunction, or <6 mo old	Proof of vaccination may be required **before** flying directly from an infected or endemic country in South America or Africa
Immunity: 10 y	

Poliomyelitis vaccine:

Recommended **before** travel to some countries

Immunity: One-time inactivated injectable adult booster needed if childhood series was completed

(*Continues*)

Table 102 General Geography-Based Vaccine Recommendations for Adults Traveling Internationally[a,b] (Cont'd.)

Routine Vaccines Appropriate for All Adults Prior to Travel	Travel Only to Western Europe, Japan, Australia, or New Zealand
MMR:	
Series: 2 doses if born after 1957; live viral vaccine not suitable for immunocompromised patients	
Pneumococcal vaccine:	
For patients aged ≥65 y or who have underlying chronic medical conditions (DM, renal insufficiency, asplenia, CVD, immunosuppression)	
Human papillomavirus vaccine:	
Should be offered to women aged 9-26 y	
Varicella vaccine:	
Series: 2 doses 4 wk apart for patients with no immunity to varicella; live viral vaccine not suitable for immunocompromised patients	
Shingles vaccine:	
Series: 1 dose for patients aged >60 y; live viral vaccine not suitable for immunocompromised patients	

[a] These are general guidelines for healthy persons and do **NOT** apply to immunocompromised persons.

[b] Before any vaccination is administered, patients should consult with a health care professional to review their personal medical history and discuss the contraindications and risks of vaccines.

Travel to Countries in South America, Africa, or the Middle East	Travel to Eastern Europe, the Former USSR, or Asia

Typhoid vaccine:

Oral or injectable; oral formulation is a live attenuated bacterial vaccine not suitable for immunocompromised patients

Immunity: 5 y (oral) or 2 y (injectable)

Rabies pre-exposure vaccine:

Series: 3 doses before prolonged travel to developing countries

Immunity: 5-10 y; vaccinated patients who are exposed to rabid animals still require 2 additional rabies vaccine doses (the 1st on the day of the bite and the 2nd 3 days later) but do not need the rabies immunoglobulin (which is sparsely available in developing countries)

Hepatitis B vaccine:

Series: 3 doses (advisable for travelers making repeated trips, taking prolonged trips, or involved in overseas missionary or volunteer work, health care delivery, or medical tourism)

Immunity: Lifelong after 3 doses and seropositivity

Traveler's Diarrhea Prevention and Self-Treatment

- Food and water precautions are advisable
- Primary prophylaxis (eg, ciprofloxacin, rifaximin, or bismuth subsalicylate) is not needed but could be considered for severely immunocompromised persons traveling for a relatively short time (<2 weeks)
- Self-treatment with a course of antibiotics may be advisable for moderate to severe traveler's diarrhea
  - A fluoroquinolone such as ciprofloxacin 500 mg oral bid for 3 days or 750 mg as a single dose; or levofloxacin 500 mg oral once a day for 3 days or 500 mg as a single dose
  - azithromycin 500 mg oral daily for 3 days or 1 g oral as a single dose (for children or for travelers to southeast Asia where resistance to fluoroquinolones is increasing)
  - rifaximin 200 mg oral tid for 3 days
- Patients with persistent or bloody diarrhea should be advised to seek immediate medical attention and to avoid the use of antiperistaltic agents such as loperamide if there is blood in the stool

Suggested Reading

Centers for Disease Control and Prevention (travelers' health information) http://www.cdc.gov/travel/travel.html
World Health Organization (international travel and health) http://www.who.int/ith/en/index.html
American Society of Tropical Medicine and Hygiene http://www.astmh.org
International Society of Travel Medicine http://www.istm.org
Hill DR, et al. Clin Infect Dis. 2006 Dec 15;43(12):1499-1539. Epub 2006 Nov 8. (http://www.journals.uchicago.edu/doi/pdf/10.1086/508782/)